ADVANCEMENTS AND BREAKTHROUGHS IN ULTRASOUND IMAGING

Edited by **Gunti Gunarathne**

Advancements and Breakthroughs in Ultrasound Imaging
http://dx.doi.org/10.5772/46053
Edited by Gunti Gunarathne

Contributors

Philip Njemanze, G P P Gunarathne, Prakash S. Hiremath, Prema T. Akkasaligar, Sharan Badiger, Fenster, Chih-Yen Tu, Wei-Chih Liao, Chuen-Ming Shih, Wu-Huei Hsu, Hung-Jen Chen, Chia-Hung Chen, Lindseth, David Romero, Timm Westhoff, Nikolaos Pagonas, Stergios Vlatsas, Steven L. Orebaugh

Published by InTech

Janeza Trdine 9, 51000 Rijeka, Croatia

Publishing Process Manager Ana Pantar
Technical Editor InTech DTP team
Cover InTech Design team

Additional hard copies can be obtained from orders@intechopen.com

Advancements and Breakthroughs in Ultrasound Imaging, Edited by Gunti Gunarathne
p. cm.
ISBN 978-953-51-1159-7

For EU product safety concerns:
IN TECH d.o.o., Prolaz Marije Krucifikse Kozulić 3, 51000 Rijeka, Croatia,
info@intechopen.com or visit our website at intechopen.com.

Meet the editor

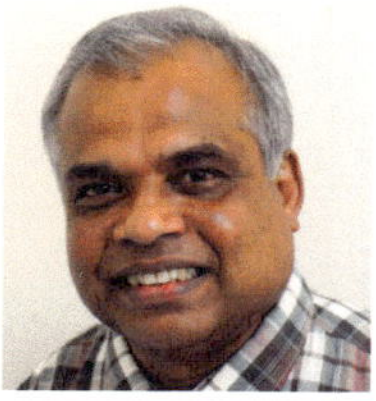

Dr Gunarathne is a Reader at the School of Engineering, Robert Gordon University (RGU), UK. He received his PhD in electrical engineering from Loughborough University of Technology, UK, in 1985, developing a patented ultrasound imaging system. At RGU, Dr Gunarathne formed the Industrial & Biomedical Instrumentation Research Group. He is also the founder and Director of the LabVIEW Academy & Centre of Excellence for Industrial Instrumentation at RGU. Dr Gunarathne has gained over 40 years of combined experience in high-speed electronic circuit design, ultrasonic engineering, industrial and biomedical instrumentation, quality control, and Non-destructive-testing research. Dr Gunarathne has chaired many national and international events and his work has been widely published with developments receiving media coverage in television, radio and in the press.

Contents

Preface

Ultrasonic imaging is a powerful diagnostic tool available to medical practitioners, engineers and researchers today. Due to the relative safety, and the non-invasive nature, ultrasonic imaging has become one of the most rapidly advancing technologies. These rapid advances are directly related to the parallel advancements in electronics, computing, and transducer technology together with sophisticated signal processing techniques. This book focuses on state of the art developments in ultrasonic imaging applications and underlying technologies presented by leading practitioners and researchers from many parts of the world.

Applications of ultrasound imaging in medicine, industry and research are extensive and wide-ranging. In medical diagnostics, ultrasonic imaging of anatomical structures and moving tissue in real-time is routine. Ultrasonic imaging is also now widely used in image guided medical intervention procedures and in aiding therapeutic applications. Industrial applications of ultrasound imaging are also wide spread and growing, e.g. in Non-destructive-evaluation (NDE) and underwater acoustics (Sonar). Acoustic microscopy at GHz frequencies can be used to visualise sub-surface microscopic structures that can yield information not possible with light.

It is important to note that imaging as applied to the application domains mentioned above; namely, medical diagnostics, NDE and Sonar have fundamental similarities and differences. Similarities in imaging modalities have greatly helped researchers working in different domains to benefit from each other, while the differences have led to the evolution of intriguing technologies exclusive to those applications.

The 10 chapters in this book are organised in such a way that Chapters 1 – 5 are focused on state-of-the-art applications and developments in ultrasound imaging systems for medical diagnostics and image guided interventional and therapeutic procedures. Chapter 6 presents research developments in the use of Functional Transcranial Doppler Spectroscopy for evaluating Neurocognitive functions and their differences between genders. Chapter 7 focuses on the detection of follicles and ovarian classification using ultrasound images. Chapter 8 presents a study on the use of various algorithms to reduce speckle noise in ultrasound images.

Chapter 9 presents techniques and strategies for hardware reduction at the design stage of portable ultrasound systems. Chapter 10, entitled "Breaking through the Speed Barrier" investigates primary performance bottlenecks of conventional ultrasonic imaging technology and presents work done in developing an unconventional imaging system that has the potential to reach the maximum theoretical limits of speed of imaging and resolution.

I sincerely hope that you will enjoy and gain much benefit in reading this book. I would like to take this opportunity to thank all the authors who worked so hard and gave a lot of time in contributing to this book. The professional support given by the editorial board and the officials of InTech at every stage of this project was excellent. Finally, I would like to extend my sincere gratitude to my dear friend and colleague, Mr Andrew Fairhead, Honorary lecturer and Former ultrasound Engineer at NHS Grampian, for his valuable comments and support throughout this project.

Gunti Gunarathne (PhD, FIET)
School of Engineering,
Robert Gordon University, UK.

Chapter 1

3D Ultrasound Imaging in Image-Guided Intervention

Aaron Fenster, Jeff Bax, Hamid Neshat,
Nirmal Kakani and Cesare Romagnoli

Additional information is available at the end of the chapter

http://dx.doi.org/10.5772/55230

1. Introduction

Soon after the discovery of x-rays, physicians recognized the importance of using imaging to guide interventional procedures. As imaging technology became more advanced with the development of fluoroscopic, CT, MR and ultrasound systems, image-guided interventions have become a critical tool for physicians in dealing with complex interventional and surgical procedures. Today, image-guided procedures make use of computer-based systems to provide real-time three-dimensional (3D) information of the anatomy of the patient being treated. The information is presented in various ways, such as virtual graphical image overlays, or multi-screen approaches to help the physician precisely visualize and target the anatomical site.

Since the development of Computed Tomography (CT) in the early 1970s, the availability of 3D anatomical information has revolutionized diagnostic radiology by providing physicians with 3D images of anatomical structures. The pace of development has continued with the development of 3D magnetic resonance imaging (MRI), positron Emission Tomography (PET), and multi-slice and cone beam CT imaging. These imaging modalities have stimulated the development of a wide variety of image-guided interventional procedures.

Although 2D ultrasound (2D US) imaging has been used extensively for interventional procedures, such as biopsy and guidance of ablation procedures, 3D ultrasound is slowly growing in clinical applications [1]. Today, the majority of US-based diagnostic and interventional procedures are still performed using conventional 2D imaging. Over the past two decades, university-based investigators and commercial companies have utilized both 1D and 2D arrays while developing 3D ultrasound (3D US) imaging techniques. 3D US techniques have been increasingly used in diagnosis, minimally invasive image-guided interventions and intra-operative use of imaging [2-4]. Today, most US system manufacturers provide 3D US imaging capability as part of the systems. Advances in 3D US imaging technology have resulted in high quality 3D images of complex anatomical structures and pathology, which are used in diagnosis of disease and to guide interventional and surgical procedures [5-9].

In this chapter we focus on the recent development of 3D US imaging as it applies to image-guided interventions. The chapter will briefly review how 3D US images are obtained and then will provide two examples of recent development of 3D US- guided interventional procedures.

2. 3D ultrasound imaging systems

2.1. Benefits of 3D ultrasound imaging

Conventional 2D US imaging systems making use of 1D transducer arrays allow users to manipulate the hand-held US transducer freely over the body in order to generate images of organs and pathology. While this capability is sufficient for many interventional procedures such as breast biopsy, some interventional procedures require 3D image visualization, which 3D US imaging attempts to provide. More specifically:

- Freely manipulating the conventional US transducer during the interventional procedure over the anatomy to generate 2D US images requires that users mentally integrate many 2D images to form an impression of the anatomy and pathology in 3D. In cases of interventions of complex anatomy or pathology, this approach leads to longer procedures and may result in variability in guidance of the interventional procedures.
- Since the conventional 2D US imaging transducer is held and manipulated manually, it is difficult to relocate the 2D US image at the exact location and orientation in the body at a later time. Since monitoring the progression of the interventional procedure often requires imaging of the same location (plane) of the anatomy, manual manipulation of a 2D US image is suboptimal.
- Conventional 2D US imaging does not permit viewing of planes parallel to the skin – often called C-mode. This approach is, at times, suboptimal since interventional procedures sometimes require an arbitrary selection of the image plane for optimal viewing of the pathology and guiding the interventional procedure.
- Planning the interventional procedure and therapy monitoring often require accurate lesion volume measurements. Since conventional 2D US imaging only provides a cross-section of the lesion, measurements of organ or lesion volume is variable and at times inaccurate.

The following sections review approaches used in generation of 3D US images based on 1D. An emphasis is placed on the geometric accuracy of the generated 3D images as well as the use of this technology in interventional and quantitative monitoring applications.

2.2. Mechanical 3D US scanning systems

Mechanical 3D US systems make use of mechanisms using motors to translate, tilt, or rotate a conventional 2D US transducer. A sequential digitized series of 2D US images and their relative positions and orientation are acquired rapidly by a computer as the 2D US transducer is moved, while the 3D US image is reconstructed. Since the scanning geometry in mechanical 3D US systems is predefined and precisely controlled by a mechanical motorized system, the relative position and orientation of the acquired 2D US images are known accurately and precisely.

These mechanical 3D scanning systems allow the user to optimize the image resolution by adjusting the angular or spatial interval between the acquired 2D image [10].

Two approaches have been used in the development of mechanical 3D US scanning systems: integrated 3D US transducers with the scanning mechanism within the transducer housing; and external mechanical fixtures that hold the housing of a conventional 2D US transducers. Both approaches have been successfully used for a variety of clinical applications including interventional applications.

2.2.1. *Wobbling or tilting mechanical 3D US scanners*

Most US system manufacturers offer integrated 3D US transducers that are based on a mechanically-swept transducer or "wobbler". In these systems a 1D US array is wobbled or swept back and forth inside the 3D transducer housing. Digital 2D US images that are generated while the 1D US array is wobbled, which are used in the 3D US image reconstruction. These 3D transducers are larger than conventional 2D US transducers. These types of 3D US transducers are convenient to use but require a special US machine that can control the 3D scanning and reconstruct the acquired 2D images into a 3D image.

Many interventional 3D US-guided interventional systems are currently using external fixtures for mechanical 3D scanning since researchers typically do not get access to the control of the US system for development of novel interventional systems. In this approach, a motorized custom made fixture is used to house the conventional 2D US transducer. A computer is used to control the motor to cause the US transducer to tilt or "wobble". The video stream from the US machine is digitized using an analogue or digital frame grabber. Since the relative angle between the acquired 2D images is known, a 3D image can be reconstructed as the 2D images are acquired.

Although the external mechanical 3D scanning fixtures are bulkier than integrated 3D transducers, they can be used with any US manufacturer's transducer, obviating the need to purchase a special 3D US machine. In addition, the external fixture approach can take advantage of improvements in the US machine (e.g., image compounding, contrast agent imaging) and flow information (e.g., Doppler imaging) without any changes in the scanning mechanism.

Both approaches used in mechanical 3D US scanning allow short imaging times, ranging from about 3 to 0.2 3D images/s. The 3D images are of high quality and also include B-mode and Doppler information.

Figure 1a is a diagram of the mechanical tilt approach of a conventional 1D array US transducer about an axis parallel to the face of the transducer, and 1b shows the tilting axis away from the face of the transducer. The latter approach is typically used in integrated 3D scanning mechanisms. In both approaches, the acquired 2D US images are arranged as a fan with an adjustable angular spacing, e.g., 1.0°. To generate a 3D image, the housing of the 3D probe or external fixture remains fixed on the skin of the patient while the US transducer is wobbled. The time required to generate a 3D US image depends on the 2D US image update rate and the number of 2D images needed to generate the 3D image. The 2D US image update rate depends on the US machine settings (i.e., depth setting and number of focal zones) and number of acquired 2D US images is determined by the chosen angular separation between the acquired 2D images, and the total scan angle needed to cover the desired anatomy. Typically, these parameters can be adjusted to optimize scanning time, image quality and the size of the volume imaged [11-16]. The most common integrated 3D transducers using the wobbling technique are used for abdominal and obstetrical imaging [17-19].

The 3D image resolution will not be isotropic. The resolution in the 3D US image will degrade in the axial direction away from the transducer due to the increasing US beam spread in the lateral and elevational directions of the acquired 2D US images. Since the acquired 2D images used to generate a 3D image are arranged as a fan, the distance between the acquired US images increases with increasing axial distance. Increasing axial distances result in decreasing spatial sampling resulting in further loss of spatial resolution in the elevational direction of the acquired 2D US images of the reconstructed 3D image [20].

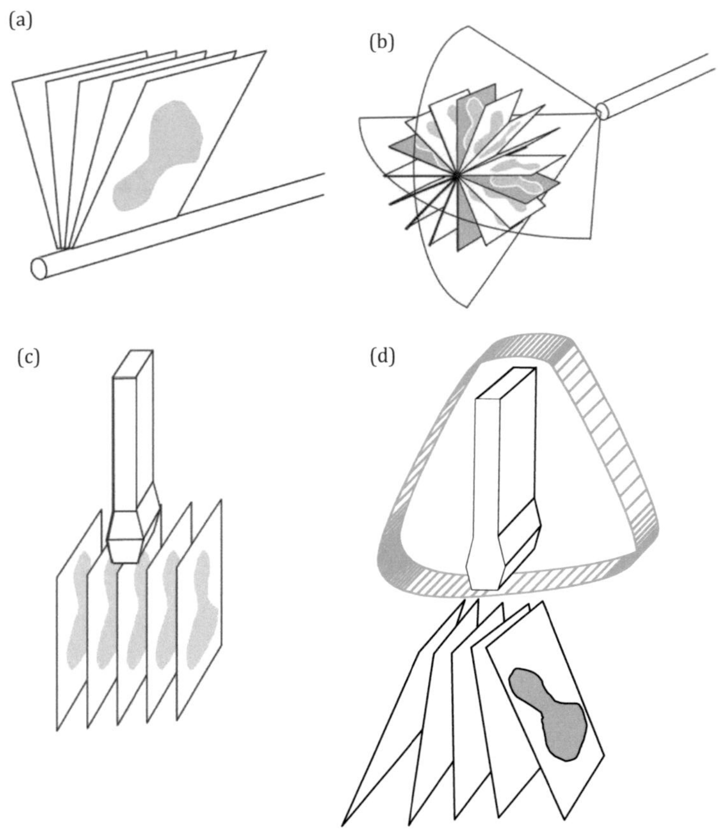

Figure 1. Schematic diagrams of 3D US mechanical scanning methods. (a) A side-firing TRUS transducer is mechanically rotated and the acquired images have equal angular spacing. The same approach is used in a mechanically-wobbled transducer. (b) A rotational scanning mechanism using an end-firing transducer, typically used in 3D TRUS guided prostate biopsy. The acquired images have equal angular spacing. (c) A linear mechanical scanning mechanism, in which the acquired images have equal spacing. (d) The mechanically tilting mechanism, but integrated into a 3D US transducer. The US transducer is "wobbled" inside the housing of the transducer.

2.2.2. *Linear mechanical 3D scanners*

Linear scanners mechanisms use an external motorized fixture to move the conventional 2D transducer across the skin of the patient. The 2D transducer can be fixed to be perpendicular to the surface of the skin or at an angle for acquiring Doppler images. The spacing between the acquired 2D images is adjustable but constant during the scan so that the acquired 2D images are parallel and uniformly spaced (see Fig. 1c). The velocity of the transducer as it is being scanned is adjusted to obtain 2D images with an appropriate spatial interval for generating high quality 3D images [10].

The predefined spacing between the acquired 2D US images allows 3D images to be reconstructed while the 2D US images are being acquired. In the direction parallel to the acquired 2D US images the resolution of the reconstructed 3D US image will be the same as the original 2D US images. However, in the direction of the 3D scanning, the resolution of the reconstructed 3D image will be equal (if spatial sampling is appropriate) to the elevational resolution of the acquired 2D US images. Thus, the resolution of the 3D US image will be poorest in the 3D scanning direction due to greater spread of the US beam in the elevational direction [21].

This scanning approach is not typically used in interventional applications; however, it has been successfully implemented in many vascular B-mode and Doppler imaging applications, particularly of for carotid arteries [11, 22-30] and tumor vascularization [25, 31-33].

2.2.3. *Endo-cavity rotational 3D scanners*

The endo-cavity rotational 3D scanning approach has been used extensively in 3D US-guided prostate interventional procedures. In this approach an external fixture or internal mechanism is used to rotate an endo-cavity transducer (*e.g.*, a transrectal ultrasound (TRUS) probe, see Fig. 1b) about its long axis. Endo-cavity transducers using an end-firing approach are typically used for prostate biopsy. When these types of conventional transducers are rotated by the motorized fixture, the set of acquired 2D images will be arranged as a fan (Fig. 1b), intersecting in the center of the 3D US image, resulting in an image as shown in Fig. 2. To obtain a 3D image of the prostate as in Fig. 2, an end-firing transducer is typically rotated by 180° [16].

Endo-cavity transducers using a side-firing 1D array are typically used in prostate brachytherapy, cryotherapy and focal therapy. When using these types of conventional transducers, the acquired images will also be arranged as a fan, but intersect at the axis of rotation of the transducer (see Fig. 1a). The side-firing transducer is typically rotated from 80° to 110° to obtain a 3D TRUS image of the prostate [16, 34, 35]. Figure 2 shows that endo-cavity scanning transducer used to image the prostate for 3D US-guided therapy [6, 9, 11, 25, 34, 36-39]

For scanning systems used for 3D US-guided prostate biopsy, the end-firing transducer is rotated by at least 180° about a fixed axis that perpendicularly bisects the transducer array. In this approach, the resolution of the 3D image will not be isotropic. Since the spatial sampling is highest near the rotation axis of the transducer and the poorest away from the axis of rotation of the transducer, thus the resolution of the 3D US image will degrade as the distance from the rotational axis of the transducer is increased. In addition, the axial and elevational resolution will decrease as the distance from the transducer is increased, as discussed above. The combination of these effects will result in a 3D US image resolution that is best near the transducer and the rotational axis, while being poorest away from the transducer and rotational axis.

3D rotational scanning with an end-firing transducer is most sensitive to the motion of the transducer and patient since the axis of rotation is in the center of the 3D US image. Any motion during the 3D scan will cause a mismatch in the acquired 2D US images, resulting in artifacts in the center of the 3D US image. Artifacts in the center of the 3D US image will also occur if the axis of rotation is not accurately known; however, proper calibrations can remove this source of potential error. Thus, for interventional applications such as 3D US-guided prostate biopsy or brachytherapy, the rotational scanning mechanism is typically supported by a stabilization apparatus [16, 34, 40].

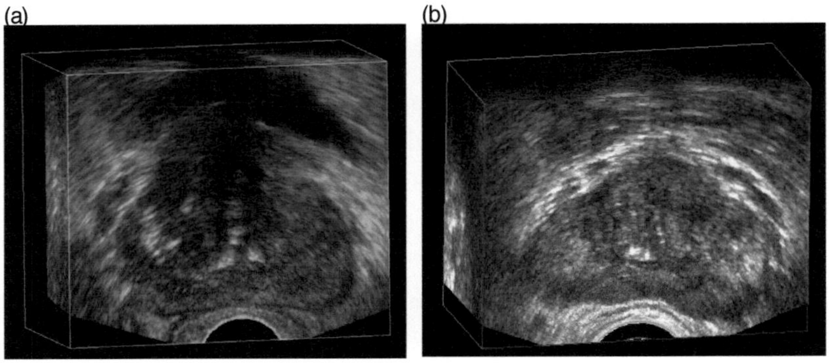

Figure 2. The 3D US of the prostate displayed using the multi-planar reformatting approach: (a) An end-firing TRUS prostate cube-view 3D image, allowing the sides to be translated and angles to reveal the desired anatomy. (b) A 3D TRUS image acquired using a side-firing transducer using the mechanical rotation approach.

2.2.4. Free-hand scanning with position sensing

Some 3D US-guided interventional procedures are making use of 3D scanning techniques that do not require a mechanical scanning device. In this approach, the user holds and manipulates a conventional US transducer to cover the patient's anatomy being investigated. Since construction of a 3D US image requires that the position and orientation of the conventional transducer be known, free-hand scanning requires a method to track the positions and orientations of the transducer as it is being moved. All methods to accomplish this task require a sensor to be mounted on the transducer to allow measurement of the conventional 2D transducer's position and orientation as it is moved over the body.

Over the past 2 decades, several approaches for free-hand scanning have been developed: tracked 3D US with articulated arms, free-hand 3D US with acoustic sensing, free-hand 3D US with magnetic field sensing, and image-based sensing (speckle decorrelation). The method used most commonly is the magnetic field sensing approach with several companies providing the sensing technology: Ascension – Bird sensor [3] Polhemus – Fastrack sensor [41] and Northern Digital – Aurora sensor [4].

The most successful free-hand 3D US scanning approach used in interventional procedures makes use of magnetic field sensors, as well as applications such as echocardiography, obstetrics, and vascular imaging [3, 4, 41-51]. To track the transducer during generation of a 3D US image, a small receiver is mounted on the transducer containing three orthogonal coils allowing six-degrees-of-freedom sensing. The small receiver mounted on the transducer measures the strength of the magnetic field in three orthogonal directions, which is generated by a time-varying 3D magnetic field transmitter placed near the patient. The position and orientation of the transducer is calculated by continuously measuring the strength of the three components of the local magnetic field.

Since magnetic field sensors are small and unobtrusive devices, they allow the transducer to be tracked without the need for bulky mechanical devices, and without the need to keep a clear line of sight as required by optical tracking methods. Since magnetic field sensors are sensitive to electromagnetic interference or ferrous (or highly conductive) metals located nearby, geometric tracking errors can occur leading to distortions in the 3D US image. Thus, metal beds used in procedures, or surgical rooms can cause significant distortions. However, modern magnetic field sensors have been produced to be less susceptible to these sources of error, particularly ones that use a magnetic transmitter placed between the bed and the patient.

3. 3D Ultrasound-guided focal liver ablation

3.1. Clinical problem

Hepatocellular carcinoma (HCC) is the fifth most common diagnosed malignancy and the third most frequent cause of cancer related deaths worldwide [52]. Incidence is particularly high in Asia and sub-Saharan Africa due to the large incidence of hepatitis B and C, both of which are complicated by hepatic cirrhosis, which is the greatest risk factor for HCC. Recently, increasing trends in HCC have been reported from several Western countries [53]. Furthermore, the liver is the second most common site of metastatic cancer arising in other organs.

When feasible, surgical resection or liver transplant is the accepted standard therapeutic approach, and currently has the highest success rate of all treatment methods for primary and metastatic liver cancer. Unfortunately, only 15% of patients are candidates for surgery [54, 55]. Patients who do not qualify for surgery usually are offered other therapeutic solutions such as chemotherapy and radiotherapy, but unfortunately have variable limited success rates.

Minimally invasive percutaneous techniques, such as radio-frequency (RF) and microwave (MW) ablation of malignant tissue in the liver is a rapidly expanding research field and treatment tool for those patients who are not candidates for surgical resection or transplant. In some cases this acts as a bridge to liver transplantation [54, 56]. Due to low complications rates and shorter recovery times, the indications for these minimally invasive procedures are constantly increasing. However, these methods have a higher local recurrence rate than surgical resection, mostly due to insufficient or inaccurate local ablation of cancerous cells [56, 57].

Microwave energy-induced tissue heating by near-field probes is emerging as a common thermal treatment of liver tumors [58]. Application of MW for tumor ablation has multiple advantages over other techniques, including higher treatment temperatures and the ability to create larger uniformly shaped ablation zones in shorter time periods. However, the accurate placement of the probe is critical in achieving the predicted treatment goal [59]. The current standard of care uses CT images for planning and 2D US image guidance for intra-operative guidance of the ablation probe(s) into the target lesion. However, this approach suffers from several disadvantages, such as: (1) 2D US imaging requires physicians to mentally integrate many 2D images to form an impression of the anatomy and pathology, leading to more variability in guidance during interventional procedures; (2) 2D US does not permit the viewing of planes parallel to the skin, (3) liver deformation and motion artifact due to breathing reduces targeting accuracy, (4) 2D US-based for measurement of tumor volume needed for the treatment plan is variable and at times inaccurate, and (5) the detection and tracking of the needle delivering the thermal energy in the liver is crucial for accurate placement of the needle relative to the tumor, but can be difficult using 2D US. 3D US imaging of the liver and target may help to overcome these disadvantages resulting in improved accuracy of probe placement and improved ablation of the lesion.

The use of 3D US-guidance for focal liver tumor ablation is based on the fact that the use of 3D US will show the features of liver masses and the hepatic vasculature more clearly, allow guidance of the ablation probes to the target more accurately, and allow more accurate monitoring of the ablation zone during the procedure and at follow up.

3.2. 3D US Scanner for focal liver tumor ablation

We have developed 3D US guidance systems for improving cancer diagnosis and treatment by introducing hardware and software innovations [21, 60-64]. Our previous efforts have been extended to the development of a 3D US-guidance system for treating HCC. Specialized hardware and software tools are used that allow 3D acquisition of 3D US images, real-time registration of the pre-operative CT to intra-operative 3D US images, and tracking of the ablation probes during insertion into the target. This is accomplished by registering previously acquired contrast CT images that show the location of the target lesion to near real-time 3D US images, plus providing visualization and guidance tools to guide the procedure.

The 3D US scanning system consists of: a hand-held electro-mechanical motor/encoder assembly to move a conventional 2D US imaging transducer in a fan shaped, linear or hybrid motion to a maximum angular limit of 60 degrees and/or 30 mm linear extent to acquire a series of 2D US images; and, a PC equipped with a digital frame grabber and software components to control the motor assembly, acquire 2D images, reconstruct them in 3D, and visualize them in 3D.

3.2.1. Mechanical design

The handheld 3D scanning device is motorized and constructed with two mechanical systems for generating a linear and tilt scanning motions of the transducer is shown schematically and photographically in Figs. 3 and 4. The linear scanning system is operated with a geared DC motor and lead screw providing linear translation. The tilt motion is generated via a parallelogram linkage, which is mounted on the carriage of the linear slide. A second geared DC motor is used to generate the tilt motion, allowing for independent control of the two systems.

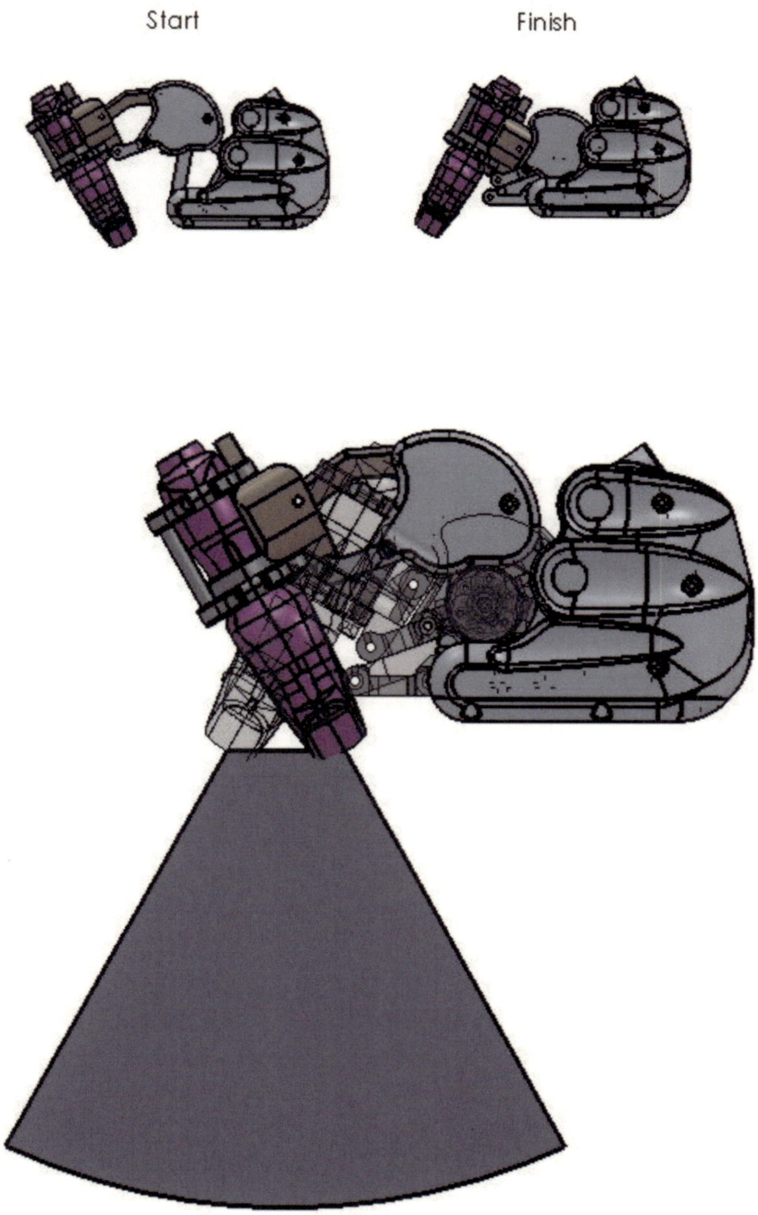

Figure 3. Schematic diagram of the hybrid 3D US scanner for used in the focal liver ablation procedure. The diagram shows the start and end positions of the hybrid (linear and tilt) scan.

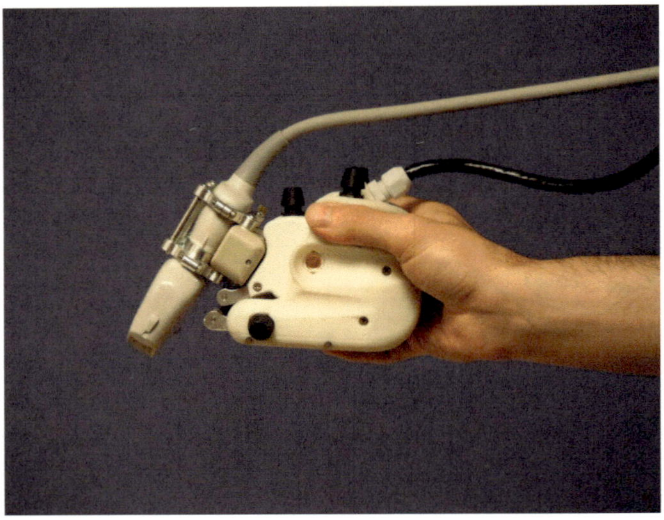

Figure 4. Photograph of hybrid scanner with abdominal ultrasound transducer mounted and ready for scanning.

The 3D scanning device has three modes of operation: a linear translation, in which the transducer (oriented perpendicular to the surface or at an angle for Doppler imaging) is translated along a straight line parallel to the patient's surface. This motion generates a rectangular volume shown in Fig. 5a. The second mode generates a tilt motion (or wobbling), in which the transducer is rotated about its face resting on the patient's skin surface (Fig. 5b). The third mode is a combination of the first two modes that creates a combined (or hybrid) motion. The transducer is rotated as it is moved along a surface covering a larger volume than either of the first two modes (Fig. 5c). For example, if transducer with linear array is used at 15cm depth setting on the ultrasound machine (typical depth for abdominal imaging), hybrid scanning gives a volume that is three times larger than the linear mode and 47% larger than the tilt mode only.

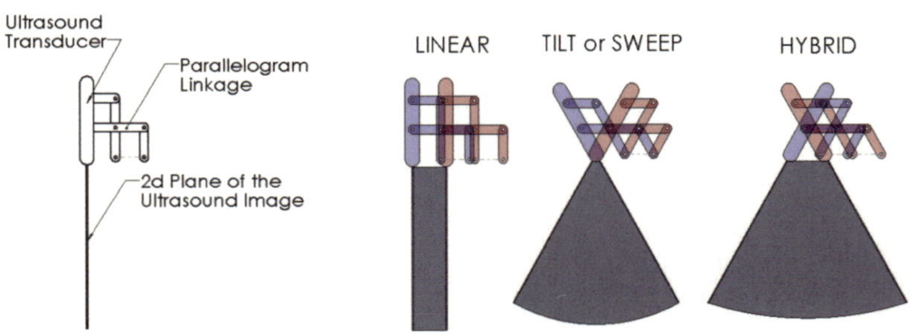

Figure 5. Schematic diagrams showing the three modes of operation of the mechanical compound 3D US scanning device. On the left is the schematic of the linkage and the right are the linear, tilt and hybrid motions.

http://dx.doi.org/10.5772/55230

The 3D scanning system parameters can be set by the user: *Scanning mode:* Three different modes of linear, tilt and combined (or hybrid, a combination of both linear and tilt imaging modes to maximize the field-of-view) are available depending on the anatomy of body parts being scanned and the image requirements. *Scan Extent:* Maximum extent of linear translation (typically 2.5 cm) or tilt angle (typically 60 deg) can be set individually to the extremes values. *Scan Spacing:* Elevational linear and angular spacing can be set to optimize the trade-off between the scanning time and the scan spacing. *Frame-Rate:* The rate at which images are digitized by the frame grabber is set (typically 15 frames/s). *Scanning Depth:* Maximum scanning depth can be set prior to each scan for accurate reconstruction of the volumes.

3.2.2. Validation methods

Since the hybrid scanning mode involves coordination between two acquisition methods, it was tested in terms of accuracy of 3D image generation. We used two custom made phantoms with known geometry. The validation experiments where performed using the handheld 3D US scanning device in hybrid scanning mode using a two-dimensional conventional curved array ultrasound transducer used for abdominal applications (Toshiba, PVT-375BT).

Geometrical Error in 3D reconstruction: This test was designed to measure the accuracy of the 3D reconstruction of the 3D hybrid scanner in three directions. The test phantom was made of a grid of known dimensions made with 0.1 mm thick nylon monofilament threads wrapped around an accurately machined frame to form a 4-layer grid. Each layer was slightly shifted from the layer above to avoid acoustic shadowing. The distance between any two layers was 1cm. The phantom was submerged in a 15% glycerol solution [61] and imaged at different depth settings. The acquired 3D US images were then viewed and analyzed by measuring the distances between the images of the monofilaments and comparing them to the expected values.

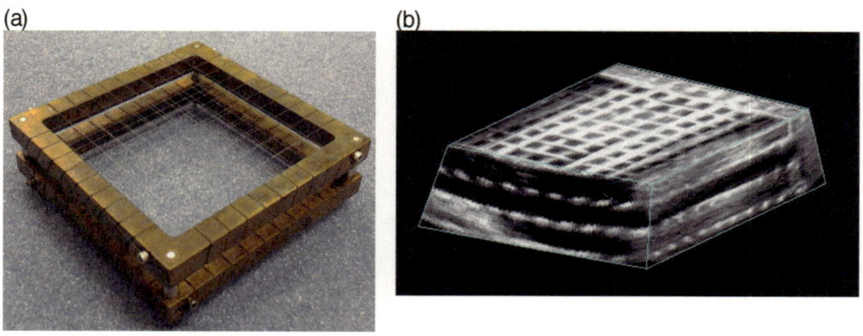

Figure 6. (a) Photograph of the 3D monofilament thread grid, which was used to validate the 3D reconstruction of the ultrasound image. (b) The 3D ultrasound image of the phantom, showing the grid of threads.

Error in 3D volume measurements: In the second test, we assessed the accuracy in measuring volumes using our system. For this experiment, several spherical phantoms with different sizes were made of tissue mimicking agar [65]. The volume of each of these spherical phantoms was measured prior to embedding them in a cube of tissue mimicking agar phantom. The spherical phantoms were then imaged with our hybrid scanner, viewed in the 3D visualization software, and manually segmented. The volume of spherical structures were calculated and compared with the expected values.

3.2.3. Validation results

Testing the 3D hybrid scanner with the 3D thread phantom showed that mean error in the measured values of the distances in the X, Y and Z directions were 3.6%, 2.5% and 5.7% respectively. A one-sample t-test was performed to compare the measured distance values with the known distance value of 1cm, showed there was no statistical significant difference between the measured values and expected values between the threads.

Validation of volume measurements using the hybrid scanner were carried out by imaging a tissue mimicking agar sphere with a volume of 10 cm^3 embedded in a block of tissue mimicking agar phantom. The measurements were performed at two different depth settings on the ultrasound machine (10 and 15 cm). The mean errors of the volume measurement were 5.7% and 4.4% for the 10cm and 15cm depth settings respectively, demonstrating that the hybrid scanner can be used to make sufficiently accurate volumetric measurements.

In-vivo experiments: After obtaining institutional research board (IRB) approvals, we investigated the use of the scanner in thermal ablation treatment of primary hepatic tumors. Figure 7 shows a 3D US image acquired during the microwave ablation procedure of a primary (hepatocellular) tumor. It shows application of the hybrid mode in acquiring volumes large enough to include both the ablated tumor region as well as all ablation needles in two different views.

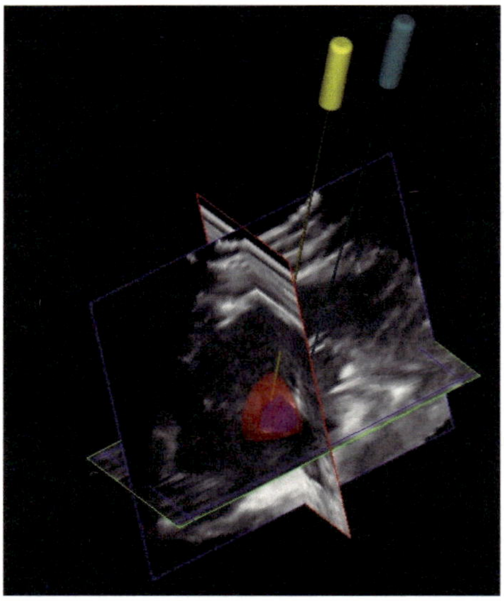

Figure 7. 3D ultrasound image of a primary (hepatocellular) tumor with two microwave applicators in place. The applicators and tumor have been segmented and displayed in 3D allowing the interventional radiologist to examine the placement accuracy of the applicators in the tumor. In addition, the ablation zone has also been superimposed.

http://dx.doi.org/10.5772/55230

4. 3D ultrasound guided prostate biopsy

4.1. The clinical problem

Prostate Cancer (PCa) is the most commonly diagnosed malignancy in men, and is found at autopsy in 30% of men at age 50, 40% at age 60, and almost 90% at age 90 [66, 67]. Worldwide, it is the second leading cause of death due to cancer in men, accounting for between 2.1% and 15.2% of all cancer deaths [68, 69]. Symptoms PCa are generally absent until extensive local growth or metastases develop. When diagnosed at an early stage, the disease is curable [70, 71], and even at later stages treatment can be effective [72]; however, once the tumor has extended beyond the prostate, the risk of metastases and locally aggressive cancer increases. Clearly, early diagnosis, accurate staging of prostate cancer, and appropriate therapies are critical to the patient's well-being.

In managing patients with possible PCa, the challenges facing physicians are to: (a) diagnose clinically relevant cancers at a curable stage; (b) stage the disease accurately; (c) apply appropriate therapy accurately to optimize destruction of cancer cells while preserving normal tissues and function; and (d) follow patients to assess side effects and therapy effectiveness. This section focuses on improving early PCa diagnosis and staging with the use of 3D ultrasound-guided prostate biopsy.

Since not all cancers are palpable by digital rectal exam (DRE), PCa diagnosis is established by histological examination of prostate tissue obtained most commonly by trans-rectal ultrasound (TRUS)-guided biopsy. Prostate needle biopsy is the only definitive diagnostic modality capable of confirming malignancy, and is now always performed with TRUS guidance.

Since many small tumors are not detected by TRUS or DRE, biopsy samples are obtained from predetermined regions of the prostate known to have a high probability of harboring cancer. These are typically in the peripheral zone (PZ), which harbors 80% of all PCs and a higher proportion of clinically significant ones, and close to the capsule, as most cancers are thought to start within 5*mm* of the prostate capsule. Most centers are now taking 8-12 cores or more as part of their routine assessment [73-76].

TRUS biopsies are now performed with a thin, 18-gauge needle mounted on a spring-loaded gun connected to the TRUS probe, forcing the needle to stay in the imaging plane. Each core is separately identified as to the prostate region from which it was drawn, so that the pathologist can report the extent and grade of the cancer within each region.

Since prostate volume sampled by the biopsy is small, and PCa is often multi-focal, involving only a small volume of the prostate in the early stages of the disease [77, 78], the probability for obtaining a sample of the tumour on biopsy is small. Thus, a negative biopsy may be, in fact, false, and the patient may be harbouring cancer at an early and curable stage. Various reports have shown that the false negative rate ranges from 10% to 25% [73, 74]. Since cancer is still present in 1/10 to 1/4 of patients with a negative first biopsy, the current biopsy procedure is still suboptimal [74, 79]. Clearly, an improved procedure with improved planning and recording of biopsy locations is necessary to resolve these issues.

Due to the increasing number of younger men with early and potentially curable PCa undergoing repeated prostate biopsy, it is therefore vital not to re-biopsy the same area if the original biopsy was negative, and it is particularly vital to re-biopsy the same area if a possible abnormal area was detected on first biopsy as ASAP [80]. Thus, the locations of the cores obtained from the prostate must be known accurately to help guide the physician during the repeat biopsy [81, 82], to help in correlating any imaging evidence of the disease, and to provide improved planning for subsequent therapy.

4.2. Multi-modality directed prostate biopsy

A variety of imaging techniques and molecular imaging probes are being investigated to improve early detection of PCa. Different magnetic resonance imaging (MRI) techniques have been evaluated using body and endo-rectal coils, contrast enhancement, and different pulse sequences [83-85] resulting in disease detection sensitivity and specificity of 80-88% and 75-95%, respectively [84, 86, 87]. Positron emission tomography (PET) (combined with CT or MRI) is used to detect early disease, with the newer PET imaging probes proving to be the more promising [88-90]. Although progress has been made with improved PET and MRI techniques, they do not yet have ideal specificity or sufficient accuracy to assess the grade of the cancer; thus a biopsy of suspicious lesions on MRI or PET is required to provide a definitive diagnosis and grade of the disease. Systems have been developed to perform biopsies in the MRI suite; however, the cost of the equipment and prolonged use of the MRI is extremely expensive and likely prohibitive given the large number of patients requiring biopsy. Unfortunately, conventional 2D TRUS guidance of the biopsy procedure limits the physician's ability to target locations identified as suspicious on other modalities.

As we currently do not have a highly sensitive and specific imaging test for local staging of PCa, there is a growing belief that the optimal method to guide prostate biopsy will involve not just one, but a combination of imaging modalities. 3D TRUS imaging combined with functional or molecular imaging from another imaging modality such as radiopharmaceutical imaging (PET, SPECT), or magnetic resonance imaging (MRS, MRI) may provide the best approach for guiding prostate biopsy.

4.3. 3D TRUS-guided prostate biopsy system

Since ultrasound imaging is the clinical standard for image-guided biopsy of the prostate, we have developed a 3D TRUS-based navigation system that provides a reproducible record of the 3D locations of the biopsy targets throughout the procedure and allows fusion with MR images with identified lesions for targeting.

The system we have developed is a mechanical 3D biopsy system that maintains the procedural workflow, minimizing costs and physician retraining. This mechanical system has 4 degrees-of-freedom (DOF) and has an adaptable cradle that supports commercially available end-firing TRUS transducers used for prostate biopsy [16]. It also allows real time tracking and recording of the 3D position and orientation of the biopsy needle as the physician manipulates the TRUS transducer. The following describes the components of the system, including hardware, modeling and segmentation algorithms, and system validation using a multi-modal US/CT prostate phantom.

Our approach involves the use of a device composed of two mechanisms shown as a schematic in Figure 8. The system is composed of an articulated multi-jointed stabilizer and a transducer tracking mechanism.

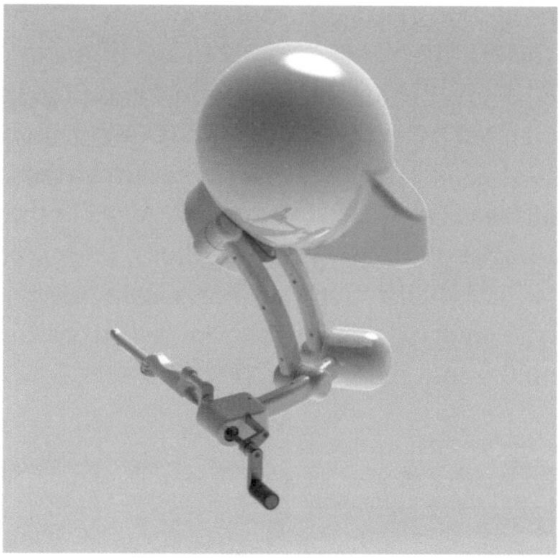

Figure 8. A schematic diagram of the mechanical tracker, which supports the TRUS transducer and attached cradle. This configuration constrains the TRUS probe motion to three degrees-of-freedom and one degree of translation along the axis of the probe. The system is mounted at the base of a stabilizer while the linkage allows the TRUS transducer to be manually manipulated about a remote center of motion (RCM), which is at the center of the ultrasound transducer tip.

The end-firing TRUS transducer with the biopsy needle guide in place is mounted to the mechanical tracking mechanism in a manner where the US probe is free to rotate around its longitudinal axis (Fig. 8). The tracking assembly is attached to a stabilizer, which is mounted on a free-standing cart. Thus, the physician can manipulate the tracking mechanism freely, insert the transducer through the anus, and rotate the transducer in order to acquire a 3D image of the prostate. The tracking linkage contains angle-sensing encoders mounted to each joint in order to transmit to the computer the angles between the arms. This arrangement allows the computer to determine the relative position of the transducer as it is being manipulated. Since the biopsy gun is mounted onto the transducer and its position relative to the transducer is calibrated, the needle location can be calculated.

The mechanical tracking device is a spherical linkage assembly, in which the axis of the joints converge to a common point on the remote center of motion (RCM). The RCM design minimizes targeting errors within the prostate. As the TRUS transducer is constrained through a stationary point, the physician's movements are replicated at a scaled down rate (minified through the RCM), minimizing changes in morphology and dislocation of the prostate. In addition, the RCM enables a precision equivalent to that of robotic assisted machines. Thus, the system improves the physician's ability to accurately biopsy a point of interest within the patient's prostate.

4.4. Prostate biopsy procedure

To perform a 3D US-guided prostate biopsy, the end-firing US transducer is mounted onto the tracking assembly such that the tip of the probe is initially set to the RCM point of the tracker linkage. The physician inserts the TRUS transducer into the patient's rectum and aligns the prostate to the center of the 2D TRUS image. A 3D image of the prostate is then acquired by rotating the transducer 180 degrees about its longitudinal axis (Fig. 1b) [91]. A graphical model of the prostate is then generated by a semi-automatic 3D segmentation algorithm [61, 92-94]. After the prostate model has been constructed, the physician can then manipulate the 3D image on the computer screen and select locations to biopsy. After all of the biopsy targets have been selected, the system then displays the 3D needle guidance interface (Fig. 9), which facilitates the systematic targeting of each biopsy location previously selected. Other images or information (*e.g.*, MRI or PET/CT images), if available, are registered to the 3D TRUS image and displayed as an overlay on the computer screen (Fig. 10).

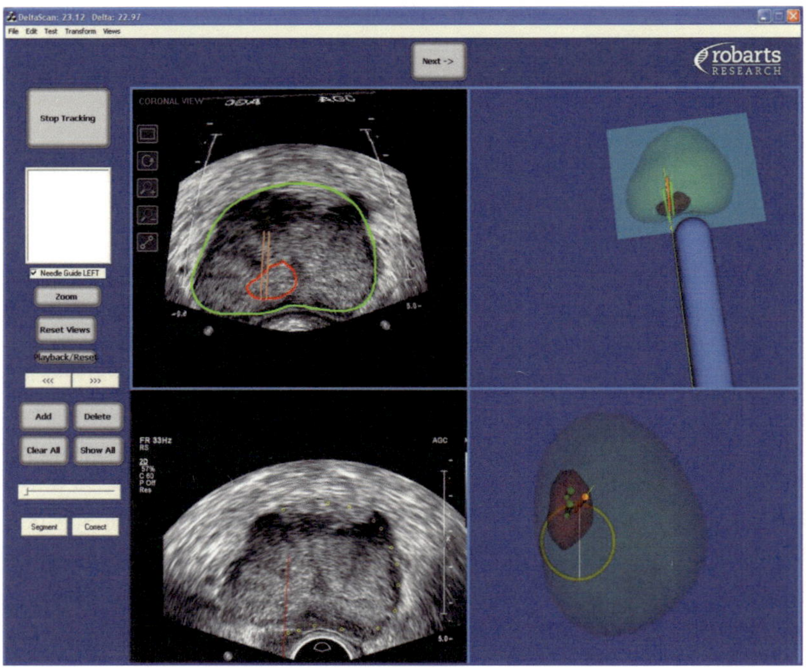

Figure 9. The 3D US-guided prostate biopsy system interface is composed of 4 windows: (top left) the 3D TRUS image dynamically sliced to match the real-time TRUS probe 3D orientation, (bottom left) the live 2D TRUS video stream, (right side) and the 3D location of the biopsy core is displayed within the 3D prostate models. The targeting ring in the bottom right window shows all the possible needle paths that intersect the preplanned target by rotating the TRUS about its long axis. This allows the physician to move the TRUS probe to the target (highlighted by the red dot) in the shortest possible distance. The segmented tumor to be targeted is outlined and rendered in red.

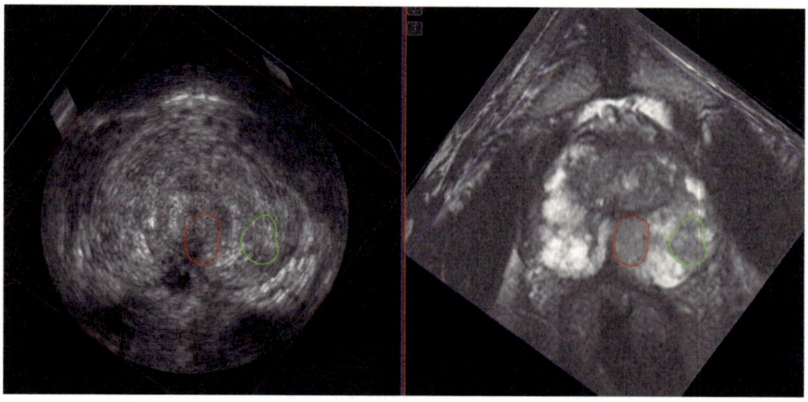

Figure 10. Registered 3D TRUS and MRI images of the same patient showing delineated suspicious lesions identified in the MR images (right panel). The MR images were then registered with the 3D TRUS images (left panel) and the delineated two regions (red and green) superimposed on the 3D TRUS images. These regions were then targeted with the 3D TRUS-guided biopsy system shown in Figs. 8 and 9.

As the physician manually manipulates the TRUS transducer, the 3D location and orientation of the transducer and needle trajectory are tracked in real-time throughout the procedure on the computer screen. Figure 9 illustrates the biopsy interface, which is composed of 4 windows: the live 2D TRUS video stream, the 3D TRUS image, and two 3D model views. The 2D TRUS window displays the real-time 2D TRUS image from the US machine. The 3D TRUS window contains a 2D slice of the 3D static model in real-time to reflect the expected orientation and position of the TRUS probe. This correspondence allows the physician to compare the 3D image with the real-time 2D image to determine if the prostate has moved or deformed to a prohibitive extent. After each biopsy, the biopsy location is recorded in 3D from the tracker orientation, and the system is ready for the next biopsy. After the needle is withdrawn, a 3D image may be obtained to determine if there is any movement or swelling of the prostate.

4.5. Clinical evaluation of 3D TRUS/MRI-guided biopsy

Clinical studies are being performed at a number of centers to evaluate the clinical impact of fusion of MRI to intra-biopsy 3D TRUS for 3D US-guided targeted biopsy of suspicious MRI lesions on prostate cancer detection and grading. At the London Health Sciences Centre in London, Canada, prostate MR imaging was performed on 31 patients with clinical suspicion for prostate cancer in advance of their 3D TRUS-guided biopsy. T2, diffusion-weighted and dynamic-contrast enhanced MR sequences were collected in a 3T MRI system with an endo-rectal RF coil. All suspicious lesions in the MR images were then identified and delineated on the images, which were then registered to the 3D TRUS image obtained during the biopsy procedure (see Figure 10). Using the 3D TRUS-guided biopsy system, prostate biopsy cores were targeted toward each suspicious delineated MRI lesion, which were displayed on the 3D TRUS image. A standard 12-core set of random biopsies was also performed on each patient and used as an internal control.

The results of this study showed that MRI-3D TRUS fusion was successfully performed and the targeted biopsy needle cores had a significantly higher rates of prostate malignancy (30.0%) compared to random, sextant cores (10.0%). In total, prostate cancer was biopsy confirmed in 11 patients; however, only 7 of these patients had abnormal MRI findings (even in retrospective analysis) and were sampled with targeted MRI-3D TRUS fusion. Random sampling detected the remaining four patients. A significantly higher percentage of the targeted biopsy cores (47+/-26%) contained cancer compared to the randomly sampled cores (28+/-26%), and for 3 patients, the MRI-targeted cores detected a higher Gleason cancer grade than the random cores, modifying potential treatment modalities. This study showed that MRI-3D TRUS fusion allows for superior sampling of prostate cancer visible on MRI. This technology may benefit both cancer detection and accurate malignancy grading for appropriate therapeutic management; however, further testing is needed to establish the full utility of this technology.

5. Conclusions

Clinical evaluation of the mechanical tracking systems for use in 3D ultrasound guidance for focal liver ablation and prostate biopsy have been found to be easy to use. The tracker permits manual motions identical to the current conventional procedure, where restricted movements are produced by the US probe in the patient's rectum.

Reconstruction of 3D TRUS images using the hybrid approach for focal liver ablation, and rotational approach for prostate biopsy can produce accurate 3D images without significant visible discontinuity or artefacts. Volume calculations from the 3D TRUS image have shown that the 3D US systems can generate accurate volume measurements.

The patient studies have demonstrated that it is possible to minimize the effects of liver and prostate motion through a variety of mechanical and software mechanisms. However, improved solutions, which correct any patient motion automatically are still needed. It is not possible to control all patient/organ motion during the procedures, particularly if the patient moves during the prostate biopsy procedure after the firing of the prostate biopsy needle. To overcome this problem, a software module would have to be developed to inform the physician that the prostate has moved and then correct for the motion and deformation. This task must be done quickly, possibly in real-time, using an implementation of the software in a graphical processing unit (GPU).

Acknowledgements

The authors gratefully acknowledge the financial support of the Canadian Institutes of Health Research, the Ontario Institute for Cancer Research, the Ontario Research Fund, the National Science and Engineering Research Council, and the Canada Research Chair program.

Author details

Aaron Fenster[1,2,3], Jeff Bax[1,2], Hamid Neshat[1,2], Nirmal Kakani[3] and Cesare Romagnoli[3]

1 Robarts Research Institute, University of Western Ontario, London, Canada

2 Biomedical Engineering Department, University of Western Ontario, London, Canada

3 Department of Medical Imaging, University of Western Ontario, London, Canada

References

[1] Elliott ST. Volume ultrasound: the next big thing? Br J Radiol. 2008;81(961):8-9.

[2] Downey DB, Fenster A, Williams JC. Clinical utility of three-dimensional US. Radiographics. 2000;20(2):559-71.

[3] Boctor EM, Choti MA, Burdette EC, Webster Iii RJ. Three-dimensional ultrasound-guided robotic needle placement: an experimental evaluation. Int J Med Robot. 2008;4(2):180-91.

[4] Hummel J, Figl M, Bax M, Bergmann H, Birkfellner W. 2D/3D registration of endoscopic ultrasound to CT volume data. Phys Med Biol. 2008;53(16):4303-16.

[5] Carson PL, Fenster A. Anniversary paper: evolution of ultrasound physics and the role of medical physicists and the AAPM and its journal in that evolution. Med Phys. 2009;36(2):411-28.

[6] Wei Z, Wan G, Gardi L, Mills G, Downey D, Fenster A. Robot-assisted 3D-TRUS guided prostate brachytherapy: system integration and validation. Med Phys. 2004;31(3):539-48.

[7] Smith WL, Surry K, Mills G, Downey D, Fenster A. Three-dimensional ultrasound-guided core needle breast biopsy. Ultrasound in Med and Bio. 2001;27(8):1025-34.

[8] Chin JL, Downey DB, Onik G, Fenster A. Three-dimensional prostate ultrasound and its application to cryosurgery. Tech Urol. 1996;2(4):187-93.

[9] Chin JL, Downey DB, Mulligan M, Fenster A. Three-dimensional transrectal ultrasound guided cryoablation for localized prostate cancer in nonsurgical candidates: a feasibility study and report of early results. J Urol. 1998;159(3):910-4.

[10] Smith WL, Fenster A. Optimum Scan Spacing for Three-Dimensional Ultrasound by Speckle Statistics. Ultrasound in Medicine and Biology. 2000;26(4):551-62.

[11] Fenster A, Tong S, Sherebrin S, Downey DB, Rankin RN. Three-dimensional ultrasound imaging. SPIE Physics of Medical Imaging. 1995;2432:176-84.

[12] Delabays A, Pandian NG, Cao QL, Sugeng L, Marx G, Ludomirski A, et al. Transthoracic real-time three-dimensional echocardiography using a fan-like scanning approach for data acquisition: methods, strengths, problems, and initial clinical experience. Echocardiography. 1995;12(1):49-59.

[13] Downey DB, Nicolle DA, Fenster A. Three-dimensional orbital ultrasonography. Can J Ophthalmol. 1995;30(7):395-8.

[14] Downey DB, Nicolle DA, Fenster A. Three-dimensional ultrasound of the eye. Administrative Radiology Journal. 1995;14:46-50.

[15] Gilja OH, Thune N, Matre K, Hausken T, Odegaard S, Berstad A. In vitro evaluation of three-dimensional ultrasonography in volume estimation of abdominal organs. Ultrasound Med Biol. 1994;20(2):157-65.

[16] Bax J, Cool D, Gardi L, Knight K, Smith D, Montreuil J, et al. Mechanically assisted 3D ultrasound guided prostate biopsy system. Med Phys. 2008;35(12):5397-410.

[17] Goncalves L, Nien J, Espinoza J, Kusanovic J, Lee W, Swope B, et al. Two-Dimensional (2D) versus three- and four-dimensional (3D/4D) us in obstetrical practice: Does the new technology add anything? American Journal of Obstetrics and Gynecology. 2005;193(6):S150-S.

[18] Peralta CF, Cavoretto P, Csapo B, Falcon O, Nicolaides KH. Lung and heart volumes by three-dimensional ultrasound in normal fetuses at 12-32 weeks' gestation. Ultrasound Obstet Gynecol. 2006;27(2):128-33.

[19] Kurjak A, Miskovic B, Andonotopo W, Stanojevic M, Azumendi G, Vrcic H. How useful is 3D and 4D ultrasound in perinatal medicine? J Perinat Med. 2007;35(1): 10-27.

[20] Blake CC, Elliot TL, Slomka PJ, Downey DB, Fenster A. Variability and accuracy of measurements of prostate brachytherapy seed position in vitro using three-dimensional ultrasound: an intra- and inter-observer study. Med Phys. 2000;27(12):2788-95.

[21] Fenster A, Downey DB, Cardinal HN. Three-dimensional ultrasound imaging. Phys Med Biol. 2001;46(5):R67-99.

[22] Downey DB, Fenster A. Vascular imaging with a three-dimensional power Doppler system. AJR Am J Roentgenol. 1995;165(3):665-8.

[23] Picot PA, Rickey DW, Mitchell R, Rankin RN, Fenster A. Three-dimensional colour Doppler imaging. Ultrasound Med Biol. 1993;19(2):95-104.

[24] Pretorius DH, Nelson TR, Jaffe JS. 3-dimensional sonographic analysis based on color flow Doppler and gray scale image data: a preliminary report. J Ultrasound Med. 1992;11(5):225-32.

[25] Downey DB, Fenster A. Three-dimensional power Doppler detection of prostate cancer [letter]. 1995;165(3):741.

[26] Landry A, Fenster A. Theoretical and experimental quantification of carotid plaque volume measurements made by 3D ultrasound using test phantoms. Medical Physics. 2002.

[27] Landry A, Ainsworth C, Blake C, Spence JD, Fenster A. Manual planimetric measurement of carotid plaque volume using three-dimensional ultrasound imaging. Medical Physics. 2007;34(4):1496-505.

[28] Landry A, Spence JD, Fenster A. Quantification of carotid plaque volume measurements using 3D ultrasound imaging. Ultrasound Med Biol. 2005;31(6):751-62.

[29] Ainsworth CD, Blake CC, Tamayo A, Beletsky V, Fenster A, Spence JD. 3D Ultrasound Measurement of Change in Carotid Plaque Volume; A Tool for Rapid Evaluation of New Therapies. Stroke. 2005;35:1904-9.

[30] Krasinski A, Chiu B, Spence JD, Fenster A, Parraga G. Three-dimensional Ultrasound Quantification of Intensive Statin Treatment of Carotid Atherosclerosis. Ultrasound in Medicine & Biology. 2009;35(11):1763-72.

[31] Bamber JC, Eckersley RJ, Hubregtse P, Bush NL, Bell DS, Crawford DC. Data processing for 3-D ultrasound visualization of tumour anatomy and blood flow. SPIE. 1992;1808:651-63.

[32] Carson PL, Li X, Pallister J, Moskalik A, Rubin JM, Fowlkes JB. Approximate quantification of detected fractional blood volume and perfusion from 3-D color flow and Doppler power signal imaging. 1993 ultrasonics symposium proceedings. Piscataway, NJ: IEEE; 1993. p. 1023-6.

[33] King DL, King DLJ, Shao MY. Evaluation of in vitro measurement accuracy of a three-dimensional ultrasound scanner. J Ultrasound Med. 1991;10(2):77-82.

[34] Tong S, Downey DB, Cardinal HN, Fenster A. A three-dimensional ultrasound prostate imaging system. Ultrasound Med Biol. 1996;22(6):735-46.

[35] Tong S, Cardinal HN, McLoughlin RF, Downey DB, Fenster A. Intra- and inter-observer variability and reliability of prostate volume measurement via two-dimensional and three-dimensional ultrasound imaging. Ultrasound Med Biol. 1998;24(5): 673-81.

[36] Downey DB, Chin JL, Fenster A. Three-dimensional US-guided cryosurgery. Radiology. 1995;197(P):539.

[37] Chin JL, Downey DB, Elliot TL, Tong S, McLean CA, Fortier M, et al. Three dimensional transrectal ultrasound imaging of the prostate: clinical validation. Can J Urol. 1999;6(2):720-6.

[38] Onik GM, Downey DB, Fenster A. Three-dimensional sonographically monitored cryosurgery in a prostate phantom. J Ultrasound Med. 1996;15(3):267-70.

[39] Wei Z, Gardi L, Downey DB, Fenster A. Oblique needle segmentation and tracking for 3D TRUS guided prostate brachytherapy. Med Phys. 2005;32(9):2928-41.

[40] Cool D, Sherebrin S, Izawa J, Chin J, Fenster A. Design and evaluation of a 3D transrectal ultrasound prostate biopsy system. Med Phys. 2008;35(10):4695-707.

[41] Treece G, Prager R, Gee A, Berman L. 3D ultrasound measurement of large organ volume. Med Image Anal. 2001;5(1):41-54.

[42] Detmer PR, Bashein G, Hodges T, Beach KW, Filer EP, Burns DH, et al. 3D ultrasonic image feature localization based on magnetic scanhead tracking: in vitro calibration and validation. Ultrasound Med Biol. 1994;20(9):923-36.

[43] Hodges TC, Detmer PR, Burns DH, Beach KW, Strandness DEJ. Ultrasonic three-dimensional reconstruction: in vitro and in vivo volume and area measurement. Ultrasound Med Biol. 1994;20(8):719-29.

[44] Hughes SW, D'Arcy TJ, Maxwell DJ, Chiu W, Milner A, Saunders JE, et al. Volume estimation from multiplanar 2D ultrasound images using a remote electromagnetic position and orientation sensor. Ultrasound Med Biol. 1996;22(5):561-72.

[45] Leotta DF, Detmer PR, Martin RW. Performance of a miniature magnetic position sensor for three-dimensional ultrasound imaging. Ultrasound Med Biol. 1997;23(4):597-609.

[46] Gilja OH, Detmer PR, Jong JM, Leotta DF, Li XN, Beach KW, et al. Intragastric distribution and gastric emptying assessed by three-dimensional ultrasonography. Gastroenterology. 1997;113(1):38-49.

[47] Nelson TR, Pretorius DH. Visualization of the fetal thoracic skeleton with three-dimensional sonography: a preliminary report. AJR Am J Roentgenol. 1995;164(6):1485-8.

[48] Pretorius DH, Nelson TR. Prenatal visualization of cranial sutures and fontanelles with three-dimensional ultrasonography. J Ultrasound Med. 1994;13(11):871-6.

[49] Raab FH, Blood EB, Steiner TO, Jones HR. Magnetic position and orientation tracking system. IEEE Transactions on Aerospace and Electronic systems. 1979;AES-15:709-17.

[50] Riccabona M, Nelson TR, Pretorius DH, Davidson TE. Distance and volume measurement using three-dimensional ultrasonography. J Ultrasound Med. 1995;14(12):881-6.

[51] Hsu PW, Prager RW, Gee AH, Treece GM. Real-time freehand 3D ultrasound calibration. Ultrasound Med Biol. 2008;34(2):239-51.

[52] Jemal A, Bray F, Center MM, Ferlay J, Ward E, Forman D. Global cancer statistics. CA Cancer J Clin. 2011;61(2):69-90.

[53] Jemal A, Siegel R, Xu J, Ward E. Cancer statistics, 2010. CA Cancer J Clin. 2010;60(5): 277-300.

[54] Solbiati L, Ierace T, Tonolini M, Cova L. Ablation of Liver Metastases: Springer, Berlin; 2004. 311 - 21 p.

[55] El-Serag HB, Marrero JA, Rudolph L, Reddy KR. Diagnosis and treatment of hepatocellular carcinoma. Gastroenterology. 2008;134(6):1752-63.

[56] Adam A, Mueller P. Interventional Radiological Treatment of Liver Tumors. Cambridge, UK: Cambridge University Press; 2009.

[57] McKay A, Fradette K, Lipschitz J. Long-term outcomes following hepatic resection and radiofrequency ablation of colorectal liver metastases. HPB Surg. 2009;2009:346863.

[58] Seki T. "Microwave Coagulation Therapy for Liver Tumors", Tumour Ablation, Principle and Practice: Springer; 2004. 218 - 27 p.

[59] Haemmerich D, Laeseke PF. Thermal tumour ablation: devices, clinical applications and future directions. Int J Hyperthermia. 2005;21(8):755-60.

[60] Cool DW, Gardi L, Romagnoli C, Saikaly M, Izawa JI, Fenster A. Temporal-based needle segmentation algorithm for transrectal ultrasound prostate biopsy procedures. Med Phys. 2010;37(4):1660-73.

[61] Wang Y, Cardinal HN, Downey DB, Fenster A. Semiautomatic three-dimensional segmentation of the prostate using two-dimensional ultrasound images. Med Phys. 2003;30(5):887-97.

[62] Ding M, Cardinal HN, Fenster A. Automatic needle segmentation in three-dimensional ultrasound images using two orthogonal two-dimensional image projections. Med Phys. 2003;30(2):222-34.

[63] Ding M, Fenster A. A real-time biopsy needle segmentation technique using Hough transform. Med Phys. 2003;30(8):2222-33.

[64] Karnik VV, Fenster A, Bax J, Gardi L, Gyacskov I, Montreuil J, et al. Evaluation of inter-session 3D-TRUS to 3D-TRUS image registration for repeat prostate biopsies. Med Image Comput Comput Assist Interv. 2010;13(Pt 2):17-25.

[65] Rickey DW, Picot PA, Christopher DA, Fenster A. A wall-less vessel phantom for Doppler ultrasound studies. Ultrasound Med Biol. 1995;21(9):1163-76.

[66] McNeal JE, Bostwick DG, Kindrachuk RA, Redwine EA, Freiha FS, Stamey TA. Patterns of progression in prostate cancer. Lancet. 1986;1(8472):60-3.

[67] Garfinkel L, Mushinski M. Cancer incidence, mortality and survival: trends in four leading sites. Stat Bull Metrop Insur Co. 1994;75(3):19-27.

[68] Silverberg E, Boring CC, Squires TS. Cancer statistics, 1990 [see comments]. CACancer J Clin. 1990;40:9-26.

[69] Abbas F, Scardino PT. The natural history of clinical prostate carcinoma [editorial; comment]. Cancer. 1997;80(5):827-33.

[70] Shinohara K, Scardino PT, Carter SS, Wheeler TM. Pathologic basis of the sonographic appearance of the normal and malignant prostate. Urol Clin North Am. 1989;16(4): 675-91.

[71] Terris MK, McNeal JE, Stamey TA. Estimation of prostate cancer volume by transrectal ultrasound imaging. J Urol. 1992;147(3 Pt 2):855-7.

[72] Rifkin MD. Ultrasound of the prostate-Imaging in the diagnosis and therapy of prostatic disease. 2 ed. Ryan JD, Patterson D, DiFrancesco R, editors. Philadelphia, New York: Lippincott-Raven Publishers; 1997.

[73] Djavan B, Zlotta AR, Ekane S, Remzi M, Kramer G, Roumeguere T, et al. Is one set of sextant biopsies enough to rule out prostate Cancer? Influence of transition and total prostate volumes on prostate cancer yield. Eur Urol. 2000;38(2):218-24.

[74] Djavan B, Remzi M, Schulman CC, Marberger M, Zlotta AR. Repeat prostate biopsy: who, how and when?. a review. Eur Urol. 2002;42(2):93-103.

[75] Matlaga BR, Eskew LA, McCullough DL. Prostate biopsy: indications and technique. J Urol. 2003;169(1):12-9.

[76] Presti JC, Jr., O'Dowd GJ, Miller MC, Mattu R, Veltri RW. Extended peripheral zone biopsy schemes increase cancer detection rates and minimize variance in prostate specific antigen and age related cancer rates: results of a community multi-practice study. J Urol. 2003;169(1):125-9.

[77] Jemal A, Thomas A, Murray T, Thun M. Cancer statistics, 2002. CA Cancer J Clin. 2002;52(1):23-47.

[78] Nelson WG, De Marzo AM, Isaacs WB. Prostate cancer. N Engl J Med. 2003;349(4): 366-81.

[79] Park SJ, Miyake H, Hara I, Eto H. Predictors of prostate cancer on repeat transrectal ultrasound-guided systematic prostate biopsy. Int J Urol. 2003;10(2):68-71.

[80] Iczkowski KA, Chen HM, Yang XJ, Beach RA. Prostate cancer diagnosed after initial biopsy with atypical small acinar proliferation suspicious for malignancy is similar to cancer found on initial biopsy. Urology. 2002;60(5):851-4.

[81] Thorson P, Humphrey PA. Minimal adenocarcinoma in prostate needle biopsy tissue. Am J Clin Pathol. 2000;114(6):896-909.

[82] San Francisco I, DeWolf W, Rosen S, Upton M, Olumi A. Extended prostate needle biopsy improves concordance of Gleason grading between prostate needle biopsy and radical prostatectomy. Urology. 2003;169:136-40.

[83] Futterer JJ, Heijmink SW, Scheenen TW, Veltman J, Huisman HJ, Vos P, et al. Prostate cancer localization with dynamic contrast-enhanced MR imaging and proton MR spectroscopic imaging. Radiology. 2006;241(2):449-58.

[84] Hricak H, Choyke PL, Eberhardt SC, Leibel SA, Scardino PT. Imaging prostate cancer: a multidisciplinary perspective. Radiology. 2007;243(1):28-53.

[85] Manenti G, Carlani M, Mancino S, Colangelo V, Di Roma M, Squillaci E, et al. Diffusion tensor magnetic resonance imaging of prostate cancer. Invest Radiol. 2007;42(6): 412-9.

[86] Heijmink SW, Futterer JJ, Hambrock T, Takahashi S, Scheenen TW, Huisman HJ, et al. Prostate cancer: body-array versus endorectal coil MR imaging at 3 T--comparison of image quality, localization, and staging performance. Radiology. 2007;244(1): 184-95.

[87] Morgan VA, Kyriazi S, Ashley SE, DeSouza NM. Evaluation of the potential of diffusion-weighted imaging in prostate cancer detection. Acta Radiol. 2007;48(6):695-703.

[88] Farsad M, Schiavina R, Castellucci P, Nanni C, Corti B, Martorana G, et al. Detection and localization of prostate cancer: correlation of (11)C-choline PET/CT with histopathologic step-section analysis. J Nucl Med. 2005;46(10):1642-9.

[89] Martorana G, Schiavina R, Corti B, Farsad M, Salizzoni E, Brunocilla E, et al. 11C-choline positron emission tomography/computerized tomography for tumor localization of primary prostate cancer in comparison with 12-core biopsy. J Urol. 2006;176(3):954-60; discussion 60.

[90] Schoder H, Gonen M. Screening for cancer with PET and PET/CT: potential and limitations. J Nucl Med. 2007;48 Suppl 1:4S-18S.

[91] Fenster A, Downey DB, Cardinal HN. Topical Review: Three-dimensional ultrasound imaging. Phys Med Biol. 2001;46(5):R67-99.

[92] Ladak HM, Mao F, Wang Y, Downey DB, Steinman DA, Fenster A. Prostate boundary segmentation from 2D ultrasound images. Med Phys. 2000;27(8):1777-88.

[93] Hu N, Downey DB, Fenster A, Ladak HM. Prostate boundary segmentation from 3D ultrasound images. Med Phys. 2003;30(7):1648-59.

[94] Cool D, Downey D, Izawa J, Chin J, Fenster A. 3D prostate model formation from non-parallel 2D ultrasound biopsy images. Med Image Anal. 2006;10(6):875-87.

Chapter 2

Ultrasound-Based Guidance and Therapy

Frank Lindseth, Thomas Langø, Tormod Selbekk,
Rune Hansen, Ingerid Reinertsen,
Christian Askeland, Ole Solheim,
Geirmund Unsgård, Ronald Mårvik and
Toril A. Nagelhus Hernes

Additional information is available at the end of the chapter

http://dx.doi.org/10.5772/55884

1. Introduction

Minimally invasive and non-invasive image guided therapy can reduce surgical traumas and improve outcome for patients suffering from a wide variety of diseases. It may also reduce hospital stays and costs. Ultrasound is an important intraoperative imaging modality for guidance and monitoring of these therapeutic methods. Ultrasound has emerged as one of the main modalities for medical imaging in healthcare, the main reason being its ability to image soft tissue, blood flow, organ function and physiology with considerably improved image quality. Furthermore, ultrasound has the unique advantages of real time imaging, equipment portability, safety, and low costs. Ultrasound is now facing a paradigm shift in technology and clinical usability over the coming 10 years. The future potential will be released through exploration in knowledge and innovation deliveries in transducer arrays, ultrasound electronics, software beam forming, parallel imaging and compressed sensing, minimum diffractive wave imaging, model powered acquisition and new technology for a wide range of methods related to physiology, tissue properties and organ function in real time and on site. High-frequency ultrasound imaging makes it possible to obtain significantly improved spatial resolution, however, with limitations related to how deep into the tissue the imaging can be performed. In many image-guided surgery and therapy applications, ultrasound is performed with probes placed directly on the tissue and organ of interest (e.g. intravascular ultrasound, open chest cardiac surgery, esophagus probes for cardiac imaging, probes dedicated to surgery of pituitary gland). These applications limit the size of the ultrasound probe head and thus also the quality of the images. However, with miniaturization based on nanomaterials and nanoelectronics technology, significant improvements in image quality may be obtained. Furthermore, new ultrasound technology can greatly enhance the detection of contrast agents and drug carriers in the tissue. Integration of imaging with navigation technologies will ease image interpretation and further improve precision and accuracy of the therapeutic procedure. Ultrasound technology may also be used for therapeutic purposes. High intensity focused ultrasound (HIFU) for ablation of tumor tissue is already a commercial product. It has also been shown that ultrasound may improve the delivery and distribution of nanoparticles and local drug delivery by enhancing the local release, improving the penetration across the capillary wall and through the extracellular matrix as well as enhance the cellular uptake. The underlying mechanisms are cavitation, radiation force and heating. The ultrasound induced transient increase in porosity and permeability of cell membranes can potentially enhance drug uptake through tissue barriers (also the blood-brain barrier) and improve local drug delivery.

Therapeutic use of ultrasound will be addressed at the end of this chapter, which is mainly about guiding instruments into the body in a safe way using ultrasound, as well as the technological solutions involved to augment ultrasound in combination with other modalities and techniques. Ultrasound has been used to guide interventional instruments into the body for a long time. Different approaches have been used. From freehand 2D guidance, via "needle" guides mounted on conventional ultrasound probes to ultrasound-based navigation using tracking technology and 3D ultrasound (see figure 1). Surgical navigation will be the focus of this chapter and the analogy to GPS-navigation in a car is clear; instead of plotting the position of the car onto electronic maps of the terrain using satellites and GPS-receivers the position of important surgical instruments are shown on medical images of the patient using highly accurate tracking systems. Systems for image-guided surgery are now well established within many clinical disciplines. Surgical tools may be tracked by positioning systems and the surgeon may accurately navigate the tools into the patient with high precision based on image information only. Intraoperative imaging has shown to be important for obtaining improved tumor resection and increased survival for cancer patients undergoing surgery. Integration of intraoperative imaging with navigation technology, providing the surgeon with *updated* image information, is important to deal with tissue shifts and deformations that occur during surgery. MR, CT and ultrasound have been presented as alternative intraoperative imaging modalities showing complementary information and having different benefits and drawbacks. These intraoperative imaging modalities are reported to be useful for accurate navigation of surgical instruments, monitoring the progression of surgery and solving the shift problem. Intraoperative imaging has been used for updating preoperative images, which may be important for accurate guidance. In recent years ultrasound has gained increased attention as a useful intraoperative imaging modality (see figure 2), due to improved image quality and relatively low price. In addition, more integrated solutions, that makes the technology user friendly and flexible has been presented. In the evolution of the next generation of ultrasound-based multimodal navigation systems, advances in ultrasound imaging, registration algorithms, visualization and display techniques and navigation accuracy are important ingredients. We will therefore start by looking into the technology that is needed in order to make ultrasound-based navigation a reality and then show key applications of the navigation technology. Recent advances in ultrasound imaging will be useful also for intraoperative imaging. Furthermore,

http://dx.doi.org/10.5772/55884

ultrasound needs to be integrated with tracking technology in order to make a navigation system with intraoperative imaging capabilities. In addition, such a system might be able to use preoperative CT/MR data, update these data to match the current patient anatomy using intraoperative ultrasound, extract important structures from the different datasets, present the available multimodal information to the surgeon in an optimal way and be able to track all the surgical tools. Last but not least we need to make sure that the navigation system is highly accurate so that we know that the navigation scene presented to the surgeon on the computer screen is a realistic representation of what's really going on inside the patient.

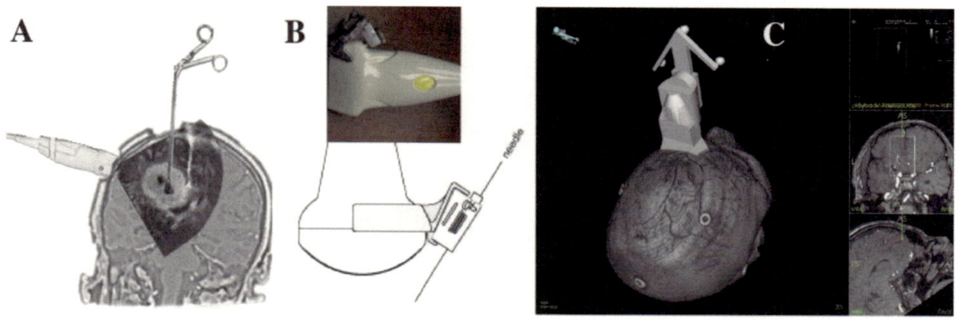

Figure 1. Ultrasound-based guidance: A) Freehand guidance: challenge to have the long axis of the instrument in the 2D ultrasound plane. B) Needle guides: an adapter mounted on the probe makes sure that the instrument is within the 2D ultrasound plane. C) Navigation: tracking technology and 3D data from modalities like CT, MR and ultrasound is used to guide relevant surgical instruments in place. Here an ultrasound probe is guided by MR during a freehand 3D ultrasound aquistion

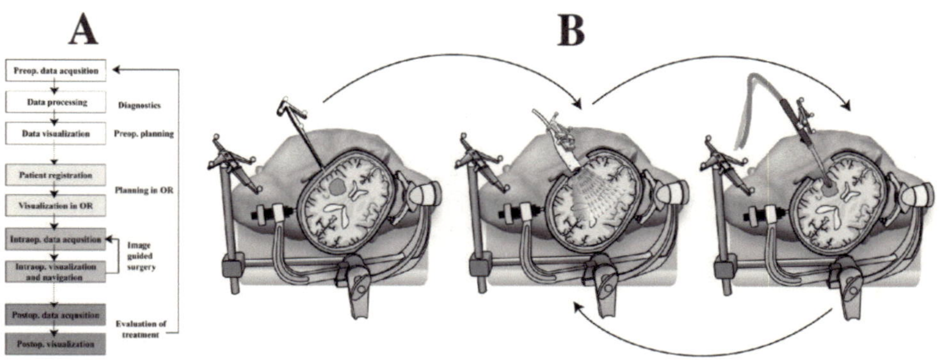

Figure 2. A) Workflow: Important steps in image-guided surgery. B) Ultrasound-based navigation example from neurosurgery: Plan using preoperative MR. Acquire intraoperative 3D ultrasound. Navigation and resection control based on updated ultrasound images. Acquire additional ultrasound data when needed.

2. Recent advances in ultrasound imaging

Sound in the human audible range have frequencies between 20 and 20 000 Hz. Ultrasound is defined as sound with frequencies above 20 kHz. In medical imaging, the ultrasound frequencies are usually between 2 and 40 MHz, with the highest frequencies currently used in intravascular ultrasound (IVUS).

The generation of an ultrasound image is based on transmission of sound pulses and receiving the echoes that have been reflected from tissue boundaries or scattered from smaller objects. In most conventional scanners today, a narrow ultrasound beam is transmitted from the ultrasound transducer. When the transmitted pressure pulse meets a hinder in form of a boundary between different soft tissues, or scatter points within the tissue with different acoustic properties, some of the energy of the transmitted sound pulse is echoed back to the transducer. This pulse-echo principle forms the basis of all ultrasound-imaging techniques, such as conventional brightness mode (B-mode) imaging of organs, imaging of blood flow using Doppler techniques and exploration of mechanical tissue properties using ultrasound elastography techniques.

2.1. Advances in ultrasound hardware and transducer technology

The ultrasound machines and ultrasound probes have gone through massive improvements in the last decade. The general increase in computer power is opening new possibilities for implementing sophisticated methods for beam forming. This may lead to higher resolution and better image quality than for existing solutions [1]. The general trend with miniaturization of components has also strongly influenced the size of the ultrasound imaging systems. Small handheld ultrasound devices have been developed, which makes ultrasound an extremely portable imaging technology. One example of such a pocket sized ultrasound device is the Vscan from GE Healthcare (figure 3), which has been explored for use in echocardiography [2]. The ultrasound transducer technology has made tremendous progress the last decade. The number of elements used by a transducer is increasing and the trend is to go from a single row of elements (1D) to multi-row arrays (1.25D / 1.5D) and 2D matrix arrays. The latter provides the possibility to perform 4D ultrasound imaging, in which a 3D ultrasound volume is acquired and displayed in real time. 4D ultrasound imaging may also be used for monitoring of treatment, e.g. radiofrequency ablation [3].

Ultrasound arrays today are mostly based on piezoelectric materials. The research activities in MUT (Micromachined Ultrasound Transducer) technology, and perhaps especially CMUT (capacitive MUT) transducers, pave the way for silicon-based arrays [4]. This may introduce probes that are cheaper, more customizable and have higher frequencies and bandwidth compared to piezoelectric transducers. In combination with the everlasting trend of miniaturization, the CMUTs may in a long-term perspective allow complete ultrasound systems to be seamlessly integrated with surgical tools. It may very well be that the future surgical instrument has an ultrasound transducer integrated on the tip, and a display unit integrated in the handle.

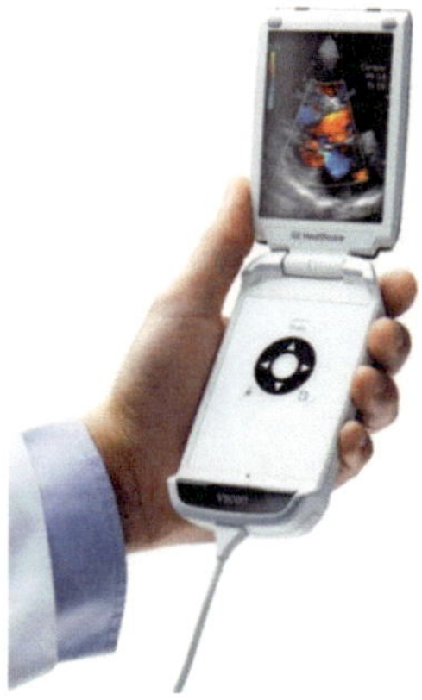

Figure 3. Pocket-sized ultrasound (Vscan from GE Healthcare)

2.2. Ultrasound elastography

The concept of ultrasound imaging of tissue strain or elasticity is often referred to as ultrasound elastography and the corresponding 2D images are frequently called elastograms. The imaging technique is often explained to be analogue to palpation, where the physician uses the fingers to apply a slight pressure in order to examine the stiffness of the tissue. If a organ is vibrating or excited, ultrasound elastography methods can in a similar fashion be used to map areas with differences in strain (figure 4).

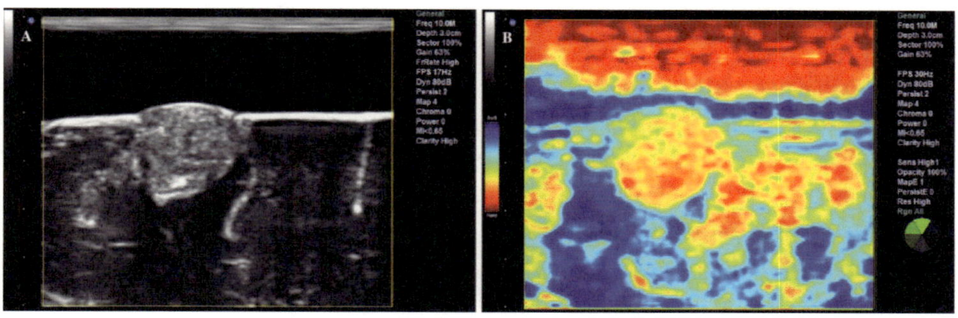

Figure 4. Elastography. A) Ultrasound B-mode image of a small meningioma, and B) the ultrasound elastogram of the tumour as displayed on an Ultrasonix MDP scanner.

The theoretical framework for the study of behavior of vibrating soft tissue was established in the early 1950ies. Von Gierke et al. published *"Physics of vibrations in living tissues"* in 1952 [5], for example. However, it was not until 30 years later that tissue movement was first measured for clinical purposes by using ultrasound in a study of tissue motion in the liver caused by vascular pulsation [6, 7]. In the late 1980ies, techniques for vibration elastography imaging, also known as vibration amplitude sonoelastography or simply sonoelasticity imaging was developed [8]. In this technique a low frequency vibration (20-1000 Hz) is applied externally to the skin surface to investigate the subcutaneous structures. The internal motion of the tissue is investigated with a pulsed Doppler technique. Stiff tissue responds differently to the vibrations than softer tissue, and can therefore be distinguished in the real-time images.

In the early 1990ies, the development of compression elastography, also referred to as quasi-static elasticity imaging, begun. Ophir published a paper in 1991 where ultrasound radio frequency (RF) data before and after applying compression were compared and processed using cross-correlation to obtain the time-shifts of the echoes. This allowed the subsequent calculation of elastograms [9]. The quasi-static elasticity imply that the force is applied for a sufficiently long time for the tissue strain to stabilize, and the resulting difference in echo travel time between ultrasound data acquired before and after compression can be calculated. The tissue may also be excited by applying forces at the surface (manually or by electromechanical devices) or by physiological processes within the organ, as for example the pulsation of the arteries. The generated elastograms are usually displayed as a color-coded overlay on the conventional ultrasound brightness mode image. The color mapping may cover a range of unit-less strain values as percentages from minimum (negative) strain to maximum (positive) strain. Alternatively, it may also be mapped from "soft" to "hard" tissue, thereby not quantifying the strain range displayed. Quasi-static elasticity imaging has been evaluated in a broad range of clinical applications. It has been reported used in diagnostics of tumors in for example breast, prostate, liver, the thyroid gland and in the brain (figure 4) [10-15]. Quasi-static elasticity imaging is an emerging ultrasound imaging modality, now becoming more and more available as an option on commercial ultrasound systems.

As previously explained, the elastography methods require that the tissue is excited. The tissue movement can be caused by physiological processes internally in the organ such as the pulsation of the arteries. The tissue can also be externally excited by manually pushing the tissue or by using an electromechanical vibrating device. An alternative approach is to use the acoustic radiation force of an ultrasonic focused beam to generate displacements in the tissue with subsequent detection of the mechanical properties. One example of such an approach is the Acoustic Radiation Force Impulse (ARFI) method developed at Duke University [16]. In this technique, short duration acoustic pulses (push pulses) are used to generate small localized displacements deep in the tissue. These displacements are tracked by ultrasonic cross correlation, in a similar fashion as for the quasi-static elasticity imaging. The method has been investigated for imaging of focal liver lesions, prostate and breast [17-19].

Another example is the innovative Supersonic Shear Imaging (SSI) method developed by the research group at the Laboratoire Ondes et Acoustique [20]. In SSI the acoustic radiation force is used to generate low-frequency shear waves (50-500 Hz) remotely in the tissue. The shear modulus of the tissue can be quantified by imaging the share wave propagation in the tissue by using ultrasound frame rates of several kHz. The method has been explored for diagnosis of liver fibrosis, breast lesions and cornea [21-23].

For a more detailed overview about methods for ultrasound elasticity imaging and its clinical use we recommend to read the review papers by Wells and Liang [24] and Parker, Doyley and Rubens [25].

2.3. Nonlinear acoustics and contrast agents

In 1980, Carstensen and Muir published two papers describing the importance of nonlinear acoustics within the field of medical ultrasound imaging [26, 27]. These papers predicted and demonstrated nonlinear acoustical effects relevant for intensities and frequencies common in biomedical imaging. There has been an increasing interest with respect to nonlinear biomedical acoustics during the last 30 years. This interest was further escalated by the introduction of ultrasound contrast agents in the form of microbubbles and the study of these microbubbles was the main impetus for the introduction of the tissue harmonic imaging technique.

Nonlinear effects can be important in the forward wave propagation. The back-scattered pressure levels of the echoes are typically too low to induce any significant nonlinear effects. One source of nonlinear terms is produced by the deformation of tissue volume elements during compression and expansion with strongly curved phase fronts. It is, however, common to use transmit beams with relatively smooth phase fronts. Consequently, this nonlinear source is usually not the most dominant. The other important nonlinear source is nonlinear terms in the tissue elasticity and hence in the relation between acoustic pressure and tissue compression/expansion. Nonlinear terms in the tissue elasticity are responsible for the fact that the tissue becomes stiffer during compression and softer during expansion. The compression also increases the mass density of the tissue, but this effect is inferior to the increased stiffness and the propagation velocity and will therefore be pressure dependent and will increase with increasing compressions and thus with increasing pressure. The resulting distortion of the transmit pressure field produces harmonic components which today are utilized in tissue harmonic imaging, especially in transcutaneous cardiac and abdominal imaging to suppress multiple scattering [28-31].

Ultrasound imaging is based on several assumptions, and one important assumption is that multiple scattering is neglected. For many organs, this approximation is valid. However, for the body wall, where larger variations in material parameters often are found, this assumption can be inadequate. Interfaces between soft tissue components with significant differences in material parameters give so strong echoes from the transmitted acoustic pulses that multiple scattering can get significant amplitudes. Such multiple scatterings are usually termed pulse reverberations [32, 33]. These reverberations reduce the ratio of the strongest to the weakest scatterer that can be detected in the neighborhood of each other, defined as the contrast resolution in the image. Reduced contrast resolution is in particular a problem when imaging hypo-echoic structures such as the heart chambers, the lumen of large blood vessels, some atherosclerotic lesions, cysts, some tumors, the gallbladder as well as in fetal imaging. The contact interface between the ultrasound transducer itself and the soft tissue is also a strong reflector enhancing the problem with multiple scattering.

Ultrasound contrast agents are made as a suspension of gas microbubbles encapsulated in thin stabilizing shells made from lipid or albumin. Typical bubble size is in the 1-5 μm range and the contrast bubbles are intravenously injected to increase the scattering from blood, which is weak compared to the scattering from soft tissues. Commercially available contrast bubbles are stable and small enough to enable transpulmonary passage and the blood half-life is typically in the range of 1-10 minutes. Scattering from microbubbles occurring within a liquid is resonant through an interaction between a co-oscillating liquid mass around the bubble and the bubble compression elasticity [34] with typical resonance frequencies of 1-7 MHz. With adequately flexible shells, the gas bubble has a very high compliance relative to the surrounding blood and when driven by ultrasound pulses at frequencies below or around the bubble resonance frequency, large bubble radius excursions on the order of one micrometer is achieved due to mainly shear deformation and limited volume compression of the blood surrounding the bubble. This bubble radius displacement is then between one and two orders of magnitude larger than typical particle displacements obtained within soft tissues. The radius oscillation of a bubble may be obtained from the Rayleigh-Plesset equation [35, 36]:

$$\rho\left(a\ddot{a} + \frac{3}{2}\dot{a}^2\right) = -B(a, \dot{a}) - p_i(t) \tag{1}$$

where ρ is the mass density of the surrounding liquid, a is the bubble radius (where the time dependence has been omitted for convenience), B is the pressure produced by the gas and the encapsulating shell, p_i is the incident drive pressure and the dots represent differentiation with respect to time so that $\dot{a}$ and $\ddot{a}$ represent the velocity and acceleration of the bubble wall, respectively. The terms on the left-hand side represent acceleration forces of the co-oscillation liquid mass whereas the terms on the right-hand side represent pressure terms due to gas and shell elasticity in addition to the drive pressure. The bubble pressure B can be written

$$B(a, \dot{a}) = -\left(p_0 + \frac{2\sigma}{a_0}\right)\left(\frac{a_0}{a}\right)^{3\kappa} - S(a_0, a) + p_0 + \frac{2\sigma}{a} + \mu\frac{\dot{a}}{a} \tag{2}$$

where the first term is the gas pressure and where κ is the polytropic exponent of the gas and a_0 is the equilibrium bubble radius. The second term S is the pressure contribution from the encapsulating shell and p_0 is the ambient hydrostatic pressure. The fourth term accounts for surface tension due to the gas-liquid interface and the last term accounts for damping effects. When a contrast bubble is insonified by frequencies below or around its resonance frequency, the local nonlinear scattering from the contrast bubble is usually much larger than from soft tissues [37, 38]. This has resulted in several nonlinear ultrasound contrast agent detection techniques with the purpose to suppress the linear part of a received signal while maintaining as much as possible of the nonlinear part of a received signal. This is then used for low transmit pressure levels. The forward wave propagation is close to linear whereas the scattering from microbubbles can be highly nonlinear. Common techniques in use today are Pulse Inversion methods that detect even harmonic components [39, 40]. Amplitude Modulation methods are also in use [41], often in combination with Pulse Inversion methods [42-44].

The equations describing the bubble oscillations can be solved numerically. An example of a bubble with equilibrium radius of 2 μm is shown in figure 5. An incident drive pulse with center frequency around 2 MHz is displayed in the time and frequency domain in the upper panel. In the middle panel, the resulting bubble radius oscillation is depicted and in the lower panel, the resulting normalized far-field component of the scattered pressure from the bubble is displayed. It can bee seen that the response is highly nonlinear and several harmonic

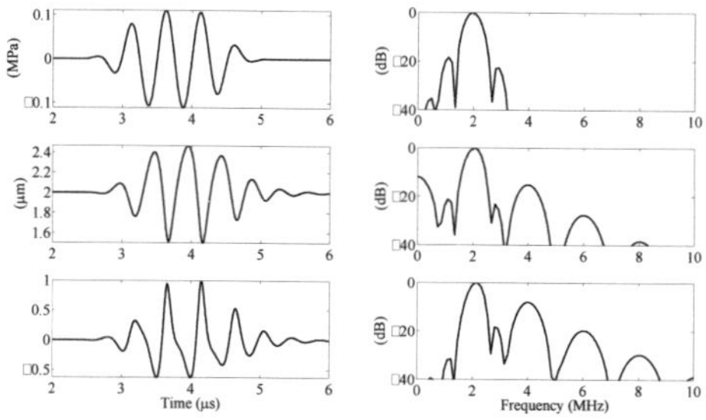

Figure 5. Numerical simulation of oscillation for a bubble with equilibrium radius of 2 μm and resonance frequency of 2.5 MHz. The upper panels show the drive pulse, the middle panels show the resulting bubble radius oscillation and the lower panels show the far-field component of the scattered pressure from the bubble. The left panels display the pulses in the time domain whereas the modulus of the Fourier Transform is displayed in the right panels.

components are present in the scattered pressure from the bubble. This response is obtained with an incident drive pulse having a mechanical index equal to 0.07, which is very low compared to what is used for regular tissue imaging. At such low transmit pressure levels, the forward wave propagation will be close to linear and distortion of the transmit field due to nonlinear tissue elasticity will thus be very low. The harmonic components can then be used to differentiate bubble echoes from tissue echoes through Pulse Inversion and Amplitude Modulation pulsing schemes. In most clinical applications of ultrasound contrast agents, it is desirable to assess the micro-circulation or the tissue perfusion which cannot be done without the use of contrast agents and which often is related to various diseases. It is then necessary to obtain a strong suppression of the tissue signal for detection of the contrast bubble signal.

An example of the use of ultrasound contrast agents in relation to minimally invasive interventions is radiofrequency ablation of liver tumors where contrast-enhanced ultrasound is used for improved detection and imaging of the lesions, for planning and guidance of multiple needle electrodes and finally for immediate evaluation of the treatment [45].

SURF (Second order UltRasound Field) imaging is a nonlinear ultrasound imaging technique being developed in Trondheim [46-50]. It is based on transmission of dual frequency band pulse complexes consisting of a low frequency manipulation pulse and a high frequency imaging pulse that are co-propagating. Two transmit pulse complexes that may be used with the SURF technique are displayed in figure 6. With the use of conventional single frequency band transmit pulses, nonlinear effects are mainly restricted to the generation of harmonic components of the imaging pulse. With dual frequency band transmit pulses, other nonlinear effects also come into play. SURF imaging aims at further utilizing nonlinear acoustics for improved imaging of various tissues and ultrasound contrast agents.

For imaging of ultrasound microbubbles, conventional techniques relies on driving the bubble into strong nonlinear oscillations with the imaging pulse at relatively low mechanical indexes. This is typically feasible when the imaging frequency is below or around the bubble resonance frequency (as in the example of figure 5) and conventional contrast agents typically have resonance frequencies below 7 MHz. However, when the imaging frequency is above the bubble resonance frequency a much higher mechanical index is required to obtain significant

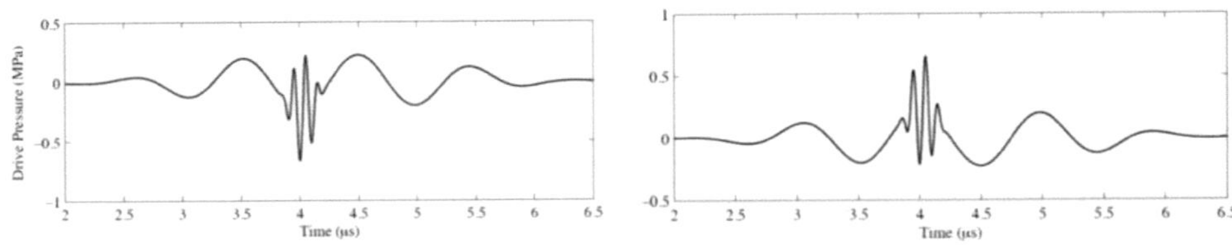

Figure 6. Example of SURF transmit pulse complexes where a low frequency manipulation pulse at 1 MHz is co-propagating with a high frequency imaging pulse at 10 MHz. The high frequency imaging pulse is in the left and right panel placed at low and high manipulation pressure, respectively.

nonlinear back-scattering from the bubble. At higher mechanical indexes the tissue will also respond nonlinearly and it then becomes difficult to differentiate the tissue signal from the bubble signal. For contrast imaging at high frequencies, such as 10 – 30 MHz, that can be used in minimal invasive interventions where the probe can be close to the object being imaged, conventional contrast imaging techniques often have limitations. The dual band SURF technique then has some advantages where the low frequency manipulation pulse can be tuned to match the bubble resonance frequency (typically around 2-3 MHz) whereas the high frequency imaging pulse can be optimized for the object being imaged and can for example be 20 MHz. The low frequency then manipulates the bubble oscillation and back-scattering which is interrogated by the high frequency pulse. The high frequency imaging pulse is hence decoupled from the resonance properties of the contrast bubbles.

3. Ultrasound-based navigation — Enabling technologies

State of the art ultrasound imaging is crucial for guiding interventions. But unlike freehand guidance and guidance based on ultrasound guides (figure 1) having optimal images on the ultrasound scanner is not enough to enable surgical navigation. In order to use ultrasound-based navigation to guide such procedures we usually have to:

- Get the images out of the ultrasound scanner and into the navigation software in real-time.
- Track the position and orientation of the ultrasound probe at all times.
- Synchronize the image and tracking streams (temporal calibration) and find the transformation between the tracking sensor mounted on the ultrasound probe and the ultrasound scan plane (spatial calibration), which is the interesting part to track.
- Reconstruct all the position tagged ultrasound frames from a conventional 2D ultrasound probe into a regular 3D volume that can be used in the same way as preoperative MR or CT is.

3.1. Streaming of ultrasound data

Convenient ultrasound-based navigation of surgical instruments requires real-time access to the ultrasound data in the navigation software (figure 7). This is required in order to tag the ultrasound frames with position and orientation data from the tracking system (alternatively the tracking data could be directed directly into the scanner and the ultrasound frames could be used off-line, e.g. to generate a 3D volume from the tagged 2D frames). The traditional way of getting real-time access to ultrasound frames is to connect the analog output (e.g., composite video, S-video) of the ultrasound scanner to a frame-grabbing card on the navigation computer. Using the analog output might affect the image quality due to the double digital-to-analog-to-digital conversion and no metadata (e.g. depth) follow the ultrasound images. Alternatively digital data can be streamed directly from the ultrasound scanner and into the navigation computer. Traditionally this has required some kind of research collaboration between the ultrasound manufacturer and the user but open ultrasound scanners are becoming available (e.g. the Ultrasonix scanner). These systems usually provide just a one-way streaming interface but two-way communication protocols where the scanner can be controlled (e.g. depth) by the navigation system exists making more integrated solutions possible (figure 7). Either way, the protocol (or interface / API) used is typically proprietary, although proposals for real-time standards are starting to emerge (e.g. OpenIGTLink, DICOM in surgery (WG24)). When the link between the ultrasound scanner and navigation system is digital, ultrasound data at different stages in the processing chain on the scanner can be transferred (e.g. scan-converted, scan-line and RF-data). Furthermore, a digital streaming interface will be required in order to use the real-time 3D scanners that are now becoming available also for navigation. It's difficult to capture the 3D content in the scanner display using a frame grabber so the data needs to be transferred in real-time or tagged with a tracking reference on the ultrasound scanner.

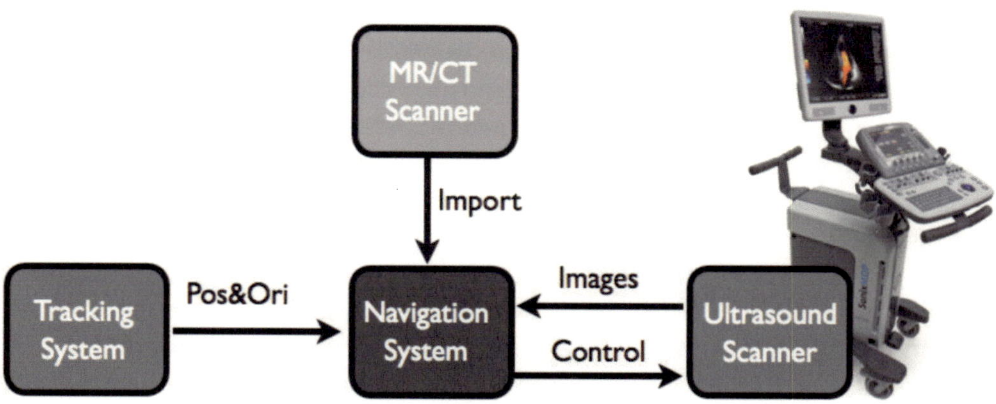

Figure 7. Streaming ultrasound data into the navigation system. The interface can either be analog using a frame grabber or digital using a direct link and a proprietary protocol. A digital interface can either be one-way (i.e. streaming) or two-way (i.e. optionally control the scanner from the navigation system as well). In any case the image stream must be tagged with tracking data and in order to do that the two streams need to be synchronized.

3.2. Tracking of ultrasound probes

In order to use ultrasound to guide surgical procedures the ultrasound probe must be tracked. Several tracking technologies have been proposed over the years (mechanical, acoustical, optical and electromagnetic), but currently the most widely used solutions are optical or electromagnetic systems (see figure 8). Choosing the best tracking technology depends on the application at hand and the ultrasound probes used. If possible optical tracking systems should be preferred as magnetic tracking in the operating room can be challenging due to disturbances from metallic objects and the accuracy is close but not as good as optical systems under favorable conditions. For flexible us-probes or probes that are inserted into the body magnetic tracking is required as the transformation between the sensor and the scan plane must be rigid and optical tracking demands clear line of sight to the cameras. In addition the magnetic sensors are very small, crucial in order to be embedded in instruments and put into the body. When the ultrasound probe is tracked it becomes one of several tools and the streamed ultrasound data can either be shown in real time at the right spot in the patient or made into a 3D volume and shown together with other images to the surgeon. A brief description of the two main tracking technologies can be found below [51, 52]:

- *Optical tracking systems*: The basic idea is to use one or more cameras with markers distributed on a rigid structure where the geometry is specified beforehand (figure 8A). At least three markers are necessary to determine the position and orientation of the rigid body in space. Additional markers allow a better camera visibility of the tracked object and improve the measurement accuracy. The markers can be infrared light-emitting diodes (active markers), infrared light reflectors (passive markers) or some kind of pattern (usually a checker board) that can be identified using visual light and image analysis.

- *Electromagnetic tracking systems*: A receiver (sensor) is placed on the ultrasound probe and the system measures the induced electrical currents when the sensor is moved within a magnetic field generated by either an alternating current (AC) or direct current (DC) transmitter / generator (figure 8B). The AC and DC devices are both sensitive to some types of metallic objects placed too close to the transmitter or receiver, and to magnetic fields generated by power sources and devices such as cathode-ray tube monitors. Therefore, both types of electromagnetic systems are challenging to use in an environment such as an operating room, where various metallic objects are moved around in the field [53]. The two metal related phenomena that influence the performance of electromagnetic tracking systems are ferromagnetism and eddy currents [54]. Ferromagnetic materials (e.g., iron, steel) affect both AC and DC systems, because they change the homogeneity of the tracker-generated magnetic field, although the DC systems may be more sensitive to these effects. In contrast, the AC technology is more affected by the presence of conductors such as copper and aluminum because of distortions caused by eddy currents [53, 55]. DC systems minimize the eddy-current related distortions by sampling the field after eddy currents have decayed.

- *Comparisons between optical and magnetic tracking systems - pros and cons:* The main advantages with optical tracking systems are their robustness and high accuracy and the challenges are line of sight problems and the relatively big sensor frames. For electromagnetic tracking system it's basically the other way around.

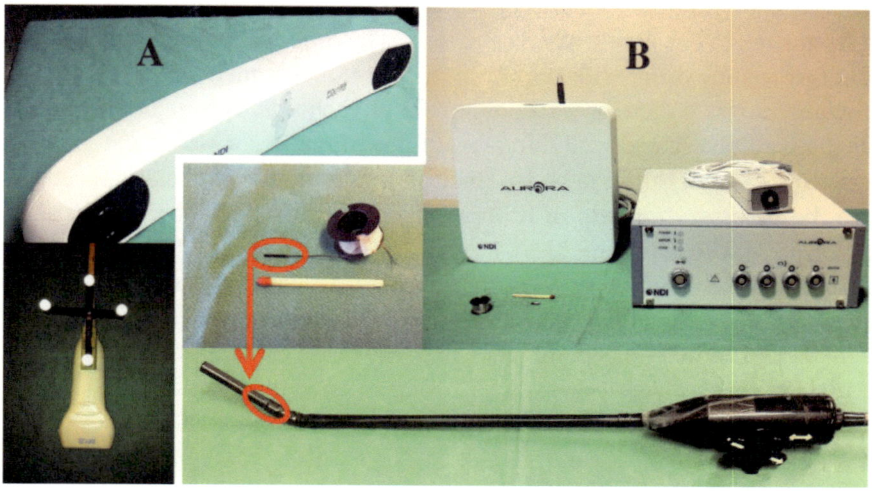

Figure 8. Optical (A) and electromagnetic (B) tracking of ultrasound probes.

3.3. Ultrasound probe calibration

After streaming ultrasound data into the navigation software and tracking the ultrasound probe, calibration is needed in order to integrate the image stream with the tracking stream. Ultrasound probe calibration is an important topic as this is the main error source for ultrasound-based navigation (see section on accuracy). Two types of calibration are necessary; temporal calibration to find the lag between the image and tracking streams and spatial calibration [56, 57] to find the transformation between the ultrasound scan plane and the tracking sensor mounted on the ultrasound-probe (see figure 9):

- *Temporal calibration (find the time lag between the image stream and the tracking stream, see figure 9A)*: The most common way to do this is to move the ultrasound probe up and down in a water bath and extract some feature in the generated us-images (or correlate the images and measure the displacement). This gives us two sinus-like curves, one for the vertical position of the extracted feature in the images and one for the vertical component in the tracking data. The two curves are compared and one of them is fitted to the other to find the time lag between the two streams.

- *Spatial calibration (find the transformation between the image and the sensor, see figure 9B)*: Considerable effort has been spent on probe calibration over the last decade, and it still seems to be a hot research topic. Maybe because it is a challenging task to make it accurate, especially if the same method / phantom is to be used for substantially different probes. It is not possible to measure this transform with a ruler because the orientation of the scan plane relative to the sensor frame is unknown, we do not know the origin of the us-plane inside the probe housing and magnetic sensors do not have a known origin. A commonly used approach for probe calibration is to acquire 2-D images of a phantom with known geometry and to identify distinct features in the images. Because the location of the same features are known in the global coordinate system, the probe calibration matrix can be found from a relatively simple matrix equation. The probe calibration methods reported in the literature mainly differ with respect to the phantom geometry, whereas the processing of the acquired data is more or less common for all methods. The majority of probe calibration methods can be categorized into one of three different classes: single- point or line; 2-D alignment; and freehand methods. The calibration matrix can be calculated as follows. Acquire the necessary amount of calibration images and find the coordinates of all the calibration points in each image. Next, we transform the corresponding physical points from global reference coordinates into sensor frame coordinates by using the inverse of the tracking matrix. The rigid body transformation that minimizes the mean Euclidian distance between the two homologous point sets will be the probe calibration matrix. The matrix can be calculated using a direct least squares error minimization technique [58].

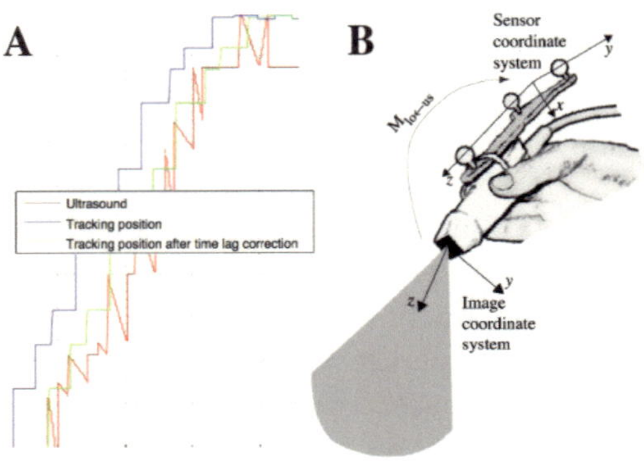

Figure 9. Temporal (A) and spatial (B) calibration of the ultrasound probe.

3.4. 3D Ultrasound

It is difficult to guide an instrument into place using conventional 2D ultrasound only (freehand guidance): in order to know where the instrument is we need to see it in the ultrasound image and to reach the target we have to know where to go from there, a challenging hand-eye coordination task. It's much more convenient to acquire a 3D ultrasound volume first and let the tracked instrument extract slices from the volume that can be annotated with the position and / or orientation of the instrument (see section on visualization).

3D ultrasound data can be acquired in different ways [59]. A conventional 1D array probe (2D +t) can be moved over the area of interest, either by freehand motion or by a motor. If freehand movement is used all the ultrasound frames can be put together into a volume using tracking data (figure 10) or correlation. A motor inside the probe hosing or external to it can also be used to cover the ROI by tilt, translation or rotation of the 1D array (figure 11). Furthermore, with a 2D matrix probe the ultrasound beam can be steered in the elevation direction in addition to the lateral (azimuth) direction so that the ROI can be covered while the probe is standing still making real-time 3D ultrasound imaging possible (figure 12).

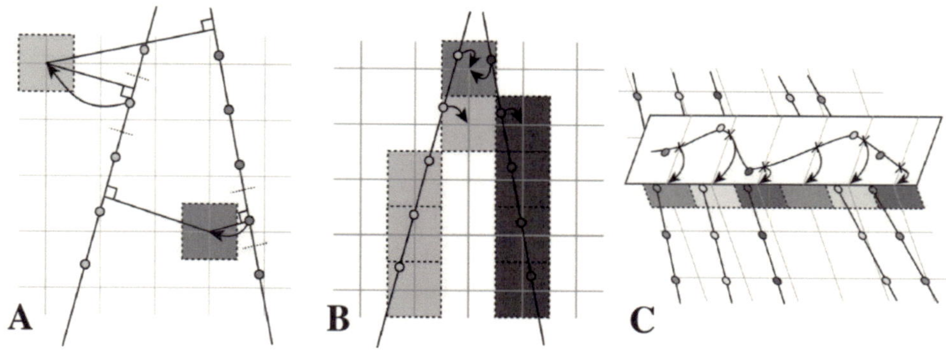

Figure 10. Reconstruction methods: A) Voxel Nearest Neighbor (VNN), B) Pixel Nearest Neighbor (PNN), Distribution Step (DS) and C) Functional Based Methods (FBM).

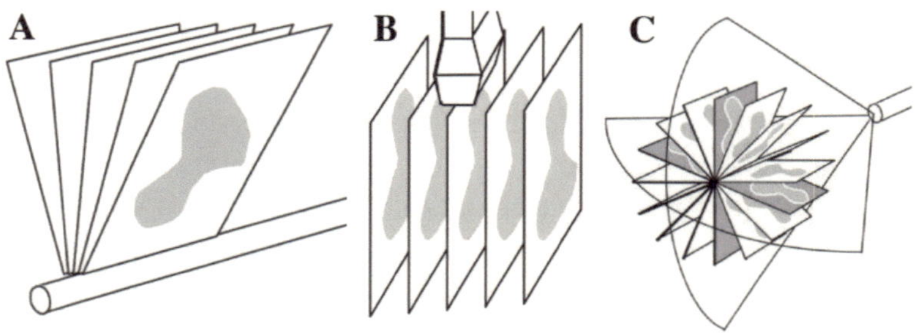

Figure 11. Motorized / mechanical tilting (A), translation (B) and rotation (C). Source: Fenster [59]

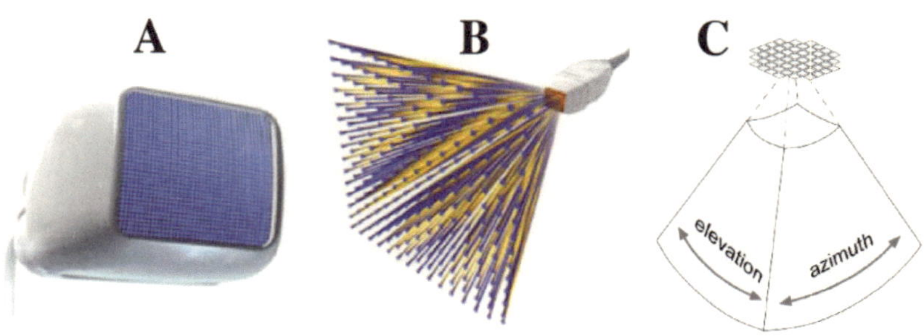

Figure 12. Matrix probes. Using a 2D array of elements (A) the beam can be steered in two directions (B) and a truncated pyramid of data is acquired (C).

In practice the following methods are in use:

- *Freehand 3D ultrasound:* This is still the most wildly used method (mainly because of its flexibility) and usually the method works in the following manner: *Scan* the area of interest using a conventional 2D probe that is tracked and *reconstruct* the position tagged ultrasound frames into a regular 3D volume that can be used in the same way as preoperative MR or CT. The ultrasound probe is usually tracked by optical or electromagnetic sensors, but other methods have been proposed. Furthermore, different methods exist to reconstruct all the 2D frames into a regular 3D volume. The methods can be categorized into tree main groups [60]:
  - *Voxel-based methods (VBM)*: VBM traverse each voxel in the target voxel grid and gather information from the input 2D images to be placed in the voxel. One or several pixels may contribute to the value of each voxel. The simplest method in this category is Voxel Nearest Neighbor (VNN), which traverses each voxel in the target volume and assigns the value of the nearest image pixel (see figure 10A).
  - *Pixel-based methods (PBM)*: PBM usually consists of two steps: a Distribution Step (DS) where the input pixels are traversed and applied to one or several voxels and a Hole-Filling Step (HFS) where the voxels are traversed and empty voxels are being filled. The simplest method in this category is Pixel Nearest Neighbor (PNN) that runs through each pixel in all the 2D input images and assigns the pixel value to the nearest voxel in the target volume (see figure 10B).
  - *Function based methods (FBM)*: FBM choose a particular function (like a polynomial) and determine the coefficients to make the functions pass through the input pixels. Afterwards, the function can be used to create a regular voxel array by evaluating the function at regular intervals (see figure 10C). These methods produce reconstructed volumes with the highest quality but are very computational intensive and are in limited use today.
- *Motorized (or mechanical) 3D ultrasound*: Instead of using freehand movement of the ultrasound probe over the area of interest a motor can cover the same region by tilting (figure 11A), translating (figure 11B) or rotating (figure 11C) a conventional 1D ultrasound array. Motorized probes have existed for a long time and the motor can either be mounted inside the probe housing (easy to use but requires a specially build ultrasound probe) or be applied externally (more flexible as conventional probes can be used). Many of the benefits with freehand scanning also apply to motorized scanning, e.g. the possibility to use high frequency probes with higher spatial resolution, also in the elevation direction (1.25D/1.5D probes). Motorized scanning can use the same kind of reconstruction methods as freehand scanning but usually more optimized methods are used as the movement is known and the probe do not need to be tracked during the acquisition. Compared to freehand ultrasound the motorized probes are easier to use in an intraoperative setting, but on the other hand, they are not as flexible in general.
- *Real-time 3D ultrasound using 2D matrix probes* [61-65]: Instead of using a conventional 1D array transducer that is moved by freehand or by a motor to sweep out the anatomy of interest, transducers with 2D phased arrays (figure 12A) that can generate 3D images in real time have been developed. Electronics is used to control and steer the ultrasound beam

(figure 12B) and sweep out a volume shaped like a truncated pyramid (figure 12C). The main challenge with this technology is the large and heavy cable that would be required to connect all the elements in the array to a wire. Fortunately technological achievements in terms of multiplexing, sparse arrays and parallel processing over the last decade have made these systems commercially available. They are used extensively in echocardiology, which requires dynamic three-dimensional imaging of the heart and its valves.

3.5. Integrated ultrasound-based navigation solutions

Ultrasound and navigation can be integrated in different ways as we have seen. Complete systems can usually be categorized as follows:

- *Two-rack systems:* Where the navigation computer with tracking system etc. and the ultrasound scanner are two separate systems. This is most common, especially in a research environment. The main reason for this is flexibility, in principle any ultrasound scanner with an analog output can be used together with a navigation system that is equipped with ultrasound-based navigation software. An example of such a configuration is our in house research system for us-based navigation called CustusX (figure 13A). The system is used for different clinical applications (e.g. neurosurgery and laparoscopy), each navigation rack is equipped with both optical and magnetic tracking and can be connected to a variety of ultrasound scannersusing analog and digital interfaces.

- *One-rack systems:* Here the ultrasound scanner and the navigation computer have been integrated in the same system. These systems are more convenient to use in the operating room but are less flexible. Most commercial solutions belong to this category. Two variations exists:

  - *An ultrasound scanner with navigation software integrated.* The PercuNav system from Philips, an integrated solution for navigation and intraoperative imaging, is an example of this (figure 13B).

  - *A navigation system with an ultrasound scanner integrated*: The SonoWand system (Trondheim, Norway), where an ultrasound scanner has been embedded in the navigation rack, is an example of this (figure 13C). The system can be used in three distinct ways: 1) as a navigation system based on preoperative MR/CT data, 2) as a standalone ultrasound scanner and 3) as an ultrasound-based navigation system with intraoperative imaging capabilities, its main use.

4. Registration and segmentation in ultrasound-based navigation

Registration is the process of transforming an image into the coordinate system of a patient, or another image. After registration, the same anatomical features have the same coordinates in both the image and the patient, or in both images. Image-to-patient registration is one of the cornerstones of any navigation system, and is necessary for navigation using pre-operative

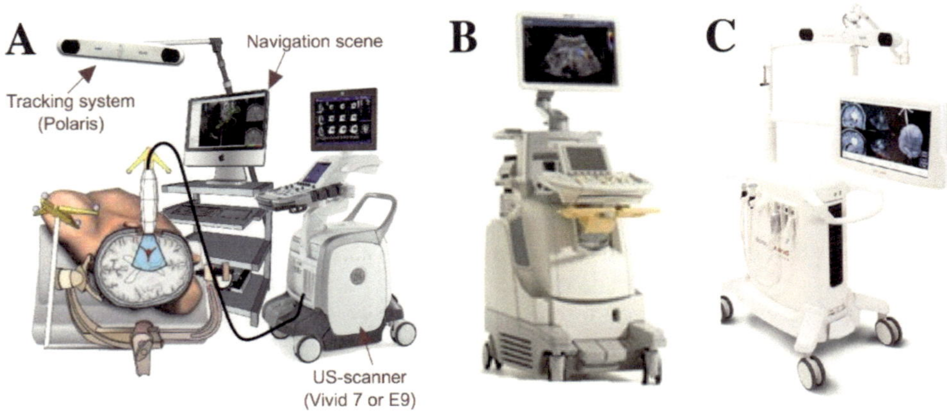

Figure 13. Different approaches to integrating (3D) ultrasound and navigation. A) A two-rack solution and examples of one-rack solutions (B and C).

images such as MR and/or CT. Image-to-image registration is useful to align pre-operative images before registration to the patient, and also to update the pre-operative images during surgery using for example intra-operative US. Only the latter involves US and will be the focus in this section, but image-to-patient registration is important for proper initialization of the MR/CT-to-US registration. The main motivation behind image-to-image registration is that different images contain different and complimentary information about the patient at a given point in time. When we bring the images into the same coordinate system and into the coordinate system of the patient, we can take advantage of more of the useful information in the different images. Such information can be the size and location of the surgical target, important blood vessels, critical structures that should be avoided etc. The registration method used in each case depends heavily on the type of images we want to register. The type of spatial transformation, how we measure the similarity between the images and how this measure is optimized are key components of any registration procedure.

4.1. Registration of preoperative images to the patient

Image-to-patient registration is a necessary and crucial step in order to use pre-operative images for guidance. Intraoperative ultrasound only shows a limited portion of the surgical field and might require some experience to appreciate. Preoperative data can therefore be used for overview and interpretation. In neurosurgery, for example, it is not possible to acquire ultrasound images before opening of the dura. Pre-operative images are therefore necessary for planning the craniotomy.

One of the most frequently used registration methods consists in using self-adhesive markers, also called fiducials. The fiducials are glued to the patient's skin before MR or CT imaging. The markers can be identified in the images and the corresponding markers can be identified on the patient using a tracked pointer once the patient is immobilized on the operating table (figure 14). A spatial transformation can then be computed transforming the image into the coordinate system of the patient. The surgeon can then point on the patient using a tracked pointer and see the corresponding location in the images on the computer screen. The use of markers for image-to-patient registration presents some limitations both for the patient and the hospital staff. First, fiducial based registration requires an imaging session shortly before surgery to minimize the risk for markers to fall off or be displaced. In many cases this imaging session comes in addition to an initial session needed for diagnosis. Any displacement of the fiducial markers between the imaging session and surgery will compromise the image-to-patient registration accuracy. The placement of fiducials also represents an inconvenience for patients and hospital staff in the preparations for the procedure.

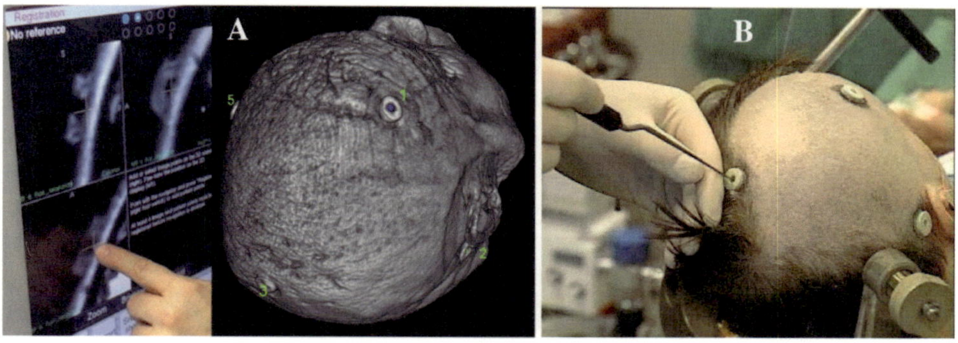

Figure 14. Image-to-Patient registration using corresponding points between image space (A) and physical space (B).

In order to avoid the use of fiducial markers, natural anatomical landmarks can be used for patient registration. Typical features in the context of neurosurgery are the medial and lateral corners of the eyes, the nose and ears. Like fiducial based registration, an image-to-patient registration framework using natural anatomical landmarks requires identification of points in the pre-operative images. The typically used landmarks are almost coplanar, and they are all located in a relatively small area around the face and ears. This might compromise the registration accuracy in other parts of the head, and possibly close to the surgical target [66]. A number of groups have presented surface matching techniques to address this issue. The skin surface of the patient is segmented from pre-operative data and registered to a set of surface points acquired in the operating room. Techniques to acquire surface points in the operating room include cameras [67, 68], laser surface scanners [69-71] and tracked pointers [72]. The accuracy of the different methods has been evaluated and compared [71, 73-75]. Both landmarks and surface based registration alone are less accurate than fiducial based registration. Different approaches combining registration based on anatomical landmarks and alignment of surfaces have therefore been developed.

As surgery proceeds, tissue will shift and deform due to gravity, retraction, resection and administration of drugs. Consequently, the pre-operative images do not correspond to the patient anymore. In this case, intraoperative ultrasound can be used for direct guidance and to update the location of the pre-operative data according to the surgical reality at a given point in time.

4.2. Ultrasound-based update of preoperative data

As surgery proceeds the pre-operative images no longer reflect the reality and updated information is necessary for accurate navigation. Intra-operative ultrasound can be acquired when needed during the procedure and be used for direct guidance and resection control, but also as a registration target for pre-operative images in order to update their position. This is particularly important for images such as functional MRI (fMRI) and diffusion tensor imaging (DTI) in neurosurgery because the information contained in these images cannot be easy re-acquired during the procedure. By performing MR/CT-to-US registration, the information contained in the pre-operative images can be shifted to the correct position at any given point in time (figure 15). Registration of MR/CT to US is a challenging task due to differences in image appearance and noise characteristics. The existing methods can be divided into two main categories:

- *Intensity-based methods*: These methods take the original images (MR/CT and B-mode US) as input, and the optimization of the registration parameters is computed from the image intensities, either directly or indirectly (blurring, gradients etc.). Some of the existing methods use well-known similarity measures such as mutual information and cross-correlation, while others have developed similarity measures particularly adapted to the registration of MR/CT and ultrasound [76-82].
- *Feature-based methods*: These methods require segmentation or "enhancement" of particular features in the images to be registered. The registration algorithm will then align the corresponding features in each image. In MR/CT-to-US registration such feature might be the vascular tree [83-85]. Blood vessels are relatively easy to identify and segment in both MR angiography and Doppler ultrasound images, and are present in nearly any region of interest. A centerline or skeleton can be computed from the segmented vessels and be used for registration. The most commonly used method for feature-based registration is the iterative closest point algorithm (ICP) [86]. In the case of vessel registration, all the points in the moving dataset are paired with the closest point in the fixed dataset. Based on these point correspondences, the registration parameters can be computed using the least squares method. The resulting transformation is then applied to the moving dataset and new point correspondences can be computed. The process is then iterated until convergence.

Several methods within the two main categories have been validated using retrospective clinical data [12, 14, 15]. So far no automatic method has been thoroughly validated intraoperatively (figure 15). The use of automatic registration methods in the operating room requires high quality data and straightforward, accurate, robust and fast image processing. With all this in place, image registration using intraoperative ultrasound will be able to correct the position of pre-operative data and thereby provide updated and reliable information about anatomy, pathology and function during surgery.

4.3. Motion correction using 4D ultrasound

Intensity based registration of ultrasound images can also be used to track the motion of an organ of interest. In the case of high-intensity focused ultrasound (HIFU or FUS) or radiotherapy, the

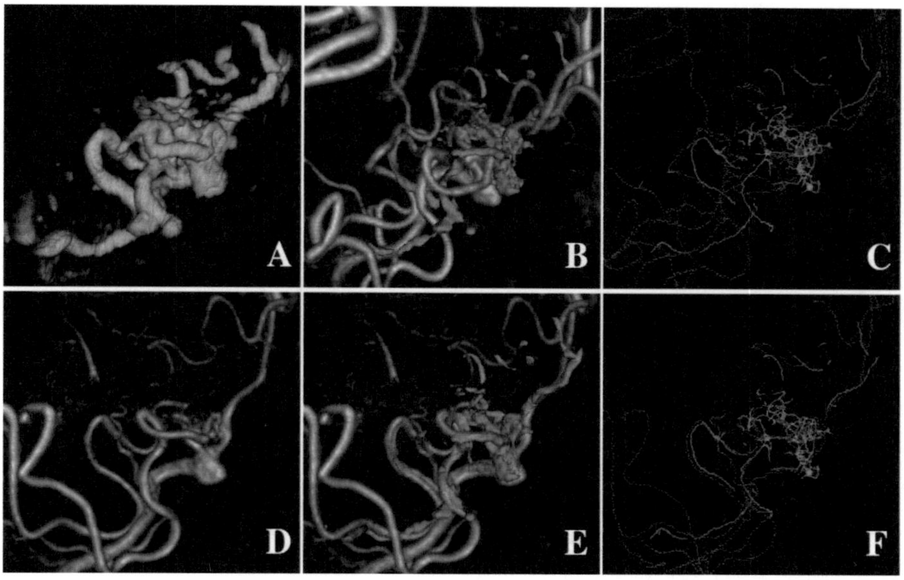

Figure 15. Ultrasound-based shift correction of preoperative MR data during an AVM operation. Top and bottom row shows the situation before and after the MR-to-US registration respectively. A) Ultrasound. D) MR. MR (gray) and US (green) before (B) and after (E) registration. Centerlines from US (green) and MR (red) before (C) and after (F) registration.

organ can be imaged using 4D ultrasound (3D + time or real-time 3D) in order to monitor the temporal changes in anatomy during the imaging, planning and delivery of treatment. The consecutive 3D images can then be registered in order to estimate the organ motion (figure 16). The positioning of the HIFU or radiation beam can then be modified accordingly in order to hit the target at any point in time. We have validated automatic motion estimation from 4D ultrasound in the liver using a non-rigid registration algorithm and a group-wise optimization approach as part of an ongoing study to be published in the near future. The offline analysis was performed using a recently published non-rigid registration algorithm that was specifically designed for motion estimation from dynamic imaging data [87]. The method registers the entire 4D sequence in a group-wise optimization fashion, thus avoiding a bias towards a specifically chosen reference time point. Both spatial and temporal smoothness of the transformations are enforced by using a 4D free-form B-spline deformation model. For the evaluation, three healthy volunteers were scanned over several breath cycles from three different positions and angles on the abdomen (nine 4D scans in total). A skilled physician performed the scanning and manually annotated well-defined anatomic landmarks for assessment of the automatic algorithm. Four engineers each annotated these points in all time frames, the mean of which was taken as a gold standard. The error of the automatic motion estimation method was compared with inter-observer variability. The registration method estimated liver motion better than the individual observers and had an error (75% percentile over all datasets) of 1 mm. We conclude that the methodology was able to accurately track the motion of the liver in the 4D ultrasound data. This methodology may be used intraoperatively to guide ablation of moving targets in the abdomen if the registration method can be run in real-time and the ultrasound probe can be made MR compatible (required for MR-guided HIFU).

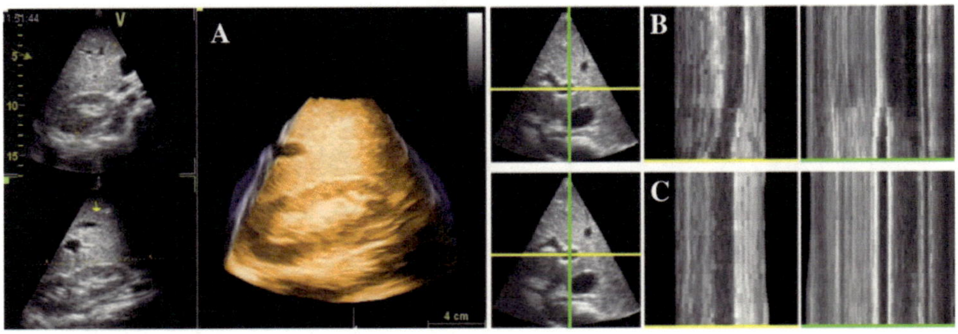

Figure 16. A) 4D (3D+t) Ultrasound of the liver. Example image before (top row B) and after (bottom row C) registration. The middle (B-C) and right panel, respectively, show the evolution over time (vertical axis) of the horizontal and vertical profile indicated by the cross in the left panel. After registration, the motion has been successfully removed from the image (streight vertical lines).

4.4. Segmentation of ultrasound data

Fully automatic segmentation of structures from B-mode ultrasound images is a challenging task. The clarity and contrast of structure boundaries depend heavily on their orientation relative to the sound wave and the acoustic properties of the surrounding tissues. Consequently, the boundaries of interest are often broken or at least unclear in parts of the image volume. It is therefore necessary to use *a priori* knowledge about the shape and appearance of the structure of interest in order to obtain reliable segmentation results. This *a priori* knowledge can be obtained by manually segmenting the structure of interest in a set of training data. Then, shape and appearance statistics can be used to segment the structure in new datasets. Akbari et al. [88] and Zhan et al. [89] used this approach for segmentation of the prostate in 3D ultrasound images of the prostate, and Xie et al. [90] used a similar approach for segmentation of the kidneys from 2D ultrasound images. The disadvantage of this method is the requirement for a database of training data with manual segmentations. This method can also be difficult to employ if the shape and appearance of the structure is unknown or presents large variations such as tumors and other pathologies. Several groups have also presented segmentation algorithms for ultrasound images of bone surfaces, and particularly the spine [91-94]. In these cases, the purpose of the segmentation process is to extract the bone surface from intra-operative ultrasound images for registration to pre-operative CT images. The ultrasound images are filtered in order to highlight the bone surface and in some cases the characteristic shadow behind the bone surface can be used for segmentation purposes as shown by Yan et al. [94]. They used backwards scan-line tracing to extract the bone surface from ultrasound images of the spine.

One of the great advantages of ultrasound is real time dynamic imaging. Methods based on shape and appearance statistics are in general not able to run fast enough to capture the dynamics of a moving organ such as the heart. Orderud et al. [95] proposed a method for real time segmentation of the beating heart. They fitted a set of control points of a model of the left ventricle to 4D ultrasound data (figure 17). The fitting process was run in real time using a state estimation approach and a Kalman filter. When the shape, appearance and localization of the structure are unknown semi-automatic or manual segmentation by an expert might be the only solution to obtain satisfactory results. Segmentation of Doppler ultrasound images, on the other hand is usually straightforward using simple thresholding methods. Vascular structures, however, often appear with a diameter that is to large in the Doppler ultrasound images causing neighboring vessels to be smeared together. Reliable segmentation of the vascular tree can therefore be challenging due to the spatial resolution of the images.

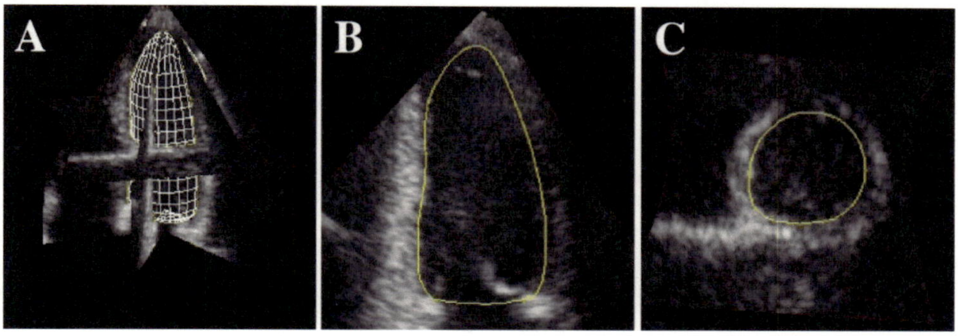

Figure 17. A 3D model of the left ventricle (A) matched in real-time to 4D Ultrasound shown here as slices in 3D (A) and 2D (B and C). Source: Orderud [95].

5. Ultrasound-based visualization and navigation

The amount of image data available for any given patient is increasing and may include pre-operative structural data such as CT and MRI (T1, T2, FLAIR, MR angiography etc.), pre-operative mapping of important gray (fMRI) and white matter (DTI), functional data from PET, intra-operative 3D ultrasound (B-mode and Doppler) in addition to images from microscopes, endoscopes and laparoscopes. All these sources of information are not equally important at all times during the procedure, and a selection of data has to be made in order to present only those images that are relevant for the surgeon at that particular point in time.

There are various ways to classify the different visualization techniques that exist. For medical visualization of 3D data from modalities like CT, MRI and US, it is common to refer to three approaches:

- *Slicing*: Slicing means extracting a 2D plane from the 3D data and can further be classified according to how the 2D slice data are generated and how this information is displayed. The sequence of slices acquired by the modality and used to generate a regular image volume is often referred to as the raw or natural slices. From the reconstructed volume we can extract both orthogonal (figure 18A) and oblique (figure 18B) slices. Orthogonal slicing is often used in systems for pre- and postoperative visualization, as well as in intraoperative

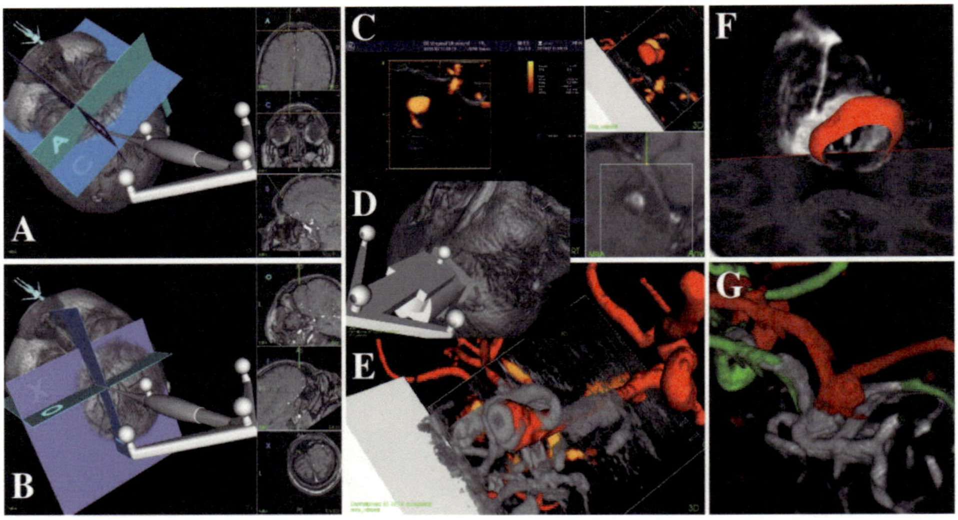

Figure 18. Multimodal visualization. Orthogonal (A) and oblique (B) slicing, the position as well as the position and the orientation of the tool are used to extract the slices respectively. The three basic visualization types are shown in each image. The head is volume rendered in a 3D view that also shows geometric representations of both the tool and slice indicators. Corresponding slices are shown in a 2D view at the right. C) Display during freehand 3D ultrasound acquisition: Real-time 2D ultrasound to the left and an indication of the us-scanplane relative to MR data in a 3D and 2D view to the top and bottom right respectively. D) Overview of probe relative to head. E) Detailed view of real-time 2D ultrasound relative to MRA (read) and 3D power Doppler data (gray). F) Slice from ultrasound (top part) and MR (bottom part), surface model in red from MR (middle part). Mismatch between US (slice) and MR (tumor model) is clearly visible. G) 3D ultrasound (gray) is used to correct MRA (moved from red to green position) during an aneurysm operation.

navigation systems, where the tip of the tracked instrument determines the three extracted slices. The slices can also be orthogonal relative to the tracked instrument or the surgeon's view (i.e., oblique slicing relative to the volume axis or patient), and this is becoming an increasingly popular option in navigation systems. When a surgical tool cuts through multiple volumes several slices are generated. These slices can then be combined in different ways using various overlay and fusion techniques.

- *Direct volume rendering*: Volume- and geometric rendering techniques are not easily distinguished. Often the two approaches can produce similar results, and in some cases one approach may be considered both a volume rendering and a geometric rendering technique. Still, the term volume rendering is used to describe a direct rendering process applied to 3D data where information exists throughout a 3D space instead of simply on 2D surfaces defined in (and often extracted from) such a 3D space. The two most common approaches to volume rendering are volumetric ray casting and 2D/3D texture mapping (figure 17 A, B, D, E, G). In ray casting, each pixel in the image is determined by sending a ray into the volume and evaluating the voxel data encountered along the ray using a specified ray function (maximum, isovalue, compositing). Using 2D texture mapping, polygons are generated along the axis of the volume that is most closely aligned with the viewing direction. The data is then mapped onto these quads and projected into a picture using standard graphics hardware.

- *Geometric surface rendering*: The technique used to render the texture-mapped quads is essentially the same technique that is used to render geometric surface representations of relevant structures (figure 17 A-F). However, the geometric representations must first be extracted from the image information. While it is possible in some cases to extract a structure and generate a 3D model of it by directly using an isosurface extraction algorithm [96], the generation of an accurate geometric model from medical data often requires a segmentation step first. The most common surface representation is to use a lot of simple geometric primitives (e.g., triangles), though other possibilities exist. Furthermore, the surfaces can be made transparent so that it's possible to see what's beneath the structure.

The challenge is to combine the available data and visualization methods to present an optimal integrated multimodal scene that shows only the relevant information at any given time to the surgeon. Multimodal visualization and various image fusion techniques can be very beneficial when trying to take advantage of the best features in each modality. It is easier to perceive an integration of two or more volumes in the same scene than to mentally fuse the same volumes when presented in separate display windows. This also offers an opportunity to pick relevant and necessary information from the most appropriate of the available datasets. Ideally, relevant information should include not only anatomical structures for reference and pathological structures to be targeted, but also important structures to be avoided. Finally, augmented reality techniques can be used to mix the virtual representation of the patient provided by 3D medical data and models extracted from these and the real representation provided by a microscope or a laparoscope for example, giving an even more realistic picture of the treatment delivered through small incisions in minimally invasive procedures.

6. Ultrasound-based navigation accuracy

The delicacy, precision and extent of the work the surgeon can perform based on image information rely on his/her confidence in the overall clinical accuracy and the anatomical or pathological representation. The overall clinical accuracy in image-guided surgery is the difference between the location of a surgical tool relative to some structure as indicated in the image information, and the location relative to the same structure in the patient. This accuracy is difficult to assess in a clinical setting due to the lack of fixed and well-defined landmarks inside the patient that can be accurately reached with a pointer. Common practice is therefore to estimate the system's overall accuracy in a controlled laboratory setting using precisely built phantoms. In order to conclude on the potential clinical accuracy, the differences between the clinical and the laboratory settings must be carefully examined.

6.1. Error sources and key points

A comprehensive analysis of the error sources involved in neuronavigation based on intraoperative ultrasound as well as preoperative MRI can be found in Lindseth et al. [97]. The overall accuracy is often referred to as the Navigation System Accuracy (NSA) and the essential points to remember can be summarized like this:

- The accuracy associated with navigation based on pre.op. MR/CT is independent of the accuracy associated with navigation based on intraoperative ultrasound, and vice versa.
- The main error sources associated with preoperative MR/CT-based navigation are related to the patient registration process in a clinical setting, and the fact that the image maps are not updated to reflect the changing patient terrain as surgery proceeds.
- In contrast, intraoperative ultrasound volumes are acquired in the same coordinate system as navigation is performed. Patient registration is therefore not necessary, and a new ultrasound volume can be acquired to reflect the current patient anatomy whenever needed. However, navigation based on ultrasound is associated with its own error chain. The main error source in this chain is the ultrasound probe calibration process. In addition, small variations in the speed of sound in different tissue types are a potential problem [97].

These points have major implications for the rational behind testing a navigation system in the lab using a phantom, and make a statement about the interesting parameter to the surgeon: the overall clinical navigation system accuracy. A lab test of a system based on preoperative MR/CT using a rigid phantom will give a very good navigation system accuracy (NSA<0.5mm, se figure 19, red line). Such a test will have limited validity in the general clinical situation, but is important to make sure that the system works as expected. The next phase in the evaluation of such a system would be to conduct a clinical study to investigate the system's ability to deal with a variety of different patient registration problems. Documenting that the system performs well in the rigid case and can deal in a satisfactory way with difficult patient registration cases is the best a system vendor can do. This does not give any information about the NSA experienced during a clinical case though. The surgeon must verify that the accuracy is acceptable after he has performed the patient registration procedure and anatomical landmarks inside the patient must be used to gain an impression about the amount of tissue shift and deformation. This shift and deformation makes systems based on preoperative MR/CT of limited use during the procedure.

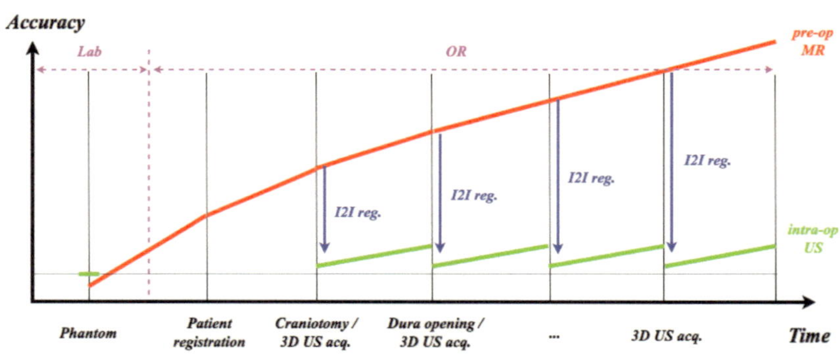

Figure 19. Navigation System Accuracy (NSA) based on preoperative (p) MR (red line) and intraoperative (i) US (green line). iUS can be used to correct pMR using various image-to-image registration techniques (blue line).

In contrast, probe calibration, the major error source associated with ultrasound-based navigation, is included in the NSA resulting from accuracy evaluations using a rigid phantom in a laboratory setting. Furthermore, the surgeon is in control of the amount of tissue shift and deformation that is acceptable in a particular clinical case. A new scan can be acquired whenever needed in order to navigate using an updated image map (se figure 19, green line). As a consequence, the NSA found in a controlled laboratory setting will also be valid in the clinical case given that navigation is based on a recently acquired ultrasound scan (real-time 3D ultrasound being the extreme case) and that the speed of sound used in the ultrasound scanner corresponds to the average speed of sound in the tissue.

A common mistake is to interpret a mismatch between MR/CT and Ultrasound in corresponding or fused displays as tissue shift. An observed mismatch between MR/CT and Ultrasound can only be interpreted as brain shift if 1a) navigation based on pre.op. data is accurate in the rigid case, 1b) the NSA, after the patient registration process, has been verified to be low, 2a) the NSA of ultrasound-based navigation in a controlled setting is low and 2b) the ultrasound data shown originate from an ultrasound volume that has recently been acquired.

Preoperative MR/CT data can be "corrected" for brain shift using intraoperative ultrasound and advanced image-to-image registration techniques [85] as can be seen in figure 19. However this is a challenging task introducing additional error sources. Therefore the NSA associated with corrected preoperative MR/CT will not be as good as the NSA for ultrasound (see figure 19, blue lines). In addition, the independence between the NSA based on MR/CT and Ultrasound will be broken (NSA for MR/CT will be dependent on NSA for Ultrasound).

The overall clinical accuracy of a navigation system will be determined by the contribution from all the individual error sources involved [97]. The net effect will not be the sum of all the error sources, but rather a stochastic contribution from all the terms. Stochastically independent contributions are summed using the following equation: $\sqrt{\sum(...)^2}$

6.2. Clinical navigation system accuracy

As stated previously, the most important parameter for the surgeon is the overall clinical Navigation System Accuracy (NSA). Although this parameter is difficult to assess, we believe that for ultrasound-based navigation an estimate can be made, based on a comprehensive laboratory evaluation and a thorough understanding of the significant additional error sources that occur in the clinical setting. Table 1 summarizes how such a calculation can be carried out assuming that a comprehensive evaluation of the system gives a NSA below 1.4 mm in a controlled laboratory setting. The error sources are assumed to be stochastically independent so that their contributions can be added on a sum-of-squares basis.

NSA using a phantom in the lab	< 1.4 mm
+ Calibration and position tracking of rigid surgical tool	< 0.5 mm
+ Interpolation of a 2D slice from a 3D volume / tool cross indication	< 0.1 mm

= Overall NSA	< 1.5 mm
+ Sound speed uncertainty	0 – 2.0 mm
+ Brain shift	0 – 10.0 mm
= Overall clinical NSA	1.5 – 10.5 mm

Table 1. Overall clinical NSA estimates

As can be seen from table 1 it is possible to achieve an overall clinical NSA close to the NSA found in the laboratory under favorable conditions, i.e., when the speed of sound used in the scanner is close to the average speed of sound in the tissue imaged, and the ultrasound volumes are frequently updated. The need for updates can be determined by real-time 2D imaging. If these conditions are not met, the accuracy becomes poorer.

6.3. Method for assessing ultrasound-based navigation accuracy

As we have seen the ultrasound-based NSA found in the lab using a phantom is valid in the OR (Operating Room) as well, under normal conditions. This makes it very interesting to develop a method that can measure the NSA automatically. We have previously suggested a method based on a phantom with 27 wire crosses and correlating an ultrasound sub-image of each cross to a synthetic template of the cross [98], and the method has been used in a thorough accuracy evaluation of a commercial navigation system [97]. We have since that developed a method that seems to be even more robust, in addition to being more flexible and more convenient to integrate in a navigation system (see figure 20). The method can be used for substantially different ultrasound probes and the phantom is easier to build and to measure accurately. The technique is based on sweeping over the single wire cross with the ultrasound probe, reconstruct all the frames into a volume containing the cross, segment and extract the centerline of the cross and register it to a centerline representation of the accurately measured physical cross, acting as a gold standard, using a modified version of the ICP algorithm [86].

7. Ultrasound-based guidance of minimally invasive procedures

While the main focus of this chapter will be navigation and image guidance using 3D ultrasound images, conventional 2D ultrasound is used for guidance in a variety of clinical applications. The simplest form of ultrasound guidance is placement of a needle inside a target using freehand 2D ultrasound imaging. First, the operator has to localize the target using ultrasound imaging, and second place the needle inside the target while keeping the needle tip in the image plane in order to verify its position. This technique requires a skilled and experienced operator due to the difficulty in keeping the needle in the image plane and the fact that the ultrasound image is not oriented relative to the patient. Despite the difficulties, this technique has been used for biopsies of the liver [99-101], lung [102] and prostate [103], placement of central vein catheters [104, 105] and for brain operations [106].

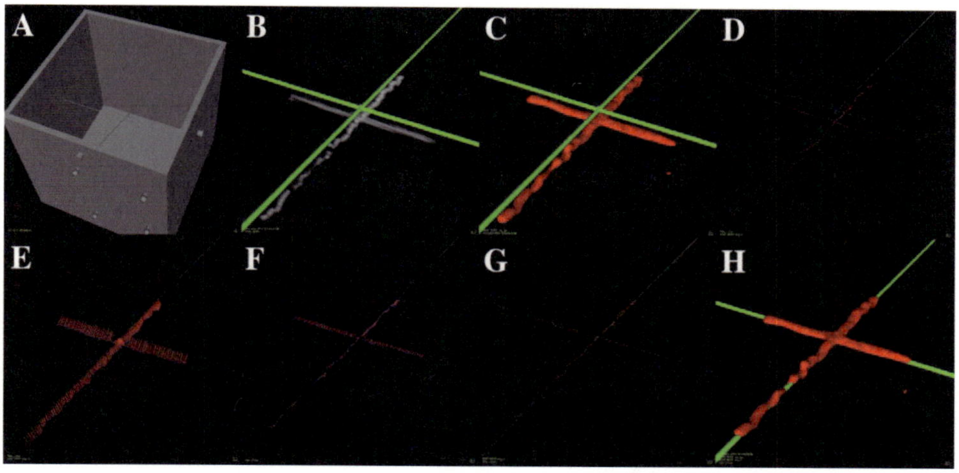

Figure 20. Automatic method for evaluating the accuracy in ultrasound-based navigation. A) The phantom with a single wire cross in the middle of the water tank and a reference frame in the front. B) Physical wire cross in green and an ultrasound volume of the wire cross in gray. C) The ultrasound data is segmented (red) and a small mismatch to the gold standard in green can be observed, i.e. small inaccuracies exist. D) Centerlines of the green and red wire crosses. E) Iterative closest point (ICP) registration between the two centerlines, initial correspondence shown. F) After some iterations. Final results showing the centerlines (G) and the wire crosses (H). The displacement is equal to the NSA.

A slightly more advanced technique for 2D ultrasound guidance includes a needle guide mounted on the ultrasound probe. The guide will ensure that the needle tip is in the image plane at a given depth depending of the ultrasound image sector and the angle of the needle guide. The angle of the needle guide has to be adapted to the depth of the target. Even though this system provides assistance in keeping the needle in the image plane, the operator has to do imaging and puncturing at the same time. In addition, the orientation issues concerning the ultrasound image relative to the patient is not solved and the anatomical overview is restricted to the current real time 2D image. However, the method is fast, does not require specialized equipment or complicated logistics, and provides sufficient guidance for a number of applications such as biopsy of thyroid nodules [107], placement of ventricular catheters in the brain [108, 109] and amniocentesis [110].

7.1. Ultrasound-based navigation in neurosurgery

Neuronavigation is the term used to describe the use of computer-assisted methods to guide or navigate instruments within the confinements of the scull (or spinal column) during surgery. A neuronavigation system should ideally provide high navigation accuracy throughout the surgical procedure. However, the anatomy of the brain is known to shift position after opening of the skull and dura due to drainage of cerebrospinal fluid (CSF), gravity effects and/or removal of tumor masses or hematomas. This shift in the position of the anatomy is often referred to as *brain shift* and has been shown to occur in the early stage of the surgery with displacement values ranging up to several centimeters [111-113]. The brain shift may therefore significantly impair the accuracy of navigation based on preoperative images as the surgery proceeds. Intraoperative ultrasound imaging provides a solution to the brain shift problem.

Compared to using only preoperative images for guidance, the navigation of instruments based on recently acquired intraoperative images can be performed with higher accuracy and precision [97].

The combined use of ultrasound imaging and navigation technology has been explored since the early 1990ies. The University of Oulu was one of the pioneers and demonstrated the clinical use of a passive mechanical arm-based navigation system, which could display reconstructions of preoperative images (CT/MR) and corresponding real-time intraoperative ultrasound images [114].

By attaching position sensors (also referred to as 3D localizers) on the ultrasound probe it is possible to establish the relative spatial position of the image pixels, and it is possible to reconstruct 2D images into an image volume, hence the term 3D ultrasound. The localizer attached to the probe is usually ultrasonic, electromagnetic or optic, and the two latter options (optic, electromagnetic) are currently the most established in commercial systems. Hata *et al* described in a paper from 1997 the initial clinical experience with a frame- and armless navigation system incorporating an ultrasound scanner and an ultrasound probe equipped with an ultrasonic positioning sensor [115]. In 1998 Jödicke *et al* presented a system for detection of brain shift, by comparing preoperative MR images and intraoperative 3D ultrasound [116]. The integration of ultrasound and navigation technology was also explored in Trondheim, Norway, and a system with the feasibility of 3D ultrasound and navigation guidance was developed. Using this system Unsgaard et al. performed the first brain tumour operation with 3D ultrasound guidance in 1996, and the system development and clinical experience was described in several papers [117-119]. The technology was further developed and commercialized by the company Sonowand AS (Trondheim, Norway), which is a spin-off company from the research activities of the National Centre for 3D Ultrasound in Neurosurgery (1995-present (2013)) at St. Olavs University Hospital. The technology has been explored for use in several neurosurgical procedures, but its predominant use is within resection of brain tumours [120]. The Sonowand system allows navigation of pre-calibrated tools equipped with an optic localizer, and it allows tools like biopsy forceps to be calibrated to the navigation system *in situ* in the operating room (figure 21) and used for image guided biopsies. The system facilitates simultaneous displays of reformatted image slices of intraoperative ultrasound and any preoperative MR series like T1, T2, FLAIR, etc. that has been registered to the patient. The position of navigated instruments is indicated in the displayed image slices.

7.1.1. 3D Ultrasound in intracranial tumour surgery

Intracranial tumours include primary and secondary tumours in the brain, pituitary gland, and meninges. Primary tumours are neoplasms originating from supportive tissue in the brain, from meninges, or from pituitary tissue. Secondary brain tumours are metastases of malignant cells that originate from a primary tumour situated in another organ of the body that spreads with the blood flow to the brain. Surgery is the primary treatment for most intracranial tumours. The patient's prognosis is in most cases related to the degree of resection of tumour. The surgical goal is usually to perform a total extirpation of the tumour, but without damaging

http://dx.doi.org/10.5772/55884

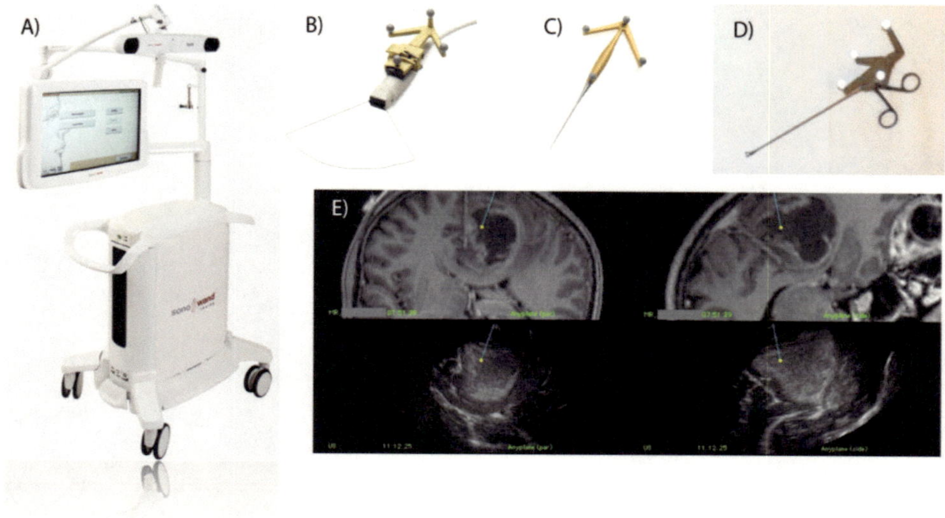

Figure 21. The Sonowand Invite® system for intraoperative ultrasound imaging and navigation (A), various tools of the navigation system equipped with optical localizer units showing one phased array ultrasound probe (B), a navigation pointer (C), a biopsy forceps (D), and a screen dump of the navigation display showing reformatted MR images in top row, and corresponding reformatted ultrasound images in bottom row (E). The tip of the navigated instrument is indicated with a bright spot in the reformatted image slices

adjacent normal brain tissue. If the tumour is located in so-called eloquent regions, harboring important functional tissue for movement, speech or vision, less extensive resections is often the result. Brain tumour surgery can therefore be a delicate balance between obtaining extensive resections and avoiding functional deficits and loss of quality of life due to the surgical trauma.

3D ultrasound is an established technique for intraoperative imaging in surgery of brain tumours, and is used for localization of the tumour and for resection control. The first acquisition of 3D ultrasound images is usually performed after opening the bone (craniotomy), but before opening the dura. Several ultrasound volumes (typically 3 to 6) are acquired during the operation to compensate for brain shift and to monitor the progress of tumour removal (figure 22).

Preoperative MR data can be displayed along with one or several ultrasound image volumes acquired at different stages of surgery. It may also be possible to import functional MR images to the navigation system. One way of doing this is to import anatomical MR images (e.g. T1/T2/FLAIR) with bold fMRI enhancements and DTI tractography overlaid as contours on the anatomical images [121-123], as shown in figure 23. The navigation system may therefore provide multimodal visualization of medical images, incorporating functional and anatomical information.

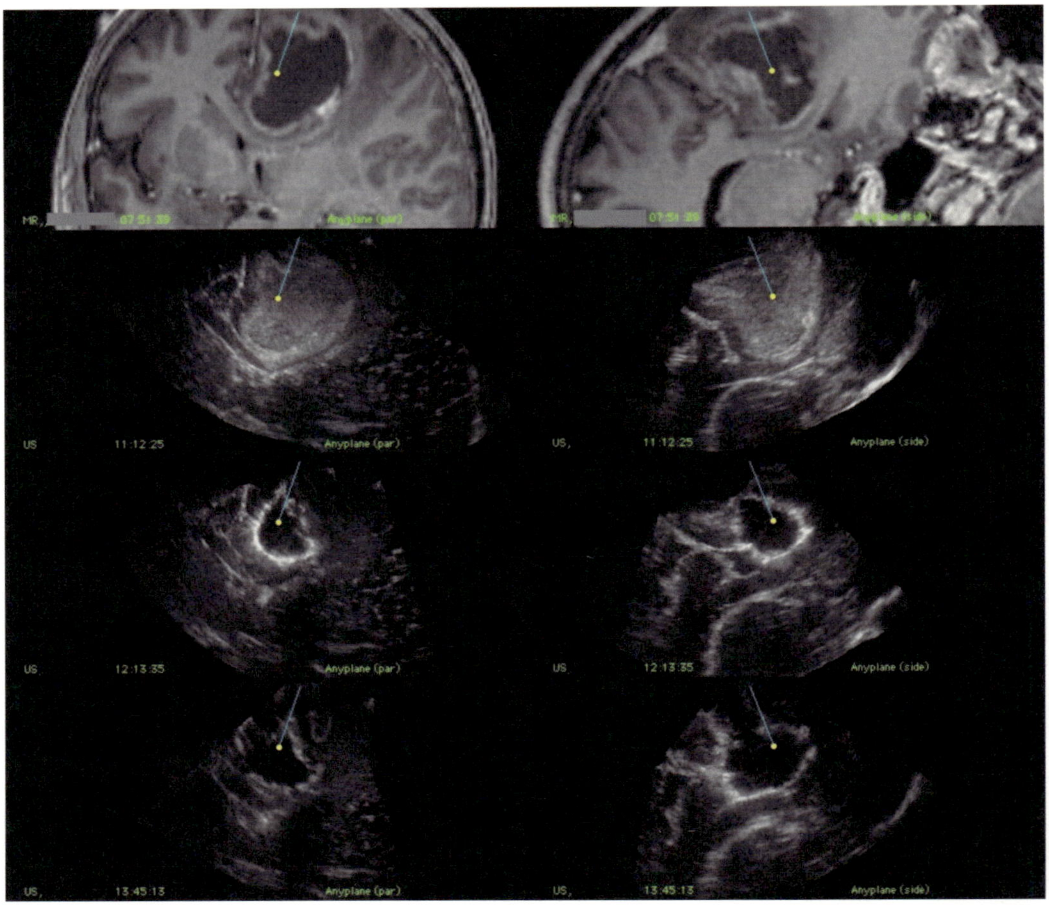

Figure 22. Navigation display showing two perpendicular reformatted image slices from each image volume. Preoperative MR slices in top row followed by slices from 3 different ultrasound volumes acquired at different stages in the operation. The ultrasound volumes in row 2, 3, and 4 were acquired prior to the resection, during the resection with some tumor tissue remaining, and after the end of the resection, respectively

Clinically, modern image technology has enabled more targeted surgical approaches, as compared to standardized explorative brain dissections that were more common two decades ago. This reduces the surgical trauma, eases anatomical orientation within the surgical field, and makes it possible for less experienced surgeons to obtain the same results as their more experienced peers. Today, even in eloquent regions where surgery is associated with increased risk, good clinical results can be obtained [121]. We have also observed that survival increased after the introduction of 3D ultrasound imaging in malignant primary brain tumour surgery [124]. Intraoperative imaging with ultrasound has also enabled more aggressive treatment strategies in tumours that microscopically resemble the brain tissue and therefore are difficult to remove with sufficient accuracy. This has improved survival without compromising risks [125]. Tailored probes designed for special surgical procedures such as the transphenoidal approach [126] through the nose can guide operations in narrow approaches with limited abilities for direct visualization. With further developments in ultrasound technology, clinical results can continue

http://dx.doi.org/10.5772/55884

to improve since good ultrasound image quality has direct consequences for the obtained clinical results, both in terms of resection grades [127] and for patient's quality of life [128].

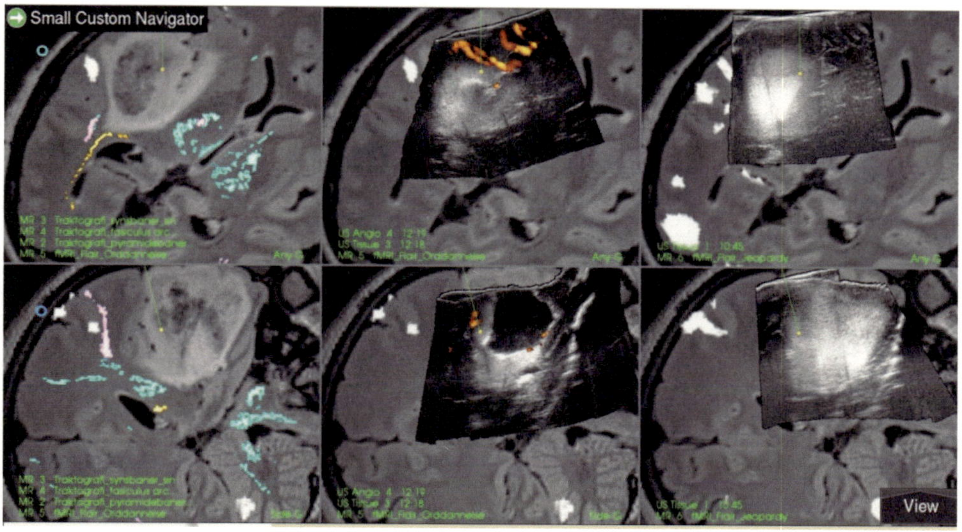

Figure 23. Example of multimodal visualization in navigation display. Left column shows anatomical MR image slices (FLAIR) with functional data shown as color overlay. The white spots indicate language area, the turquoise contours represent the pyramidal tract, the pink represent fasiculus arcuate (tract between language areas), the yellow represents the optic tract. Middle column shows preoperative MR image slices with intraoperative ultrasound acquired after some resection as overlay. Right column is identical as the middle, but with ultrasound data acquired prior to the start of the resection.

7.1.2. 3D Ultrasound in intracranial vascular surgery

It's also possible to acquire power Doppler based 3D ultrasound data of the vascular tree in the target area. This can be useful in both tumor and vascular surgery. In tumor operations the objective is to avoid injury to the vessels caused by the surgical instruments. In vascular surgery power Doppler can be useful in surgical treatment of both aneurysms (figure 18G) and arteriovenous malformations (AVMs, figure 15). For surgical treatment of aneurysms this mode is most useful for evaluating the flow in distal vessels after clipping of the aneurysm. In addition, 3D power Doppler can be used to localize peripheral aneurysms and guide direct surgical approaches. For AVM surgery intra-operative 3D power Doppler has been found to be useful in localizing deep-seated AVMs, identifying feeders and draining veins and for resection control [129]. Navigated display of 3D power Doppler based data can be used to identify and clip the larger feeders of AVMs in the initial phase of the operation, thus making it easier to perform the extirpation of the AVM.

Power Doppler based 3D ultrasound data are usually displayed in reddish color superimposed on the B-mode ultrasound slices, but the vessels are usually shown in a more optimal way using 3D rendering techniques. The power Doppler signal is often too intense and smeared out to give a sharp delineation of the small vessels. Robust acquisition of power Doppler based 3D ultrasound data of sufficient quality is essential for vessel-based shift correction and it's important to increase the spatial resolution of such data in the coming years.

7.2. Ultrasound-based navigation in laparoscopic surgery

Open surgery is the gold standard for abdominal surgeries. But over the last few decades, there has been an increasing demand to shift from open surgery to a minimally invasive approach to make the intervention and the post-operative phase less traumatizing for the patient. Advantages of laparoscopic surgery include decreased morbidity, reduced costs for society (less hospital time and quicker recovery), and also improved long-term outcomes when compared to open surgery. During laparoscopy, the surgeons make use of a video camera for instrument guidance. However, the video laparoscope can only provide two-dimensional (2D) surface visualization of the abdominal cavity. Laparoscopic ultrasound (LUS) provides information beyond the surface of the organs, and was therefore introduced by Yamakawa and coworkers in 1958 [130]. In 1991, Jakimowicz and Reuers introduced LUS scanning for examination of the biliary tree during laparoscopic cholecystectomy [131]. It seemed that LUS gave valuable information and has since expanded in use with the increase in laparoscopic procedures. LUS is today applied in laparoscopy in numerous ways for screening, diagnostics and therapeutic purposes [132, 133]. Some examples of use are screening, like stone detection or identification of lymph nodes, diagnostics, like staging of disease or assessment of operability and resection range, and therapeutic, like resection guidance or guidance of radio frequency and cryoablation. Harms and coworkers were the first to integrate an electromagnetic (EM) tracking sensor into the tip of a conventional laparoscopic ultrasound probe [134] and this made it possible to combine LUS with navigation technology, solving some of the orientation problems experienced when using laparoscopic ultrasound. The combination of navigation technology and LUS is becoming an active field of research to further improve the safety, accuracy, and outcome of laparoscopic surgery.

Navigation, as explained earlier, is the combined use of tracking and imaging technology to provide a visualization of the position of the tip of a surgical instrument relative to a target and surrounding anatomy. Various display and visualizations methods of both instruments and the medical images can be used in laparoscopic surgery. Preoperative images are useful for planning as well as for guidance during the initial phase of the procedure as long as the target area is in the retroperitoneum [135]. When preoperative images are registered to the patient, the surgeon is able to use navigation to plan the surgical pathway from the tip of the instrument to the target site inside the patient. Thus, navigation provides the intuitive correspondence between the patient (physical space), the images (image space that represent the patient) and the tracked surgical instruments. However, when the surgical procedure starts, tissue will shift and deform and preoperative data will no longer represent the true patient anatomy. LUS then makes it possible to update the map for guidance and acquire image

http://dx.doi.org/10.5772/55884

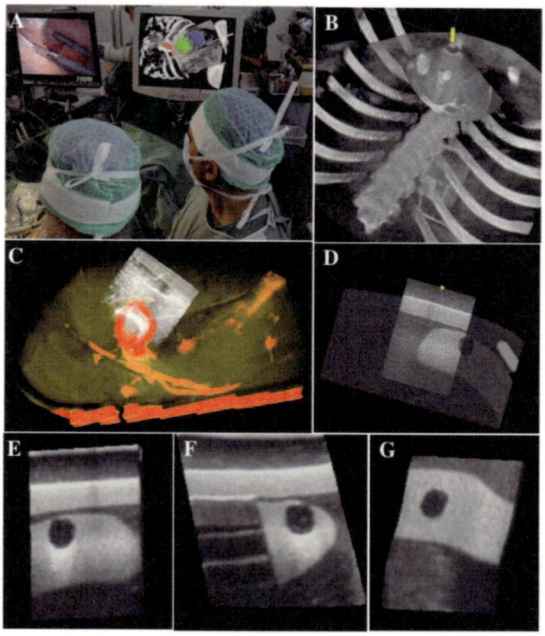

Figure 24. Illustration of visualization methods for navigation in laparoscopy. A) Navigation during adrenalectomy using preoperative CT (3D and 2D). B) Live animal model (pig) experiment showing navigated LUS combined with preoperative images (CT volume rendering). This solves the orientation problems and improves overview. C) Multimodal display of 3D LUS (volume rendering) and 3D CT from an ex vivo experiment showing that the tumor position has changed. D) Anyplane slicing from CT controlled by the LUS probe and overlaying the LUS onto the corresponding CT slice (phantom). E-G) Orthogonal slices from a 3D LUS scan (phantom).

data that display the true patient anatomy during surgery. Preoperative CT images will, however, still be useful for reference and overview as illustrated in figure 24, showing various display possibilities using LUS and navigation in laparoscopy. An example of simple overlay of tracked surgical tools onto a 3D volume rendering of computerized tomography (CT) images is shown in figure 24A. In this figure, we used the preoperative 3D CT images for initial in-the-OR planning of the procedure. The view direction of the volume was set by the view direction of the laparoscope. The LUS image could be displayed in the same scene, with an indication of the probe position in yellow. Furthermore, when 3D preoperative images are displayed together with 3D LUS, anatomic shifts can easily be visualized and measured, thereby providing updated information of the true patient anatomy to the surgical team as illustrated in figure 24C. This may improve the accuracy and precision of the procedure. Additionally, the tracked position of the LUS probe can be used to display the corresponding slice from a preoperative CT volume, providing improved overview of the position of the LUS image as shown in figure 24D. Having 3D LUS available, it is possible to display these data the same way as traditional orthogonal display of MR and CT volumes, as shown in figure 24E-G. Intraoperative augmented reality visualizations in combination with navigation technology could be valuable for the surgeons [136]. A possible future development, useful

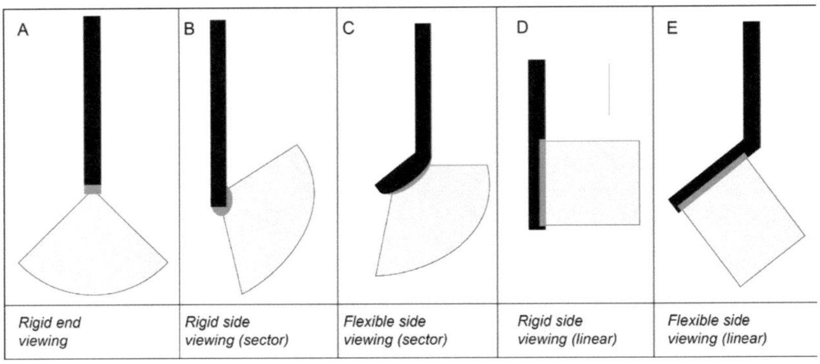

Figure 25. Different LUS probes.

for spotting the true position of lesions and vessels and hence detect anatomic shifts quickly, would be to introduce LUS data into such a multimodal display.

Intraoperative ultrasound systems are inexpensive, compact, mobile, and have no requirements for special facilities in the operating room (OR) compared to MRI or CT. Ultrasound image quality is continuously improving and for certain cases (e.g. liver) LUS could obtain image quality comparable to what is achieved in neurosurgery, as the probe is placed directly on the surface of the organ. In neurosurgery, the image quality of ultrasound has been demonstrated above. The most common LUS probe is a flexible 2- or 4-way array, linear or curved, with a frequency range of 5-10 MHz. Typical imaging depths are in the range 0-10 cm, but with 5MHz deeper imaging can be performed. The LUS transducers usually have a footprint of less than 10 mm wide to fit through trocars and 20-50 mm long. They can be manipulated at the shaft allowing real time images at user-controlled orientations and positions, depending only on the specific probe configuration. Figure 25 shows various configurations of LUS probes, while Table 2 provides an overview of currently available probes. Most LUS probes [137] can be sterilized [138].

Vendor	Probe	Frequency	Type of probe (see Fig. 2)	Transducer length, scan angle, other
Aloka	UST-52109	3-7.5 MHz	A	10 mm, 90°
	UST-5524-LAP	4-10 MHz	E	38 mm
	UST-5526L-7.5	5-10 MHz	D	33 mm
	UST-5536-7.5	5-10 MHz	E	38 mm
BK Medical	8666-RF	5-10 MHz	E	30 mm, Puncture and biopsy guide
Hitachi	EUP OL531	5-10 MHz	C	120°, Biopsy and therapy
Toshiba	PEF 704LA	5, 7.5, 10 MHz	E	34 mm
	PVM 787LA	5, 7.5, 10 MHz	B	85°

http://dx.doi.org/10.5772/55884

Vendor	Probe	Frequency	Type of probe (see Fig. 2)	Transducer length, scan angle, other
Gore	Tetrad VersaPlane	7.5 MHz (center frequency)	E	56 mm
Philips / ATL	LAP L9-5	5-9 MHz	E	NA
Esaote	LP323	4-13 MHz	E	NA

Table 2. LUS probe from various manufacturers. Relevant specifications are also given.

Being a relatively new area of research, it is interesting to note that the number of active research groups in the field of navigated laparoscopic ultrasound is approximately ten. Based on literature and almost two decades working with surgeons on developments for advanced laparoscopic surgery, a complete system designed for navigated LUS could be used according to the following clinical scenario:

- The preoperative data are imported and reconstructed into 3D volumes; several structures and organs are segmented automatically (e.g. vessels from contrast CT scan) or semi-automatically (e.g. seed point set inside the tumor).
- A quick plan is made from the visualization in the navigation system just prior to surgery, perhaps in the OR during other preparations.
- Registration is performed without fiducials using a pointer (orientation of patient) and two landmarks for a rough first approximation.
- Before mobilizing the target organ (e.g. the liver) a 3D LUS scan of major vessels near or around the tumor is performed.
- The LUS images are reconstructed in 3D and an automatic vessel based registration (CT-to-ultrasound) is performed to fine tune the patient registration.
- Augmented reality visualization, e.g. on/off overlay of preoperative data and LUS on the video laparoscope view is preformed as needed by the surgeons during the procedure
- 3D LUS scans are updated a few times during the procedure, while the real time 2D LUS image is available as either:
  - A full size image with a corresponding indication in a 3D CT rendering of its orientation and position, or
  - An overlay on the video laparoscope view with or without elements from the CT data (segmented structures for instance).

For rigid organ navigation, a single preoperative scan, highly accurate tracking (optical), and rigid surgical tools are sufficient to guide the procedure. However, for soft tissue navigation, additional tools are needed due to deformation and mobile organs in the abdominal cavity, resulting in more complex systems and additional devices in the OR. LUS can provide real time behind-the-surface information (tissue, blood flow, elasticity). When combined with advanced visualization techniques and preoperative images, LUS can enhance an augmented reality scene to include updated images of details, important for high precision surgery thus enhancing the perception for surgeons during minimal access therapy. LUS integrated with miniaturized tracking technology is likely to play an important role in guiding future laparoscopic surgery.

7.3. Other applications

One of the first, and still one of the most important applications of ultrasound imaging is in diagnostics of various heart conditions. The dynamic real-time imaging makes ultrasound the modality of choice for characterization of a moving organ such as the heart. Some examples of the use of echocardiography are evaluation of cardiovascular anomalies in fetuses and newborns [139], assessment of aortic stenosis [140], evaluation of the function of the valves and examination of the flow and function after heart attacks. These examples are purely diagnostic applications without any kind of intervention associated, but ultrasound has also been used for guidance in cardiac surgery. One example was presented by Wang et al. [141]. They evaluated 129 patients who underwent robotic cardiac surgery. Transesophageal echocardiography was used for guidance of the cannula for peripheral cardiopulmonary bypass. Ultrasound imaging can potentially also be used for guidance in minimally invasive mitral valve repair on the beating heart [123].

Intra-operative guidance during endovascular procedures is usually performed with x-ray fluoroscopy. However, some investigators have reported the use of transabdominal ultrasound for guidance. Lie et al. [142] studied the use of 2D transabdominal ultrasound during endovascular procedures. They found that ultrasound could be useful for guiding the insertion of guidewires, and control the wire position before connecting the second graft limb to the main limb of bifurcated grafts. Kaspersen et al. [143] reported a feasibility study registering ultrasound to pre-operatve CT data. This may be useful for updating the CT data used for navigation and correct for breathing motion and deformation of the blood vessels during the procedure. With recent advances in ultrasound technology, we believe that real-time 3D ultrasound have potential for further advancing the accuracy in the insertion of stentgrafts, and in particular the placement of fenestrated stentgrafts. Specifically, it is easier to track the tip of guidewires in three dimensions, while simultaneously visualizing a focused area of the 3D anatomy in real-time. A systematic review by Malkawi et al [144] concluded that percutaneous endovascular repair was associated with fewer access related complications and reduced operative time. In a study by Arthurs et al [145], it was shown that use of ultrasound guided access significantly reduced access-related complications compared to percutanous access without ultrasound guidance. Successful ultrasound guidance in secondary interventions, for sealing endoleak after endovascular repair, has also been reported. Boks et al. [146] described transabdominal embolization using duplex ultrasound guidance, and Kasthuri et al. [147] used ultrasound for guiding percutaneous thrombin injection. Navigation of stentgrafts during endovascular procedures has also been demonstrated in patients using CT imaging [148]. However, 3D or 4D ultrasound integrated with navigation technology for guidance of endovascular procedures has not yet been demonstrated in patients.

3D ultrasound has also been used to guide surgery of the spine. Kolstad et al [149] reported in 2006 a study, where spinal cord tumors were visualized using ultrasound imaging, and 3D ultrasound-guided tumor resection were performed using navigation technology. The technical application of integrating ultrasound and navigation seems feasible since it solves the orientation problem with conventional 2D ultrasound and may have the potential of improving functional outcome of spinal cord tumor surgery.

8. Ultrasound and non-invasive therapy

8.1. High Intensity Focused Ultrasound (HIFU)

High-intensity focused ultrasound (HIFU or FUS) has been known and developed for decades and can be applied to produce sharply delineated lesions in biological tissue (figure 26) [150-153]. The development of magnetic resonance (MR) thermometry enabled the thermal ablation progress to be monitored during sonication [154]. MR-guided HIFU (MRgFUS) has been approved by the FDA for the symptomatic treatment of uterine fibroids since 2004 [155]; clinical trials have been reported for breast [156, 157] and brain [158, 159] therapy, as well as pain palliation in bone [160, 161]. The MRgFUS treatment of abdominal organs, such as the kidney, pancreas or liver, poses additional technological and clinical challenges. First, for most therapeutic applications within the human body, tissue displacement caused by respiration and/or the cardiac cycle must be considered, and can be assumed to be periodic in anaesthetized patients. However, this may not be the case for free-breathing patients. This movement in addition to drift due to gravity and the intestine and bowel movement is important to account for during sonication in order to achieve accurately located FUS with respect to the target (e.g. tumour in the liver). Secondly, the presence of the rib cage affects the HIFU treatment planning and set-up. The rib cage acts as an aberrator that might affect the focusing [162, 163] and on the other hand, due to the high value of the absorption coefficient of the bone [164], the overheating on the ribs can be quite significant. These two aspects are currently the main challenges in order to achieve MRgFUS in moving abdominal organs.

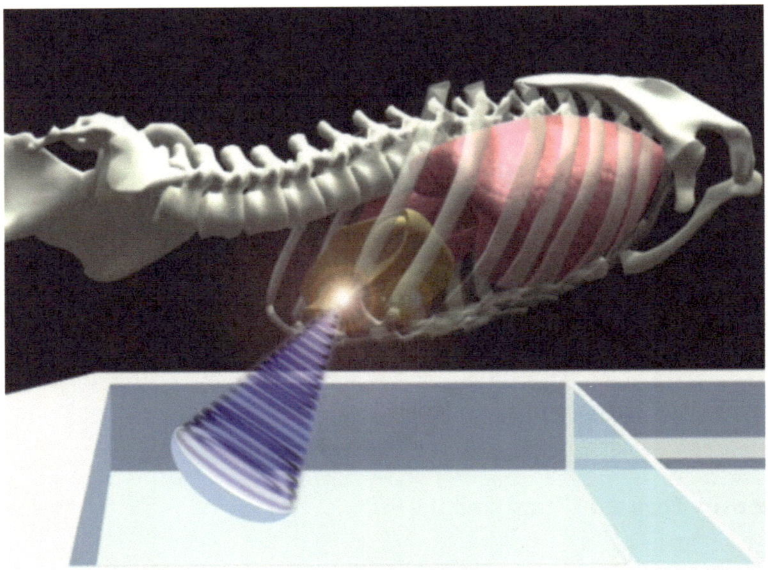

Figure 26. Illustration shows the targeting of a tumor in the liver using high intensity focused ultrasound. Currently, to perform this, the patient has to be anesthetized and breathing must be stopped during sonications. This results in long treatment times. In order to overcome this, emerging technologies in motion tracking (e.g. 4D ultrasound) can be used to track the target over time and at the same time simulate and predict the motion in order to target tumors moving due to free breathing patients.

Ultrasound is an inexpensive, flexible, real-time imaging modality, with high temporal and spatial resolution, i.e. sub-millimeter spatial resolution inplane along the beam direction. However, it provides little contrast between normal tissue and FUS-treated tissue and so far ultrasound-based temperature monitoring has not been validated under a clinical scenario.

Motion of the abdominal organs is an important issue to be accounted for during FUS treatment, but also in other therapies like radiotherapy [165, 166]. The motion estimation is useful in delineating the target and organs at risk and also determining the dosage of treatment during therapeutic irradiation. Several techniques exist and are in development to handle abdominal organ motion during FUS. A straightforward approach is to use respiratory gating. However, respiratory gating generally increases treatment time, which has been demonstrated in controlled apnea on anesthetized pigs [167, 168]. Another approach is to employ repeated breath-holds and breathing feedback to ensure a reproducible liver position [169]. De Senneville and coworkers [170] proposed a system that generates an atlas of motion fields during an initial learning phase based on magnitude data of temperature-sensitive gradient-recalled sequence acquisition. The motion field of the most similar image in the atlas is then used to correct the target position. Under the hypothesis of periodic motion, the focal point position for the next cycle is estimated. The method can only manage liver deformations caused by the periodic breathing cycle and is not capable of handling the non-rigid liver deformations, i.e. drift, caused by intestinal activity (peristalsis) or muscle relaxation [171]. Although it is established that MR imaging can provide motion estimates with a high spatial resolution, it is difficult in practice to acquire online three-dimensional (3D) isotropic images because of technical limitations, spatial and temporal resolution trade-offs, and low signal-to-noise ratio associated with fast 3D acquisition sequences [172]. In addition, the time duration between the actual target displacement and the availability of the motion information from MR data is not negligible [173]. Hence, MR information-based real-time motion compensation generally compromises spatial resolution, geometric distortion and the precision of the MR thermometry [174], of which the latter is of crucial importance during MRgFUS.

A first attempt at ultrasound-based motion tracking during MRgFUS was reported in phantoms undergoing periodic and rigid motion of small amplitude [173]. Continuous 1D ultrasound echo detection, along a direction parallel to the main axis of motion was used. This setup is not suitable for clinical applications as the external ultrasound imaging probe cannot send beams parallel to the axis of respiratory motion. Moreover, the local motion in the liver is spatially dependent and a 1D projection would not be sufficient. Truly simultaneous ultrasound and MR imaging has only been reported in literature recently [175-178]. Only one of these studies was targeted towards MRgFUS and moving abdominal organs sonication [175]. They demonstrated in moving phantoms the feasibility of ultrasound-based 2D motion-compensated sonications integrated with reference free MR temperature monitoring, using a clinical ultrasound probe and a phased-array HIFU transducer [175]. An overview of our own efforts for motion correction using 4D ultrasound can be found in section 4.3.

8.2. Ultrasound-induced drug delivery

Although diagnostic ultrasound is considered safe with no adverse effects, ultrasound can with high acoustic outputs induce significant bioeffects (e.g. HIFU) and these bioeffects are divided into thermal and mechanical effects. The thermal effect is related to energy absorption in the tissue where part of the mechanical wave energy is converted to thermal energy and hence results in an increase in tissue temperature. The mechanical effects are related to cavitation and to radiation forces. Radiation forces arise when part of the forward propagating wave is back-scattered or absorbed and result in a pushing force on the tissue along the direction of the forward propagating wave. Within fluids, such radiation forces can give rise to acoustic streaming. Cavitation is related to the oscillation and possible collapse of gas nuclei occurring naturally within the body or artificially introduced as contrast agent in the form of microbubbles. Oscillating gas bubbles will generate streaming currents in surrounding liquids and hence shear forces on nearby cells that potentially result in bioeffects. Collapsing gas bubbles can result in high local temperatures, release of free radicals, emitted shock waves and high velocity micro jets piercing into nearby cell membranes.

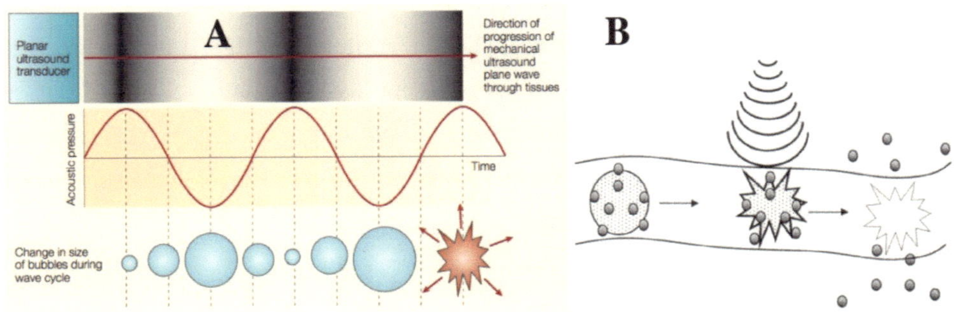

Figure 27. Ultrasound-induced drug delivery. Microbubbles carrying drugs are destructed by ultrasound (A) and the transported substances are released into the surrounding tissue (B).

The indicated bioeffects can be utilized in ultrasound induced drug delivery. The general goal of encapsulated drug delivery and targeting is to improve the efficacy of drugs within the region of diseased tissue while reducing undesired side effects in the healthy tissues. As an example, with non-encapsulated conventional chemotherapy systemic toxicity limits the drug concentration that can be obtained within the tumor and hence the efficacy of the therapy. With focused ultrasound, it is possible to obtain release of encapsulated drugs and this release can be controlled both temporally and spatially.

Ultrasound energy deposition within a localized tissue region provides a potentially efficient way of releasing drugs encapsulated in thermally sensitive carriers [179-181] by inducing a temperature increase and in sonosensitive carriers [182-184] by inducing cavitation (figure 27). The thermal and especially the mechanical cavitation effects of ultrasound also provide ways of perturbing cell membranes and thus increasing their permeability for improved drug delivery. With the introduction of microbubbles administered intraveneously that will serve as cavitation nuclei, the threshold for cavitation is significantly reduced hence facilitating this effect for endothelial cells that are close to the administered microbubbles. This effect of increased cell membrane permeability has been investigated extensively in the brain where the blood-brain barrier acts as an effective barrier for delivery of more than 95% of the drugs that potentially could be interesting for treatment of diseases in the central nervous system [185, 186]. For blood clot dissolution the combined use of ultrasound, microbubbles and thrombolytic agents have been demonstrated in several clinical trials to result in faster clot dissolution without release of large amounts of potentially hazardous clot fragments [187, 188].

9. Conclusions

Ultrasound has been used for many years as a diagnostic and interventional imaging modality, and the use is increasing in a number of different clinical areas. It is often conceded that the image quality of ultrasound is inferior to that attainable with MR or CT, but the rapid development of new ultrasound technology (scanners, transducers, specialized probes, etc.) has

http://dx.doi.org/10.5772/55884

resulted in significantly improved image quality and make ultrasound the modality of choice for several applications. Some of the obvious advantages being real-time imaging even for blood flow, portability, flexibility, safety and low cost. In addition, ultrasound images can be acquired in the coordinate system of a patient when combined with a tracking system without any need for registration. This makes surgical guidance based on intra-operative ultrasound highly accurate. The combination of several image modalities such as MR, CT and ultrasound registered to each other and to the patient make the interpretation of the individual images easier and enables the surgeon to take advantage of the complimentary information contained in each image. In this context, the ultrasound images provide real-time information in the region of interest, while MR and CT provide anatomical overview facilitating the interpretation of the ultrasound data. The use of contrast agents enhance the visualization of vessels and increase the number and types of lesions that can be detected using ultrasound. New technologies such as high-intensity focused ultrasound and the use of microbubbles for targeted drug delivery are examples of non-invasive therapeutic applications where ultrasound will play an increasingly important role in the future.

Author details

Frank Lindseth[1,2,4], Thomas Langø[1,4], Tormod Selbekk[1,2,4], Rune Hansen[1,2,4], Ingerid Reinertsen[1,4], Christian Askeland[1,4], Ole Solheim[2,3,4], Geirmund Unsgård[2,3,4], Ronald Mårvik[2,3,4] and Toril A. Nagelhus Hernes[1,2,4]

*Address all correspondence to: Frank.Lindseth@sintef.no

1 SINTEF Medical Technology, Norway

2 The Norwegian University of Science and Technology (NTNU), Norway

3 St. Olavs University Hospital, Norway

4 National Centre for Ultrasound and Image Guided Therapy, Norway

References

[1] Mehdizadeh, S., et al., Eigenspace based minimum variance beamforming applied to ultrasound imaging of acoustically hard tissues. IEEE Trans Med Imaging, 2012. 31(10): p. 1912-21.

[2] Mjolstad, O.C., et al., Assessment of left ventricular function by GPs using pocket-sized ultrasound. Fam Pract, 2012. 29(5): p. 534-40.

[3] Hotta, N., et al., Usefulness of Real-Time 4D Ultrasonography during Radiofrequency Ablation in a Case of Hepatocellular Carcinoma. Case Rep Gastroenterol, 2011. 5(1): p. 82-7.

[4] Rønnekleiv, A. Design Modeling of CMUT's for Medical Imaging. in IEEE International Ultrasonics Symposium (IUS). 2009, p. 442-450.

[5] Gierke, H.E., et al., Physics of vibrations in living tissues. J Appl Physiol, 1952. 4(12): p. 886-900.

[6] Dickinson, R.J. and C.R. Hill, Measurement of soft tissue motion using correlation between A-scans. Ultrasound in Medicine and Biology, 1982. 8(3): p. 263-71.

[7] Wilson, L.S. and D.E. Robinson, Ultrasonic measurement of small displacements and deformations of tissue. Ultrason Imaging, 1982. 4(1): p. 71-82.

[8] Lerner, R.M., S.R. Huang, and K.J. Parker, "Sonoelasticity" images derived from ultrasound signals in mechanically vibrated tissues. Ultrasound in Medicine and Biology, 1990. 16(3): p. 231-9.

[9] Ophir, J., et al., Elastography: a quantitative method for imaging the elasticity of biological tissues. Ultrason Imaging, 1991. 13(2): p. 111-34.

[10] Bae, U., et al., Ultrasound thyroid elastography using carotid artery pulsation: preliminary study. J Ultrasound Med, 2007. 26(6): p. 797-805.

[11] Emelianov, S.Y., et al., Elasticity Imaging of the Liver: Is a Hemangioma Hard or Soft? Proceedings of the 1998 IEEE Ultrasonics Symposium, 1998. 7: p. 1749-1752.

[12] Hiltawsky, K.M., et al., Freehand ultrasound elastography of breast lesions: clinical results. Ultrasound in Medicine and Biology, 2001. 27(11): p. 1461-9.

[13] Salomon, G., et al., Evaluation of prostate cancer detection with ultrasound real-time elastography: a comparison with step section pathological analysis after radical prostatectomy. Eur Urol, 2008. 54(6): p. 1354-62.

[14] Selbekk, T., J. Bang, and G. Unsgaard, Strain processing of intraoperative ultrasound images of brain tumours: initial results. Ultrasound in Medicine and Biology, 2005. 31(1): p. 45-51.

[15] Souchon, R., et al., Visualisation of HIFU lesions using elastography of the human prostate in vivo: preliminary results. Ultrasound in Medicine and Biology, 2003. 29(7): p. 1007-15.

[16] Nightingale, K., et al., Acoustic radiation force impulse imaging: in vivo demonstration of clinical feasibility. Ultrasound in Medicine and Biology, 2002. 28(2): p. 227-35.

[17] Gallotti, A., et al., Acoustic Radiation Force Impulse (ARFI) ultrasound imaging of solid focal liver lesions. Eur J Radiol, 2012. 81(3): p. 451-5.

[18] Tozaki, M., S. Isobe, and E. Fukuma, Preliminary study of ultrasonographic tissue quantification of the breast using the acoustic radiation force impulse (ARFI) technology. Eur J Radiol, 2011. 80(2): p. e182-7.

[19] Zhai, L., et al., Acoustic radiation force impulse imaging of human prostates: initial in vivo demonstration. Ultrasound in Medicine and Biology, 2012. 38(1): p. 50-61.

[20] Bercoff, J., M. Tanter, and M. Fink, Supersonic shear imaging: a new technique for soft tissue elasticity mapping. IEEE Trans Ultrason Ferroelectr Freq Control, 2004. 51(4): p. 396-409.

[21] Athanasiou, A., et al., Breast lesions: quantitative elastography with supersonic shear imaging--preliminary results. Radiology, 2010. 256(1): p. 297-303.

[22] Bavu, E., et al., Noninvasive in vivo liver fibrosis evaluation using supersonic shear imaging: a clinical study on 113 hepatitis C virus patients. Ultrasound in Medicine and Biology, 2011. 37(9): p. 1361-73.

[23] Tanter, M., et al., High-resolution quantitative imaging of cornea elasticity using supersonic shear imaging. IEEE Trans Med Imaging, 2009. 28(12): p. 1881-93.

[24] Wells, P.N. and H.D. Liang, Medical ultrasound: imaging of soft tissue strain and elasticity. J R Soc Interface, 2011. 8(64): p. 1521-49.

[25] Parker, K.J., M.M. Doyley, and D.J. Rubens, Imaging the elastic properties of tissue: the 20 year perspective. Phys Med Biol, 2011. 56(1): p. R1-R29.

[26] Carstensen, E.L., et al., Demonstration of nonlinear acoustical effects at biomedical frequencies and intensities. Ultrasound in Medicine and Biology, 1980. 6(4): p. 359-68.

[27] Muir, T.G. and E.L. Carstensen, Prediction of nonlinear acoustic effects at biomedical frequencies and intensities. Ultrasound in Medicine and Biology, 1980. 6(4): p. 345-57.

[28] Caidahl, K., et al., New concept in echocardiography: harmonic imaging of tissue without use of contrast agent. Lancet, 1998. 352(9136): p. 1264-70.

[29] Choudhry, S., et al., Comparison of tissue harmonic imaging with conventional US in abdominal disease. Radiographics, 2000. 20(4): p. 1127-35.

[30] Duck, F.A., Nonlinear acoustics in diagnostic ultrasound. Ultrasound in Medicine and Biology, 2002. 28(1): p. 1-18.

[31] Spencer, K.T., et al., Use of harmonic imaging without echocardiographic contrast to improve two-dimensional image quality. American Journal of Cardiology, 1998. 82(6): p. 794-799.

[32] Feldman, M.K., S. Katyal, and M.S. Blackwood, US artifacts. Radiographics, 2009. 29(4): p. 1179-89.

[33] Kossoff, G., Basic physics and imaging characteristics of ultrasound. World J Surg, 2000. 24(2): p. 134-42.

[34] Leighton, T.G., The Acoustic Bubble 1994, San Diego: Book from Academic Press.

[35] Plesset, M., The dynamics of cavitation bubbles. J Appl Mech, 1949. 16: p. 277–282.

[36] Rayleigh, L., On the pressure developed in a liquid during collapse of a spherical cavity. Phil Mag, 1917. 34: p. 94–98.

[37] de Jong, N. and R. Cornet, Higher harmonics of vibrating gas-filled microspheres. Part one: Simulations. Ultrasonics, 1994. 32: p. 447–453.

[38] de Jong, N. and R. Cornet, Higher harmonics of vibrating gas-filled microspheres. Part two: Measurements. Ultrasonics, 1994. 32: p. 455–459.

[39] Burns, P.N., S.R. Wilson, and D.H. Simpson, Pulse inversion imaging of liver blood flow: improved method for characterizing focal masses with microbubble contrast. Invest Radiol, 2000. 35(1): p. 58-71.

[40] Simpson, D.H., C.T. Chin, and P.N. Burns, Pulse inversion Doppler: a new method for detecting nonlinear echoes from microbubble contrast agents. IEEE Trans Ultrason Ferroelectr Freq Control, 1999. 46(2): p. 372-82.

[41] Mor-Avi, V., et al., Combined assessment of myocardial perfusion and regional left ventricular function by analysis of contrast-enhanced power modulation images. Circulation, 2001. 104(3): p. 352-7.

[42] Eckersley, R.J., C.T. Chin, and P.N. Burns, Optimising phase and amplitude modulation schemes for imaging microbubble contrast agents at low acoustic power. Ultrasound in Medicine and Biology, 2005. 31(2): p. 213-9.

[43] Haider, B. and R.Y. Chiao, Higher order nonlinear ultrasonic imaging. 1999 IEEE Ultrasonics Symposium Proceedings, Vols 1 and 2, 1999: p. 1527-1531.

[44] Phillips, P.J., Contrast Pulse Sequences (CPS): Imaging nonlinear microbubbles. 2001 IEEE Ultrasonics Symposium Proceedings, Vols 1 and 2, 2001: p. 1739-1745.

[45] Leen, E., et al., Contrast-enhanced 3D ultrasound in the radiofrequency ablation of liver tumors. World J Gastroenterol, 2009. 15(3): p. 289-99.

[46] Hansen, R. and B.A. Angelsen, SURF imaging for contrast agent detection. IEEE Trans Ultrason Ferroelectr Freq Control, 2009. 56(2): p. 280-90.

[47] Hansen, R. and B.A. Angelsen, Contrast imaging by non-overlapping dual frequency band transmit pulse complexes. IEEE Trans Ultrason Ferroelectr Freq Control, 2011. 58(2): p. 290-7.

[48] Hansen, R., et al., Utilizing dual frequency band transmit pulse complexes in medical ultrasound imaging. J Acoust Soc Am, 2010. 127(1): p. 579-87.

[49] Hansen, R., et al., Nonlinear propagation delay and pulse distortion resulting from dual frequency band transmit pulse complexes. J Acoust Soc Am, 2011. 129(2): p. 1117-27.

[50] Masoy, S.E., et al., SURF imaging: in vivo demonstration of an ultrasound contrast agent detection technique. IEEE Trans Ultrason Ferroelectr Freq Control, 2008. 55(5): p. 1112-21.

[51] Cinquin, P., et al., Computer assisted Medical Interventions. IEEE Engineering in medicine and biology, 1995. May/June: p. 254-263.

[52] Meyer, K., H.L. Applewhite, and F.A. Biocca, A survey of position trackers. Presence: Teleoperators and Virtual Environments, 1992. 1(2): p. 173-200.

[53] Birkfellner, W., et al., Systematic distortions in magnetic position digitizers. Med Phys, 1998. 25(11): p. 2242-8.

[54] Kindratenko, V., A survey of electromagnetic position tracker calibration techniques. Virtual Reality, 2000(5): p. 169-182.

[55] Birkfellner, W., et al., Calibration of tracking systems in a surgical environment. IEEE Trans Med Imaging, 1998. 17(5): p. 737-42.

[56] Lindseth, F., et al., Probe calibration for freehand 3-D ultrasound. Ultrasound Med Biol, 2003. 29(11): p. 1607-23.

[57] Mercier, L., et al., A review of calibration techniques for freehand 3-D ultrasound systems. Ultrasound Med Biol, 2005. 31(4): p. 449-71.

[58] Arun, K.S., T.S. Huang, and S.D. Blostein, Least-Squares Fitting of Two 3-D Point Sets.

[59] Fenster, A., G. Parraga, and J. Bax, Three-dimensional ultrasound scanning. Interface Focus, 2011. 1(4): p. 503-19.

[60] Solberg, O.V., et al., Freehand 3D ultrasound reconstruction algorithms--a review. Ultrasound Med Biol, 2007. 33(7): p. 991-1009.

[61] Smith, S.W., G.E. Trahey, and O.T. von Ramm, Two-dimensional arrays for medical ultrasound. Ultrason Imaging, 1992. 14(3): p. 213-33.

[62] Turnbull, D.H. and F.S. Foster, Beam steering with pulsed two-dimensional transducer arrays. IEEE Trans Ultrason Ferroelectr Freq Control, 1991. 38(4): p. 320-33.

[63] Choe, J.W., et al., Volumetric real-time imaging using a CMUT ring array. IEEE Trans Ultrason Ferroelectr Freq Control, 2012. 59(6): p. 1201-11.

[64] Wygant, I.O., et al., Integration of 2D CMUT arrays with front-end electronics for volumetric ultrasound imaging. IEEE Trans Ultrason Ferroelectr Freq Control, 2008. 55(2): p. 327-42.

[65] Oralkan, O., et al., Volumetric ultrasound imaging using 2-D CMUT arrays. IEEE Trans Ultrason Ferroelectr Freq Control, 2003. 50(11): p. 1581-94.

[66] West, J.B., et al., Fiducial point placement and the accuracy of point-based, rigid body registration. Neurosurgery, 2001. 48(4): p. 810-6; discussion 816-7.

[67] Marmulla, R., et al., New Augmented Reality Concepts for Craniofacial Surgical Procedures. Plastic and Reconstructive Surgery, 2005. 115(3): p. 1124-1128.

[68] Shamir, R.R., et al., Surface-based facial scan registration in neuronavigation procedures: a clinical study. J Neurosurg, 2009.

[69] Marmulla, R., G. Eggers, and J. Muhling, Laser surface registration for lateral skull base surgery. Minim Invasive Neurosurg, 2005. 48(3): p. 181-5.

[70] Raabe, A., et al., Laser surface scanning for patient registration in intracranial image-guided surgery. Neurosurgery, 2002. 50(4): p. 797-801; discussion 802-3.

[71] Schlaier, J., J. Warnat, and A. Brawanski, Registration accuracy and practicability of laser-directed surface matching. Comput Aided Surg, 2002. 7(5): p. 284-90.

[72] Maurer, C.R., Jr., R.J. Maciunas, and J.M. Fitzpatrick, Registration of head CT images to physical space using a weighted combination of points and surfaces. IEEE Trans Med Imaging, 1998. 17(5): p. 753-61.

[73] Hoffmann, J., et al., Validation of 3D-laser surface registration for image-guided cranio-maxillofacial surgery. J Craniomaxillofac Surg, 2005. 33(1): p. 13-8.

[74] Knott, P.D., et al., Contour and Paired-Point Registration in a Model for Image-Guided Surgery. The Laryngoscope, 2006. 116: p. 1877-1881.

[75] Schicho, K., et al., Comparison of laser surface scanning and fiducial marker-based registration in frameless stereotaxy. Journal of Neurosurgery, 2007. 106: p. 704-709.

[76] Arbel, T., et al., Automatic Non-linear MRI-Ultrasound Registration for the Correction of Intra-operative Brain deformations, in In Proc. MICCAI 20012001. p. 913-922.

[77] Arbel, T., et al., Automatic non-linear MRI-ultrasound registration for the correction of intra-operative brain deformations. Comput Aided Surg, 2004. 9(4): p. 123-36.

[78] Coupe, P., et al., 3D Rigid Registration of Intraoperative Ultrasound and Preoperative MR Brain Images Based on Hyperechogenic Structures. Int J Biomed Imaging, 2012. 2012: p. 531319.

[79] De Nigris, D., D. Collins, and T. Arbel, Multi-Modal Image Registration based on Gradient Orientations of Minimal Uncertainty. IEEE Trans Med Imaging, 2012.

[80] Ji, S., et al., Mutual-information-based image to patient re-registration using intraoperative ultrasound in image-guided neurosurgery. Med Phys, 2008. 35(10): p. 4612-24.

http://dx.doi.org/10.5772/55884

[81] Penney, G.P., et al., Deforming a Preoperative Volume to Represent the Intraoperative Scene, in Computer Aided Surgery2002. p. 63-73.

[82] Roche, A., et al., Rigid Registration of 3D Ultrasound with MR Images: A New Approach Combining intensity and Gradient Information, in IEEE Transactions on Medical Imaging2001. p. 1038-1049.

[83] Reinertsen, I., et al., Vessel Driven Correction of Brain Shift, in In Proc. MICCAI 20042004. p. 208-216.

[84] Reinertsen, I., et al., Validation of Vessel-based Registration for Correction of Brainshift. Medical Image Analysis, 2007. 11(4): p. 374-88.

[85] Reinertsen, I., et al., Clinical validation of vessel-based registration for correction of brain-shift. Med Image Anal, 2007. 11(6): p. 673-84.

[86] Besl, P.J. and N.D. McKay, A Method for Registration of 3D Shapes. IEEE Transactions on Pattern Analysis and Machine Intelligence, 1992. 14(2): p. 239-256.

[87] Metz, C.T., et al., Nonrigid registration of dynamic medical imaging data using nD + t B-splines and a groupwise optimization approach. Medical image analysis, 2011. 15(2): p. 238-49.

[88] Akbari, H. and B. Fei, 3D ultrasound image segmentation using wavelet support vector machines. Med Phys, 2012. 39(6): p. 2972-84.

[89] Zhan, Y. and D. Shen, Deformable segmentation of 3-D ultrasound prostate images using statistical texture matching method. IEEE Trans Med Imaging, 2006. 25(3): p. 256-72.

[90] Xie, J., Y. Jiang, and H.T. Tsui, Segmentation of kidney from ultrasound images based on texture and shape priors. IEEE Trans Med Imaging, 2005. 24(1): p. 45-57.

[91] Foroughi, P., et al., Ultrasound Bone Segmentation Using Dynamic Programming, in IEEE Ultrasonics Symposium2007. p. 2523-2526.

[92] Hacihaliloglu, I., et al., Non-iterative partial view 3D ultrasound to CT registration in ultrasound-guided computer-assisted orthopedic surgery. Int J Comput Assist Radiol Surg, 2012.

[93] Rasoulian, A., P. Abolmaesumi, and P. Mousavi, Feature-based multibody rigid registration of CT and ultrasound images of lumbar spine. Med Phys, 2012. 39(6): p. 3154-66.

[94] Yan, C.X., et al., Validation of automated ultrasound-CT registration of vertebrae. Int J Comput Assist Radiol Surg, 2012. 7(4): p. 601-10.

[95] Orderud, F., J. Hansgard, and S.I. Rabben, Real-time tracking of the left ventricle in 3D echocardiography using a state estimation approach. Med Image Comput Comput Assist Interv, 2007. 10(Pt 1): p. 858-65.

[96] Lorensen, W.E. and H.E. Cline, Marching Cubes: A high resolution 3D surface construction algorithm. Computer Graphics, 1987. 21(4): p. 163-169.

[97] Lindseth, F., et al., Accuracy evaluation of a 3D ultrasound-based neuronavigation system. Comput Aided Surg, 2002. 7(4): p. 197-222.

[98] Lindseth, F., J. Bang, and T. Lango, A robust and automatic method for evaluating accuracy in 3-D ultrasound-based navigation. Ultrasound Med Biol, 2003. 29(10): p. 1439-52.

[99] Matos, H., et al., Effectiveness and safety of ultrasound-guided percutaneous liver biopsy in children. Pediatr Radiol, 2012. 42(11): p. 1322-5.

[100] Copel, L., et al., Ultrasound-guided percutaneous liver biopsy: indications, risks, and technique. Surg Technol Int, 2003. 11: p. 154-60.

[101] Tzortzis, D., et al., Percutaneous US-guided liver biopsy in focal lesions using a semi-automatic device allowing to perform multiple biopsies in a single-pass. Minerva Gastroenterol Dietol, 2012. 58(1): p. 1-8.

[102] Fontalvo, L.F., et al., Percutaneous US-guided biopsies of peripheral pulmonary lesions in children. Pediatr Radiol, 2006. 36(6): p. 491-7.

[103] Pinto, F., et al., Imaging in prostate cancer diagnosis: present role and future perspectives. Urol Int, 2011. 86(4): p. 373-82.

[104] Froehlich, C.D., et al., Ultrasound-guided central venous catheter placement decreases complications and decreases placement attempts compared with the landmark technique in patients in a pediatric intensive care unit. Crit Care Med, 2009. 37(3): p. 1090-6.

[105] Palepu, G.B., et al., Impact of ultrasonography on central venous catheter insertion in intensive care. Indian J Radiol Imaging, 2009. 19(3): p. 191-8.

[106] Unsgaard, G., et al., Brain operations guided by real-time two-dimensional ultrasound: new possibilities as a result of improved image quality. Neurosurgery, 2002. 51(2): p. 402-11; discussion 411-2.

[107] Tublin, M.E., et al., Ultrasound-guided fine-needle aspiration versus fine-needle capillary sampling biopsy of thyroid nodules: does technique matter? J Ultrasound Med, 2007. 26(12): p. 1697-701.

[108] Strowitzki, M., et al., Accuracy of ultrasound-guided puncture of the ventricular system. Childs Nerv Syst, 2008. 24(1): p. 65-9.

[109] Whitehead, W.E., et al., Accurate placement of cerebrospinal fluid shunt ventricular catheters with real-time ultrasound guidance in older children without patent fontanelles. J Neurosurg, 2007. 107(5 Suppl): p. 406-10.

[110] Tonni, G., et al., 4D vs 2D ultrasound-guided amniocentesis. J Clin Ultrasound, 2009. 37(8): p. 431-5.

[111] Letteboer, M.M.J., et al., Brain shift estimation in image-guided neurosurgery using 3-D ultrasound. Ieee Transactions on Biomedical Engineering, 2005. 52(2): p. 268-276.

[112] Reinges, M.H.T., et al., Course of brain shift during microsurgical resection of supratentorial cerebral lesions: limits of conventional neuronavigation. Acta Neurochirurgica, 2004. 146(4): p. 369-377.

[113] Roberts, D.W., et al., Intraoperative brain shift and deformation: A quantitative analysis of cortical displacement in 28 cases. Neurosurgery, 1998. 43(4): p. 749-758.

[114] Koivukangas, J., et al., Ultrasound-controlled neuronavigator-guided brain surgery. J Neurosurg, 1993. 79(1): p. 36-42.

[115] Hata, N., et al., Development of a frameless and armless stereotactic neuronavigation system with ultrasonographic registration. Neurosurgery, 1997. 41(3): p. 608-613.

[116] Jodicke, A., et al., Intraoperative three-dimensional ultrasonography: An approach to register brain shift using multidimensional image processing. Minimally Invasive Neurosurgery, 1998. 41(1): p. 13-19.

[117] Grønningsæter, Å., et al., SonoWand, an Ultrasound-based Neuronavigation System. Neurosurgery, 2000. 47(6): p. 1373-1380.

[118] Hirschberg, H. and G. Unsgaard, Incorporation of ultrasonic imaging in an optically coupled frameless stereotactic system. Acta Neurochir Suppl. (Wien), 1997. 68: p. 75-80.

[119] Unsgaard, G., et al., Neuronavigation by intraoperative three-dimensional ultrasound: initial experience during brain tumor resection. Neurosurgery, 2002. 50(4): p. 804-12; discussion 812.

[120] Unsgaard, G., et al., Intra-operative 3D ultrasound in neurosurgery. Acta Neurochir (Wien), 2006. 148(3): p. 235-53; discussion 253.

[121] Berntsen, E.M., et al., Functional magnetic resonance imaging and diffusion tensor tractography incorporated into an intraoperative 3-dimensional ultrasound-based neuronavigation system: impact on therapeutic strategies, extent of resection, and clinical outcome. Neurosurgery, 2010. 67(2): p. 251-64.

[122] Gulati, S., et al., Surgical resection of high-grade gliomas in eloquent regions guided by blood oxygenation level dependent functional magnetic resonance imaging, diffusion tensor tractography, and intraoperative navigated 3D ultrasound. Minim Invasive Neurosurg, 2009. 52(1): p. 17-24.

[123] Rasmussen, I.A., Jr., et al., Functional neuronavigation combined with intra-operative 3D ultrasound: initial experiences during surgical resections close to eloquent

brain areas and future directions in automatic brain shift compensation of preoperative data. Acta Neurochir (Wien), 2007. 149(4): p. 365-78.

[124] Saether, C.A., et al., Did survival improve after the implementation of intraoperative neuronavigation and 3D ultrasound in glioblastoma surgery? A retrospective analysis of 192 primary operations. J Neurol Surg A Cent Eur Neurosurg, 2012. 73(2): p. 73-8.

[125] Jakola, A.S., et al., Comparison of a strategy favoring early surgical resection vs a strategy favoring watchful waiting in low-grade gliomas. JAMA, 2012. 308(18): p. 1881-8.

[126] Solheim, O., et al., Intrasellar ultrasound in transsphenoidal surgery: a novel technique. Neurosurgery, 2010. 66(1): p. 173-85; discussion 185-6.

[127] Solheim, O., et al., Ultrasound-guided operations in unselected high-grade gliomas--overall results, impact of image quality and patient selection. Acta Neurochir (Wien), 2010. 152(11): p. 1873-86.

[128] Jakola, A.S., G. Unsgard, and O. Solheim, Quality of life in patients with intracranial gliomas: the impact of modern image-guided surgery. J Neurosurg, 2011. 114(6): p. 1622-30.

[129] Unsgaard, G., et al., Operation of arteriovenous malformations assisted by stereoscopic navigation-controlled display of preoperative magnetic resonance angiography and intraoperative ultrasound angiography. Neurosurgery, 2005. 56(2 Suppl): p. 281-90; discussion 281-90.

[130] Yamakawa, K., S. Naito, and K. Azuma, Laparoscopic diagnosis of the intraabdominal organs. Jpn J Gastroenterol, 1958. 55: p. 741–7.

[131] Jakimowicz, J.J. and T.J.M. Ruers, Ultrasound-Assisted Laparoscopic Cholecystectomy: Preliminary Experience. Dig Surg, 1991. 8: p. 114-117.

[132] Jakimowicz, J.J., Intraoperative ultrasonography in open and laparoscopic abdominal surgery: an overview. Surg Endosc, 2006. 20 Suppl 2: p. S425-35.

[133] Richardson, W., et al., SAGES guidelines for the use of laparoscopic ultrasound. Surg Endosc, 2010. 24: p. 745–756.

[134] Harms, J., et al., Three-dimensional navigated laparoscopic ultrasonography. Surg Endosc, 2001. 15(12): p. 1459–62.

[135] Mårvik, R., et al., Laparoscopic navigation pointer for 3-D image guided surgery. Surg Endosc, 2004. 18(8): p. 1242-8.

[136] Langø, T., et al., Navigation in laparoscopy – prototype research platform for improved image-guided surgery. Minimally Invasive Therapy and Allied Technologies, 2008. 17(1): p. 17-33.

[137] Solberg, O.V., et al., Navigated ultrasound in laparoscopic surgery. Minim Invasive Ther Allied Technol (MITAT), 2009. 18(1): p. 36-53.

[138] Rutala, W.A., APIC guideline for selection and use of disinfectants. 1994, 1995, and 1996 APIC Guidelines Committee. Am J Infect Control, 1996. 24(4): p. 313-42.

[139] El Guindi, W., et al., 3D ultrasound and Doppler angiography for evaluation of fetal cardiovascular anomalies. Int J Gynaecol Obstet, 2012, http://dx.doi.org/10.1016/j.ijgo.2012.08.015

[140] Rajani, R., J. Hancock, and J.B. Chambers, The art of assessing aortic stenosis. Heart, 2012. 98 Suppl 4: p. iv14-iv22.

[141] Wang, Y., et al., Transesophageal echocardiography guided cannulation for peripheral cardiopulmonary bypass during robotic cardiac surgery. Chin Med J (Engl), 2012. 125(18): p. 3236-9.

[142] Lie, T., et al., Ultrasound imaging during endovascular abdominal aortic aneurysm repair using the Stentor bifurcated endograft. J Endovasc Surg, 1997. 4(3): p. 272-8.

[143] Kaspersen, J.H., et al., Three-dimensional ultrasound-based navigation combined with preoperative CT during abdominal interventions: a feasibility study. Cardiovasc Intervent Radiol, 2003. 26(4): p. 347-56.

[144] Malkawi, A.H., et al., Percutaneous access for endovascular aneurysm repair: a systematic review. Eur J Vasc Endovasc Surg, 2010. 39(6): p. 676-82.

[145] Arthurs, Z.M., et al., Ultrasound-guided access improves rate of access-related complications for totally percutaneous aortic aneurysm repair. Ann Vasc Surg, 2008. 22(6): p. 736-41.

[146] Boks, S.S., et al., Ultrasound-guided percutaneous transabdominal treatment of a type 2 endoleak. Cardiovasc Intervent Radiol, 2005. 28(4): p. 526-9.

[147] Kasthuri, R.S., S.M. Stivaros, and D. Gavan, Percutaneous ultrasound-guided thrombin injection for endoleaks: an alternative. Cardiovasc Intervent Radiol, 2005. 28(1): p. 110-2.

[148] Manstad-Hulaas, F., et al., Three-dimensional electromagnetic navigation vs. fluoroscopy for endovascular aneurysm repair: a prospective feasibility study in patients. J Endovasc Ther, 2012. 19(1): p. 70-8.

[149] Kolstad, F., et al., Three-dimensional ultrasonography navigation in spinal cord tumor surgery. Technical note. J Neurosurg Spine, 2006. 5(3): p. 264-70.

[150] Fry, W.J., Intense ultrasound; a new tool for neurological research. The Journal of mental science, 1954. 100(418): p. 85-96.

[151] Fry, W.J., et al., Production of focal destructive lesions in the central nervous system with ultrasound. Journal of neurosurgery, 1954. 11(5): p. 471-8.

[152] Lele, P.P., A simple method for production of trackless focal lesions with focused ultrasound: physical factors. The Journal of physiology, 1962. 160: p. 494-512.

[153] Lynn, J.G., et al., A New Method for the Generation and Use of Focused Ultrasound in Experimental Biology. The Journal of general physiology, 1942. 26(2): p. 179-93.

[154] Cline, H.E., et al., MR-guided focused ultrasound surgery. Journal of computer assisted tomography, 1992. 16(6): p. 956-65.

[155] Chapman, A. and G. ter Haar, Thermal ablation of uterine fibroids using MR-guided focused ultrasound-a truly non-invasive treatment modality. European radiology, 2007. 17(10): p. 2505-11.

[156] Furusawa, H., et al., The evolving non-surgical ablation of breast cancer: MR guided focused ultrasound (MRgFUS). Breast cancer, 2007. 14(1): p. 55-8.

[157] Huber, P.E., et al., A new noninvasive approach in breast cancer therapy using magnetic resonance imaging-guided focused ultrasound surgery. Cancer research, 2001. 61(23): p. 8441-7.

[158] Martin, E., et al., High-intensity focused ultrasound for noninvasive functional neurosurgery. Annals of neurology, 2009. 66(6): p. 858-61.

[159] McDannold, N., et al., Transcranial magnetic resonance imaging- guided focused ultrasound surgery of brain tumors: initial findings in 3 patients. Neurosurgery, 2010. 66(2): p. 323-32; discussion 332.

[160] Catane, R., et al., MR-guided focused ultrasound surgery (MRgFUS) for the palliation of pain in patients with bone metastases--preliminary clinical experience. Annals of oncology : official journal of the European Society for Medical Oncology / ESMO, 2007. 18(1): p. 163-7.

[161] Liberman, B., et al., Pain palliation in patients with bone metastases using MR-guided focused ultrasound surgery: a multicenter study. Annals of surgical oncology, 2009. 16(1): p. 140-6.

[162] Aubry, A. and A. Derode, Multiple scattering of ultrasound in weakly inhomogeneous media: application to human soft tissues. The Journal of the Acoustical Society of America, 2011. 129(1): p. 225-33.

[163] Kennedy, J.E., R.L. Clarke, and G.R. ter Haar. The effects of absorbers such as ribs in the HIFU Beam-path on the focal profile. in 2nd Intl. Symp. on Therapeutic Ultrasound. 2002.

[164] Goss, S.A., L.A. Frizzell, and F. Dunn, Ultrasonic absorption and attenuation in mammalian tissues. Ultrasound in medicine & biology, 1979. 5(2): p. 181-6.

[165] Al-Bataineh, O., J. Jenne, and P. Huber, Clinical and future applications of high intensity focused ultrasound in cancer. Cancer treatment reviews, 2012. 38(5): p. 346-53.

[166] Jenne, J.W., T. Preusser, and M. Gunther, High-Intensity Focused Ultrasound: Principles, Therapy Guidance, Simulations and Applications. Zeitschrift fur medizinische Physik, 2012. Online 9 August 2012.

[167] Kopelman, D., et al., Magnetic resonance-guided focused ultrasound surgery (MRgFUS). Four ablation treatments of a single canine hepatocellular adenoma. HPB : the official journal of the International Hepato Pancreato Biliary Association, 2006. 8(4): p. 292-8.

[168] Kopelman, D., et al., Magnetic resonance-guided focused ultrasound surgery (MRgFUS): ablation of liver tissue in a porcine model. European journal of radiology, 2006. 59(2): p. 157-62.

[169] Okada, A., et al., A case of hepatocellular carcinoma treated by MR-guided focused ultrasound ablation with respiratory gating. Magnetic resonance in medical sciences : MRMS : an official journal of Japan Society of Magnetic Resonance in Medicine, 2006. 5(3): p. 167-71.

[170] de Senneville, B.D., C. Mougenot, and C.T. Moonen, Real-time adaptive methods for treatment of mobile organs by MRI-controlled high-intensity focused ultrasound. Magnetic resonance in medicine : official journal of the Society of Magnetic Resonance in Medicine / Society of Magnetic Resonance in Medicine, 2007. 57(2): p. 319-30.

[171] von Siebenthal, M., et al., 4D MR imaging of respiratory organ motion and its variability. Physics in medicine and biology, 2007. 52(6): p. 1547-64.

[172] Ries, M., et al., Real-time 3D target tracking in MRI guided focused ultrasound ablations in moving tissues. Magnetic resonance in medicine : official journal of the Society of Magnetic Resonance in Medicine / Society of Magnetic Resonance in Medicine, 2010. 64(6): p. 1704-12.

[173] de Oliveira, P.L., et al., Rapid motion correction in MR-guided high-intensity focused ultrasound heating using real-time ultrasound echo information. NMR in biomedicine, 2010. 23(9): p. 1103-8.

[174] de Senneville, B.D., et al., Motion correction in MR thermometry of abdominal organs: a comparison of the referenceless vs. the multibaseline approach. Magnetic resonance in medicine : official journal of the Society of Magnetic Resonance in Medicine / Society of Magnetic Resonance in Medicine, 2010. 64(5): p. 1373-81.

[175] Auboiroux, V., et al., Ultrasonography-based 2D motion-compensated HIFU sonication integrated with reference-free MR temperature monitoring: a feasibility study ex vivo. Physics in medicine and biology, 2012. 57(10): p. N159-71.

[176] Feinberg, D.A., et al., Hybrid ultrasound MRI for improved cardiac imaging and real-time respiration control. Magnetic resonance in medicine : official journal of the

Society of Magnetic Resonance in Medicine / Society of Magnetic Resonance in Medicine, 2010. 63(2): p. 290-6.

[177] Tang, A.M., et al., Simultaneous ultrasound and MRI system for breast biopsy: compatibility assessment and demonstration in a dual modality phantom. IEEE transactions on medical imaging, 2008. 27(2): p. 247-54.

[178] Viallon, M., et al., Observation and correction of transient cavitation-induced PRFS thermometry artifacts during radiofrequency ablation, using simultaneous ultrasound/MR imaging. Medical physics, 2010. 37(4): p. 1491-506.

[179] Yatvin, M.B., et al., Design of liposomes for enhanced local release of drugs by hyperthermia. Science, 1978. 202(4374): p. 1290-3.

[180] Lindner, L.H., et al., Novel temperature-sensitive liposomes with prolonged circulation time. Clin Cancer Res, 2004. 10(6): p. 2168-78.

[181] de Smet, M., et al., Magnetic resonance imaging of high intensity focused ultrasound mediated drug delivery from temperature-sensitive liposomes: an in vivo proof-of-concept study. J Control Release, 2011. 150(1): p. 102-10.

[182] Evjen, T.J., et al., Sonosensitive dioleoylphosphatidylethanolamine-containing liposomes with prolonged blood circulation time of doxorubicin. Eur J Pharm Sci, 2011. 43(4): p. 318-24.

[183] Hernot, S. and A.L. Klibanov, Microbubbles in ultrasound-triggered drug and gene delivery. Adv Drug Deliv Rev, 2008. 60(10): p. 1153-66.

[184] Tinkov, S., et al., Microbubbles as ultrasound triggered drug carriers. J Pharm Sci, 2009. 98(6): p. 1935-61.

[185] Ting, C.Y., et al., Concurrent blood-brain barrier opening and local drug delivery using drug-carrying microbubbles and focused ultrasound for brain glioma treatment. Biomaterials, 2012. 33(2): p. 704-12.

[186] Hynynen, K., Ultrasound for drug and gene delivery to the brain. Adv Drug Deliv Rev, 2008. 60(10): p. 1209-17.

[187] Porter, T.R., et al., Thrombolytic enhancement with perfluorocarbon-exposed sonicated dextrose albumin microbubbles. Am Heart J, 1996. 132(5): p. 964-8.

[188] Molina, C.A., et al., Microbubble administration accelerates clot lysis during continuous 2-MHz ultrasound monitoring in stroke patients treated with intravenous tissue plasminogen activator. Stroke, 2006. 37(2): p. 425-9.

Chapter 3

Ultrasound Diagnosis of Chest Diseases

Wei-Chih Liao, Chih-Yen Tu, Chuen-Ming Shih,
Chia-Hung Chen, Hung-Jen Chen and Hsu Wu-Huei

Additional information is available at the end of the chapter

http://dx.doi.org/10.5772/55419

1. Introduction

Ultrasound (US) has been proved to be valuable for the evaluation of a wide variety of chest diseases, particularly when the pleural cavity is involved. The advantages of US are that it is a relatively inexpensive, widely available, mobile form of multi-planar imaging free from ionizing. Chest US can supplement other imaging modalities of the chest and guides a variety of diagnostic and therapeutic procedures. Under real-time US guidance the success rates of invasive procedures on pleural diseases increase significantly whereas the risks are greatly reduced. Chest US is a useful tool in the diagnosis of pleural diseases and peripheral pulmonary lesions. Moreover, endobronchial ultrasound (EBUS) is the real advance in recent chest medicine. This chapter will review the application of chest ultrasound and EBUS in chest medicine.

2. Equipment selection and patient position

The suitable probes for chest US are these equipped with 3.5- to 10-MHz linear, convex, and sector transducers. The high-frequency linear probe can exam the detailed signs of pleura and provide assessment of superficial lesions. Commonly a 3.5–5 MHz probe is used which is suitable for imaging adequate depth of penetration of lung. In some expert's opinion, the best probe to use for chest ultrasound in the 5-MHz microconvex probe because it allows access the intercostals space and facilitates to these patients unable to cooperate by sitting. During chest US examinations, patients can be in the seated (Figure 1.1) or supine position (Figure 1.2). The probe is moved along the intercostals space to avoid interference by ribs or sternum. The transducer can be moved longitudinally or horizontally in the chest wall.

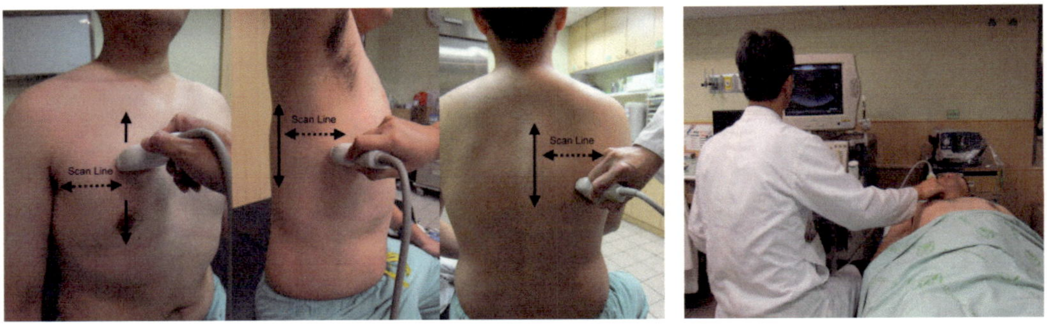

Figure 1. During chest US examinations, patients can be in the seated or supine position (Figure 1.1 on the left; Figure 1.2 on the right).

3. Chest wall: Muscle layers, bone, and pleura

Because air cannot be visualized by US, the normal lung parenchyma cannot be detected by US theoretically. The image of chest US in chest wall including muscle, fascia, bone, and pleura (Figure 2). The soft tissue echogenicity with multiple layers means muscles and fascia. The normal ribs appear hyperechoic surfaces with prominent acoustic shadows beneath the ribs. Approximal 0.5 cm below the ribs shadows, the visceral and parietal pleura appear as an enchogenic bright line. During respiratory movement, the two pleural lines glide with each other which is referred to as the "Gliding sign". Therefore, the "Gliding sign" means normal parietal and visceral pleura slide over each other during respiration and the loss of "Gliding sign" can be seen in pneumothorax or diffuse pleural thickening.

4. Pleural disease

4.1. Pleural effusion

For the purpose of investigation pleural fluid can be divided into three broad categories according to etiology: infective, malignant and miscellaneous. The infective etiologies result in either a para-pneumonic effusion or an empyema. Malignant effusions are due to primary or secondary thoracic disease, which may be pulmonary or pleural. The miscellaneous causes of pleural fluid include sterile benign effusions, haemothoraces and chylothoraces. Pleural effusions are differentiated into transudates or exudates on the basis of biochemical analysis of the aspirated fluid. The erect chest radiograph is the most common first line radiological investigation. Whereas approximately 500 ml of pleural fluid is required before an effusion can be identified clinically, as little 200 ml will blunt the costophrenic angle. US in either a standing or sitting position [1] not only is able to detect smaller volumes of pleural fluid than the erect frontal chest radiograph but it also gives useful information about the nature of the effusion. The pleural effusion images in ultrasound appearances are characterized by an echo-free space between the visceral and parietal pleura. The formulae to estimate the volume of pleural effusions are well documented [1-5], but the different variation of actual volume was found in individual condition. The classifications of the volume of pleural effusion known currently are minimal, small, moderate, and massive. The minimal effusion indicate the echo-free space is seen within the costophrenic angle; small effusion indicates the space is greater than costphrenic angle but still within a one-probe range; moderate effusion indicates the space is greater than one-probe range but within a two-probe; and massive effusion indicates the space is bigger than two-probe range.

4.2. Pleural effusion echogenicity

The strength of ultrasound lies in demonstrating characteristics of the pleural fluid itself. Four basic ultrasounds patterns of internal echogenicity of pleural effusion were identified and they can be subclassified as anechoic, complex nonseptated, complex septated, and homogenously echogenic (Figure 3). Anechoic effusion is defined as echo-free spaces between visceral and parietal pleura. Complex nonseptated effusion is defined as heterogenous echogenic materials inside the pleural effusions. Complex septataed effusion is defined as fibrin strands or septa floating inside the pleural effusions. Homogenously enchogenic effusion is defined as echogenic spots density evenly distributed within the effusion [2, 3]. A purely anechoic collection is found in exudates and transudates with equal frequency. However, internal echoes in the form of septations or focal areas of debris are due invariably to exudates. US presentations in transudative pleural effusions are not always in an anechoic pattern. Transudative pleural effusions may have a complex nonseptated pattern or an anechoic pattern [4].

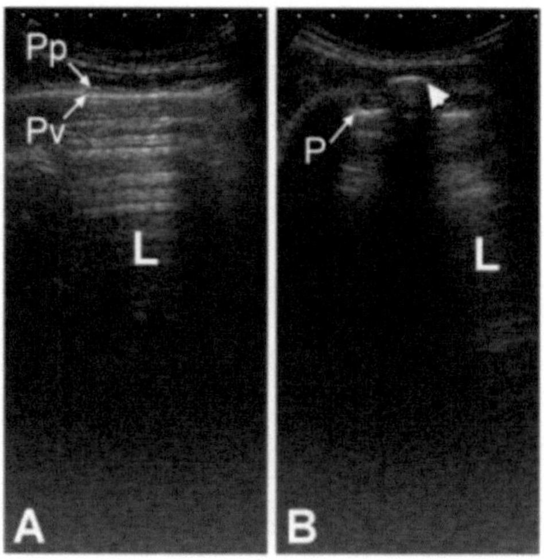

Figure 2. Sonographic images of normal pleura and chest wall using a 5-MHz convex scanner. (A) Transverse image through the intercostal space. The chest wall is visualized as multiple layers of echogenicity representing muscles and fascia. The visceral and parietal pleura appear as echogenic bright lines that glide during respiration (gliding sign). Reverberation echo artifacts beneath the pleural lines imply an underlying air-filled lung. (B) Longitudinal image across the ribs. Normal ribs are seen as hyperechoic chambered surfaces (arrowheads) with prominent acoustic shadows beneath the ribs. Pp, parietal pleura; Pv, visceral pleura; L, lung

There was no transudative pleural effusion with complex septated or homogenously echogenic pattern [5]. The ability of chest US to detect underlying disease was comparable to that of computed tomography (CT) in pleural and parenchymal lesions [6]. The applications of sonographic appearances in effusions of febrile patients in the intensive care unit (ICU) can determine the necessity of thoracentesis in high risk patients with effusion in ICU [7]. This study reported that complex nonseptated and relatively hyperechoic, complex septated and homogenously echogenic pleural effusion patterns might predict the possibility of empyema in febrile patients in the ICU. The sonographic septation in lymphocyte-rich exudative pleural effusions can help us differentiate tuberculosis pleurisy from malignant pleural effusion [8].

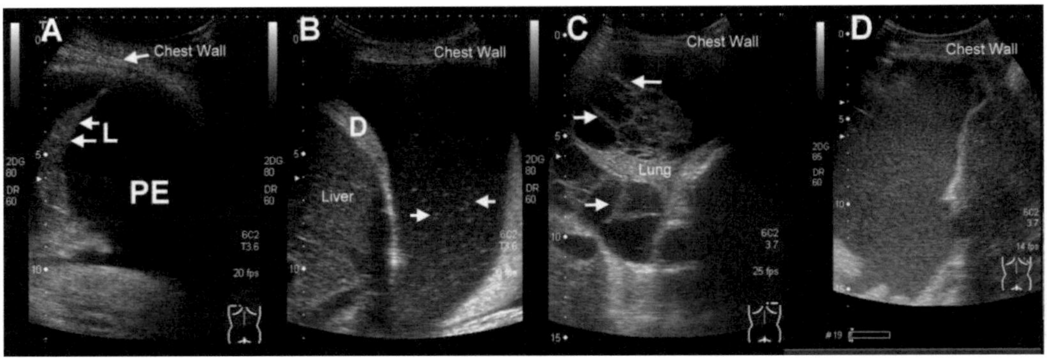

Figure 3. Sonographic appearance of pleural effusion (PE). The effusion can be subclassified as anechoic (A), complex nonseptated with spots(arrows) floating inside effusion. D, diaphragm (B), complex septated (arrows) (C), and homogenously echogenic (D)

5. Pneumothorax

Expiratory erect chest radiographs are the initial examination of choice in suspected pneumothoraces, but the sensitivity of diagnosis was ranging between 50% and 90% [9, 10]. The diagnosis of a pneumothorax on the frontal radiograph is most difficult in critically ill patients where the patient is semi-recumbent and unable to comply with expiratory breath holding. Chest US may be help in the diagnosis of pneumothoraces. Normal parietal and visceral pleura slide over each other during respiration and a pneumothorax is suspected when this 'Gliding sign' is absent in chest US [11]. A recently published systemic review, chest US had a sensitivity of 90.0% and a specificity of 98.2% [12]. The confirmation of lung gliding has a 100% negative predictive value for the absence of pneumothorax [13]. The use of M-mode can also objectify the presence or absence of lung gliding. In the normal lung, the familiar "sea-shore" or "sandy-beach" sign appearance will confirm the presence of lung gliding (Figure 4). In the pneumothorax, the "bar code" or stratosphere sign (Figure 5) is seen [14]. The "curtain sign" describes the variable obscuring of underlying structures by air-containing tissue that movement of air-fluid level denoting a hydropneumothorax (Figure 6).

http://dx.doi.org/10.5772/55419

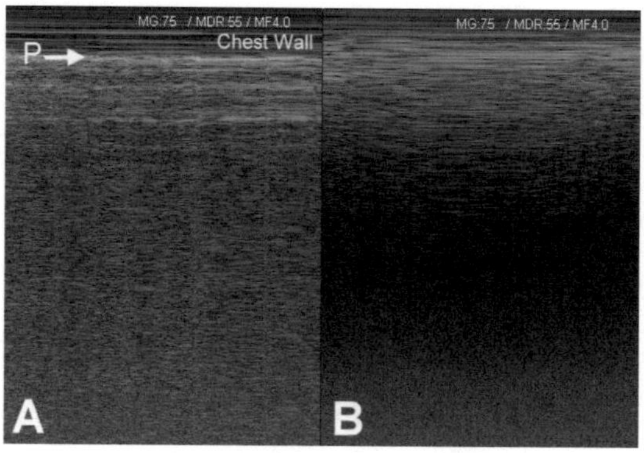

Figure 4. Lung sliding (on M-Mode sonography). P, pleura. Panel (A) shows the granular 'sea-shore' appearance of normal lung sliding. Panel (B) shows the horizontal 'bar-code' appearance that occurs with loss of lung sliding

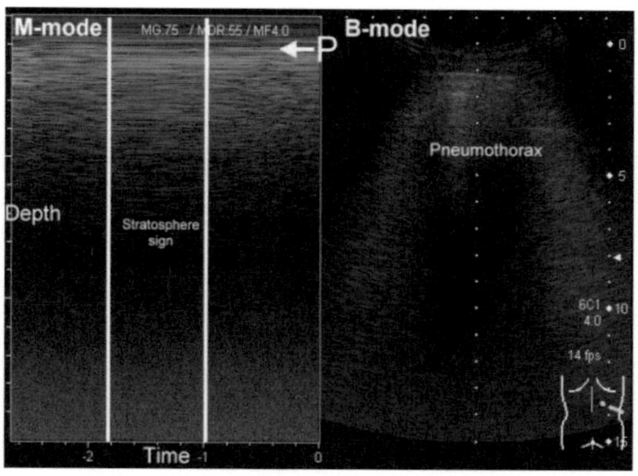

Figure 5. Pneumothorax. Chest US reveals stratosphere sign

5.1. Pulmonary lesions

The normal aerated lung is difficult to image because the dramatic change in acoustic impedance between chest wall and lung results in specular reflection of ultrasound waves at the pleura. However, consolidated lung has a tissue density and echo-texture similar to liver, analogous to pathological hepatisation. This removes the change in acoustic impedance at the pleural interface, and ultrasound waves pass directly into the affected lung. When patient with lobar or segmental pneumonia and the lesion is adjacent to pleura or in the pleural effusion, the pneumonia may be detected by chest US. A marked consolidation with air-bronchogram and treelike ramifications is easily seen (Figure 7). Within the consolidated area, hyperechoic (white) foci may be visible, again representing a change in acoustic impedance, but this time at the tissue interface between solid lung and air-filled bronchi. Subpleural nodule also can be seen in chest US (Figure 8).

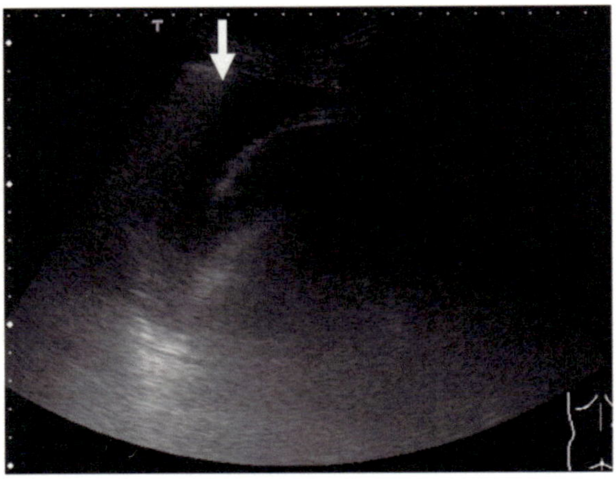

Figure 6. Sonogram of a hydropneumothorax. Notice the gas–fluid and fibrin interface (arrow) between the bright hyperechoic line dorsally representing the pneumothorax and the ventral fluid and fibrin.

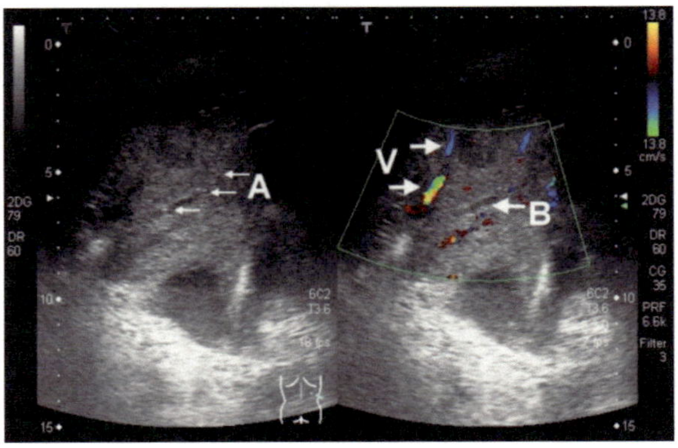

Figure 7. Air bronchogram. Notice the hypoechoic parenchyma and the small hyperechoic areas (A arrows) consistent with residual air in the bronchial tree. Color Doppler can distinguish between vessel and bronchus. V, vessel; B, bronchus.

Chest US with color Doppler is a powerful tool for differentiating the peripheral air-fluid abscess from empyema [15]. The differentiation by chest radiograph alone is difficult when the empyema presents with an air-fluid level. Thoracic CT scanning can prove valuable in differentiating lung abscess from empyema; however, the problems of radiation exposure and contrast induced renal failure sometimes limit its application. The empyema can be detected by chest US with an image of a hypoechoic lesion with complex-septated effusions, passive atelectasis, width uniformity, and smooth luminal and outer margins. Color Doppler ultrasound could not identify vessel signals in pericavitary atelectasis. The lung abscess in the US image reveals hypoechoic lesion with typical pulmonary consolidation, irregular wall width, and irregular luminal and outer margins. Color Doppler ultrasound could identify vessel signals in pericavitary consolidation (Figure 9).

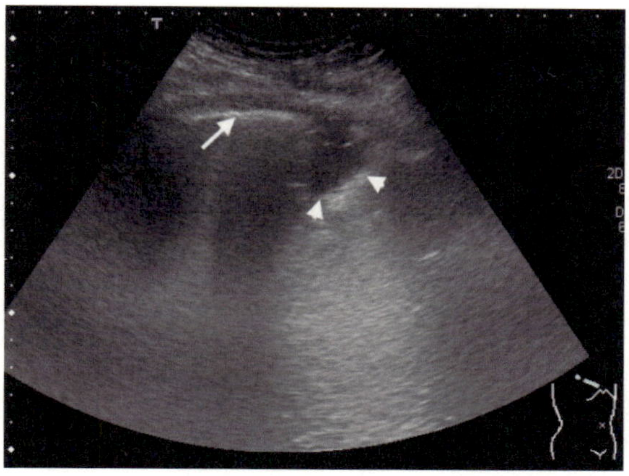

Figure 8. Transverse chest US scan shows a subpleural nodule (arrowheads). The linear hyperechoic area (arrow) represents visceral pleura.

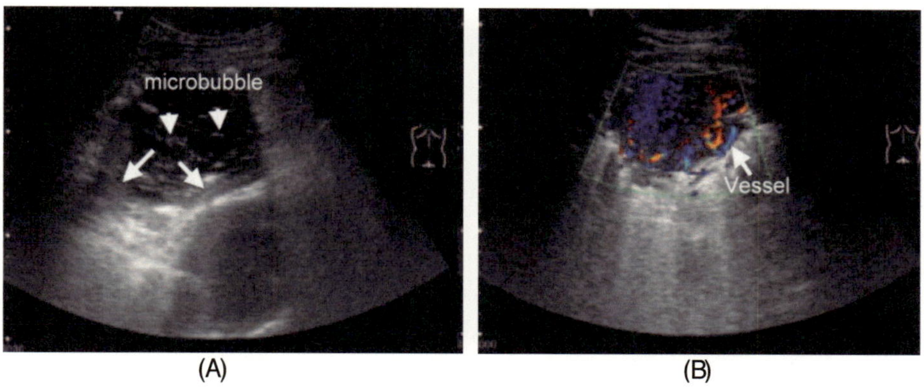

Figure 9. Lung abscess in chest US with Doppler. Chest US examination reveals a hypoechoic lesion with microbubble sign, which is surrounded by whole-lung parenchyma (arrows) (A). Color Doppler ultrasound can identify vessel signals in pericavitary consolidation in a lung abscess (B).

5.2. Alveolar interstitial syndrome

During previous studies, ultrasound imaging is not useful for pulmonary parenchyma imaging. Alveolar interstitial syndrome constitutes a group of diseases that is caused by an increase in lung fluid and/or a reduction in its air content. The result of this thickening of the interlobular septa causes a particular artifact that is seen arising from pleura line. The ultrasound appearance of alveolar interstitial syndrome is a vertical artifact, called B-line. Presence of the comet-tail artifact (Figure 10) allowed diagnosis of alveolar-interstitial syndrome by chest ultrasound [16]. The major causes of alveolar interstitial syndrome include pulmonary edema, acute respiratory distress syndrome (ARDS), and interstitial fibrosis. In the advanced study, application of chest ultrasound in the patients with respiratory failure, chest ultrasounds can help the clinician make a rapid diagnosis in patients with acute respiratory failure according the BLUE protocol [17].

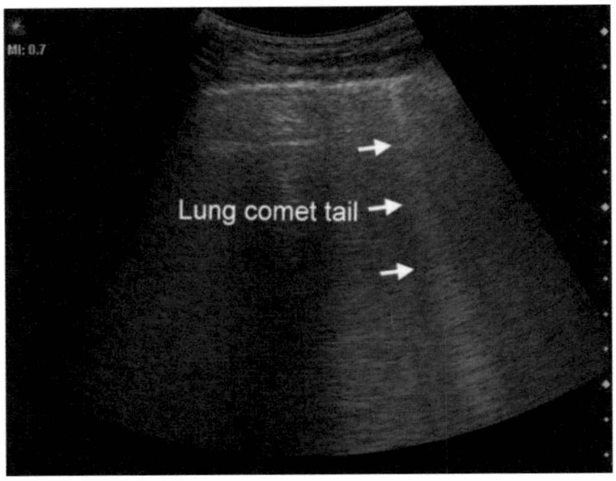

Figure 10. Lung comets. Lung comet tail, also known as 'B lines' (arrows) are indicative an alveolar interstitial syndrome.

6. Ultrasound-guided intervention

6.1. Diagnostic thoracentasis

The aim of the initial assessment of pleural fluid is to identify malignancy or infection and starts with a visual inspection of the aspirate prior to laboratory analysis. Therefore diagnostic thoracentesis is mandatory. When performed with image guidance thoracentesis provides clinically useful information in more than 90% of cases. If the pleural effusion spans three intercostal spaces and its presence can be confirmed clinically by percussion then aspiration can be performed safely at the bedside without the aid of image guidance. When the effusion is small, loculated or associated with underlying pulmonary collapse this becomes more difficult and hazardous. In all these situations US examination is required to confirm the presence of fluid and to guide thoracentesis. Moreover, bed-side procedures are sometimes necessary due to patient debilitation and can be performed satisfactorily with a portable US machine. By performing the aspiration at the time of the US examination success rates will be optimized and complication rates kept to a minimum. The most commonly reported complication for non-guided thoracentesis is that of pneumothorax with published rates varying from 11 to 12%. When US-guidance diagnostic thoracentesis is performed the complication rates fall to between 0.2% and 2.7% [18].

6.2. Ultrasound-guided small-bore chest tube insertion

Chest US also can be used guidance for small-bore catheter (pigtail tube) insertion and also provide a safe and effective method of draining various pleural diseases which includes pneumothorax, malignant pleural effusion, para-pneumonic effusion/empyema, and massive transudate effusions [19]. In primary spontaneous pneumothorax patients, ultrasound-guided pigtail catheter drainage is effective and had a shorter hospital stay than patients treated by chest tube drainage [20]. Moreover, US-guided pigtail catheter for secondary spontaneous pneumothorax (SSP) is also effective and has low complication rate. A higher treatment failure rate was noted in infectious related SSP patients [21, 22]. In mechanically ventilated patients, US-guided pigtail catheter drainage is also effective in treating iatrogenic pneumothorax [23].

6.3. Ultrasound-guided biopsy

Transthoracic needle biopsy with fluoroscopic or computed tomographic (CT) guidance is a well-established and safe method for diagnosing malignant and benign thoracic lesions. However, radiation exposure is considerable and the cost is relatively high, as compared with US guidance. US is as effective as CT for guidance of transthoracic biopsies of peripheral pulmonary lesions and mediastinal tumors and offers a number of advantages. Real-time US imaging allows for dynamic evaluation of vessels and localization of target lesions that move during respiration. In US-guided transthoracic biopsy, the tip of the needle can be monitored throughout the procedure and fine adjustments can be made quickly and precisely; this is especially beneficial for biopsy of small thoracic lesions [24, 25]. Pleural biopsy is required for unexplained pleural effusions, pleural thickening (whether focal or diffuse) and pleural masses. The advances in imaging of the pleura provided by US and CT have meant that radiologists now play an important role in pleural biopsy either directly or indirectly. In most instances biopsies are performed to establish whether or not pleural disease is due to malignancy or to evaluate a suspected inflammatory process such as tuberculosis. Because focal pleural thickening or pleural tumors can be easily identified by US, US-guided pleural biopsy is related to possible focal pleural involvement in various diseases such as pleural tumor, thickening pleura, and small amounts of pleural effusion [26]. Besides, in critically ill patients, chest US is helpful in diagnosis and is a useful diagnostic tool for critically ill patients with chest disease [27].

6.4. Endobronchial Ultrasound (EBUS)

Endobronchial ultrasound (EBUS) technology is a relatively new bronchoscopic method of visualizing the tracheobronchial tree, the surrounding pulmonary parenchyma, and the mediastinal structures, with a particular role in lung cancer diagnosis, staging, and treatment [28]. There are 2 types of probes used in EBUS: the peripheral or radial probe (RP) and the linear or convex probe (CP) EBUS, which have technical differences and distinct diagnostic abilities. Both are used for EBUS-guided biopsies and transbronchial needle aspirations (TBNA), which increases the diagnostic yield over conventional bronchoscopic techniques, thus providing advanced information on staging, diagnosis, and treatment. The 20-MHz RP-EBUS (Figure 11) is positioned inside a water-inflatable balloon and is inserted through the working channel of the bronchoscope. The RP-EBUS was first introduced to evaluate the central airway structure. With advances in technology, the small radial probes can now visualize and assist transbronchial biopsies of peripheral lung nodules without exposure to radiation. Kurimoto and colleagues [29] showed that using a guide sheath with radial probe EBUS and leaving it there to pass the forceps catheter through it could improve the diagnostic yield of specimens from peripheral pulmonary lesions/nodules, including those too small to be visualized by fluoroscopy. Nowadays, the evaluation of mediastinal lesions has been facilitated by the use of CP-EBUS probe. This type of probe incorporates a 7.5-MHz ultrasound transducer at the tip of a flexible bronchoscope. Real-time biopsies of the lymph nodes can be carried out with a 22-gauge needle inserted through the working channel. EBUS-TBNA is most commonly used for staging non-small cell lung cancer (NSCLC), but is also used for diagnosis of unexplained mediastinal lymphadenopathy (Figure 12) of other causes. The safety of this technique is well established and few serious complications have been reported, including pneumothorax, pneumomediastinum, and hemomediastinum [30, 31].

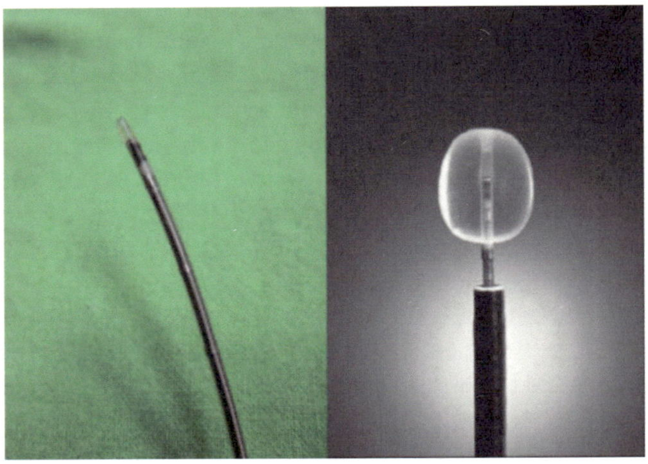

Figure 11. Radial Probe Endobronchial Ultrasound. Left, probe and deflated balloon. Right, probe within a bronchoscope with balloon inflated.

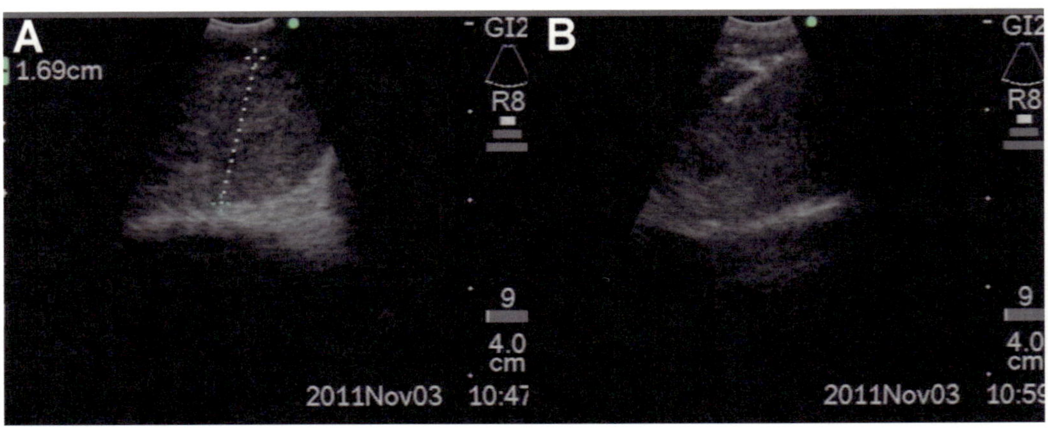

Figure 12. Image of a lymph node biopsy under endobronchial ultrasound guidance. Real-time EBUS-TBNA revealed a lymph node of 1.69 cm (A). The needle (arrows) is clearly visible in the lymph node (B).

http://dx.doi.org/10.5772/55419

7. Conclusions

Pleural US has a proven role in improving the safety of pleural procedures and should be offered as standard of care in this setting. US also offers advantages over conventional radiography in the detection, quantification and characterisation of pleural effusions. Lung US has excellent test characteristics for the diagnosis of consolidation, interstitial syndrome and subpleural pulmonary nodules. EBUS based technology may be used in the diagnosis of a lung or mediastinal lesion, staging of lung cancer, and treatment of an endobronchial abnormality.

In the future, chest sonography is likely to be an essential skill for the physician, and training requirements are likely to evolve with advances in the field.

Author details

Wei-Chih Liao[1,2], Chih-Yen Tu[1,2,3*], Chuen-Ming Shih[1,2], Chia-Hung Chen[1,2], Hung-Jen Chen[1,2] and Hsu Wu-Huei[1,2]

*Address all correspondence to: chesttu@gmail.com

1 Division of Pulmonary and Critical Care Medicine, Department of Internal Medicine, China Medical University Hospital, Taichung, Taiwan

2 China Medical University, Taichung, Taiwan

3 Department of Life Science, National Chung Hsing University, Taiwan

References

[1] Eibenberger KL, Dock WI, Ammann ME, et al. Quantification of pleural effusions: sonography versus radiography. Radiology 1994; 191:681-684

[2] Yang PC, Luh KT, Chang DB, et al. Value of sonography in determining the nature of pleural effusion: analysis of 320 cases. AJR Am J Roentgenol 1992;159 29-33.

[3] Hirsch JH, Rogers JV, Mack LA. Real-time sonography of pleural opacities. AJR Am J Roentgenol 1981;136 297-301.

[4] Chen HJ, Tu CY, Ling SJ, et al. Sonographic appearances in transudative pleural effusions: not always an anechoic pattern. Ultrasound Med Biol 2008;34 362-369.

[5] Tsai TH, Yang PC. Ultrasound in the diagnosis and management of pleural disease. Curr Opin Pulm Med 2003;9 282-290.

[6] Yu CJ, Yang PC, Wu HD, et al. Ultrasound study in unilateral hemithorax opacification. Image comparison with computed tomography. Am Rev Respir Dis 1993;147 430-434.

[7] Tu CY, Hsu WH, Hsia TC, et al. Pleural effusions in febrile medical ICU patients: chest ultrasound study. Chest 2004;126 1274-1280.

[8] Chen HJ, Hsu WH, Tu CY, et al. Sonographic septation in lymphocyte-rich exudative pleural effusions: a useful diagnostic predictor for tuberculosis. J Ultrasound Med 2006;25 857-863.

[9] Ball CG, Kirkpatrick AW, Laupland KB, et al. Factors related to the failure of radiographic recognition of occult posttraumatic pneumothoraces. Am J Surg 2005;189 541-546.

[10] Chiles C, Ravin CE. Radiographic recognition of pneumothorax in the intensive care unit. Crit Care Med 1986;14 677-680.

[11] Targhetta R, Bourgeois JM, Chavagneux R, et al. Ultrasonic signs of pneumothorax: preliminary work. J Clin Ultrasound 1993;21 245-250.

[12] Alrajhi K, Woo MY, Vaillancourt C. Test characteristics of ultrasonography for the detection of pneumothorax: a systematic review and meta-analysis. Chest 2012;141:703-708.

[13] Lichtenstein DA, Menu Y. A bedside ultrasound sign ruling out pneumothorax in the critically ill. Lung sliding. Chest 1995;108 1345-1348.

[14] Lichtenstein DA. Ultrasound in the management of thoracic disease. Crit Care Med 2007;35 S250-261.

[15] Chen HJ, Yu YH, Tu CY, et al. Ultrasound in peripheral pulmonary air-fluid lesions. Color Doppler imaging as an aid in differentiating empyema and abscess. Chest 2009;135 1426-1432.

[16] Lichtenstein D, Meziere G, Biderman P, et al. The comet-tail artifact. An ultrasound sign of alveolar-interstitial syndrome. Am J Respir Crit Care Med 1997; 56 1640-1646.

[17] Lichtenstein DA, Meziere GA. Relevance of lung ultrasound in the diagnosis of acute respiratory failure: the BLUE protocol. Chest 2008;134 117-125.

[18] Jones PW, Moyers JP, Rogers JT, et al. Ultrasound-guided thoracentesis: is it a safer method? Chest 2003;123 418-423.

[19] Liu YH, Lin YC, Liang SJ, et al. Ultrasound-guided pigtail catheters for drainage of various pleural diseases. Am J Emerg Med 2010;8 915-921.

[20] Liu CM, Hang LW, Chen WK, et al. Pigtail tube drainage in the treatment of spontaneous pneumothorax. Am J Emerg Med 2003;21 241-244.

[21] Chen CH, Chen W, Hsu WH. Pigtail catheter drainage for secondary spontaneous pneumothorax. QJM 2006;99 489-491.

[22] Chen CH, Liao WC, Liu YH, et al. Secondary spontaneous pneumothorax: which associated conditions benefit from pigtail catheter treatment? Am J Emerg Med 2012;30 45-50.

[23] Lin YC, Tu CY, Liang SJ, et al. Pigtail catheter for the management of pneumothorax in mechanically ventilated patients. Am J Emerg Med 2010;28 466-471.

[24] ang PC, Kuo SH, Luh KT. Ultrasonography and ultrasound-guided needle biopsy of chest diseases: indications, techniques, diagnostic elds and complications. J Med Ultrasound 1993;2 53–63.

[25] Yang PC. Ultrasound-guided transthoracic biopsy of peripheral lung, pleural, and chest-wall lesions. J Thorac Imaging 1997;12 272-284.

[26] Chang DB, Yang PC, Luh KT, et al. Ultrasound-guided pleural biopsy with Tru-Cut needle. Chest 1991;100 1328-1333.

[27] Yu CJ, Yang PC, Chang DB, et al. Diagnostic and therapeutic use of chest sonography: value in critically ill patients. AJR Am J Roentgenol 1992;159 695-701.

[28] Gomez M, Silvestri GA. Endobronchial ultrasound for the diagnosis and staging of lung cancer. Proc Am Thorac Soc 2009;6 180-186.

[29] Kurimoto N, Miyazawa T, Okimasa S, et al. Endobronchial ultrasonography using a guide sheath increases the ability to diagnose peripheral pulmonary lesions endoscopically. Chest 2004;126 959-965.

[30] Lazzari Agli L, Trisolini R, Burzi M, et al. Mediastinal hematoma following transbronchial needle aspiration. Chest 2002;122 1106-1107.

[31] Kucera RF, Wolfe GK, Perry ME. Hemomediastinum after transbronchial needle aspiration. Chest 1986;90:466.

Chapter 4

Diagnostic Use of Sonography in the Evaluation of Hypertension

Nikolaos Pagonas, Stergios Vlatsas and
Timm H. Westhoff

Additional information is available at the end of the chapter

http://dx.doi.org/10.5772/56171

1. Introduction

Hypertension is the most frequently treated disease in internal medicine. More than 1 billion people worldwide suffer from hypertension. Hypertension leads to cardiovascular end-organ damage increasing morbidity and mortality and is related with high costs to society, making this disease an important public health challenge. Sonography is a crucial diagnostic tool in the evaluation of a hypertensive patient. It is used both for the search of secondary forms of hypertension and for the identification of hypertensive end organ damage. There are several ultrasound examinations that may be warranted in hypertension. *Abdominal ultrasound* is recommended by several guidelines for the basic diagnostic workup in every newly diagnosed hypertensive patient. *Doppler sonography of the renal arteries* is reasonable only in a subset of hypertensives that are at increased risk of renal artery stenosis. *Echocardiography* is able to reveal cardiac end organ damage in terms of hypertensive heart disease. *Ultrasound of the carotid arteries* is frequently used to detect and evaluate in the case of hypertension-induced vascular end organ damage. The assessment of the *intima-media thickness* allows the detection of early stages of atherosclerotic wall changes. Prior to any structural vascular damage that may be visualized by ultrasound techniques, hypertension leads to functional changes of the endothelium, called endothelial dysfunction. Endothelial dysfunction encompasses a variety of changes in vascular function including a reduced endothelium-dependent vasodilation. This can be diagnosed by sonography measuring the diameter changes of the brachial artery in response to predefined endothelial stimuli. *Flow-mediated dilation* in response to hyperemia is regarded as the gold-standard in the non-invasive assessment of endothelial dysfunction. To date, it is rather used scientifically than in daily clinical practice. The present chapter provides an overview on the practical performance of all of these ultrasound techniques in the approach to hypertension.

2. Abdominal ultrasound

The use of abdominal ultrasound in the evaluation of hypertension is twofold.

- In the detection of a secondary forms of hypertension.
- In the evaluation of subclinical organ damage induced by hypertension.

In the current European Society of Cardiology/European Society of Hypertension (ESC/ESH) guidelines for hypertension the use of abdominal ultrasound is recommended as a part of the evaluation of hypertensive individuals. The abdominal ultrasound supplies information about the etiology of hypertension as well as possible end organ damages.

The main interest is the morphology of the kidneys, the adrenal glands and of the aorta. Due to their retroperitoneal position, kidneys are completely and easily detectable. A 3.5-5 MHz probe is typically used to scan the kidney. The examination from dorsolateral allows the evasion of the intestinal loops and thus allows for a non-overlapping imaging in the supine position. The formerly widely spread examination in the lateral recumbent position is nowadays used only in exceptional cases. Renal ultrasound has now almost completely replaced intravenous urography in the anatomical exploration of the kidney. While the latter requires the injection of potentially nephrotoxic contrast medium, ultrasound is non-invasive and provides the necessary anatomic data about kidney size and shape, cortical thickness, urinary tract obstruction and renal masses [1]. Renal parenchymal disease is one of the most common causes of secondary hypertension which leads to a wide spectrum of morphologic alterations. The finding of bilateral upper abdominal masses at physical examination is consistent with polycystic kidney disease and should warrant an abdominal ultrasound examination. Acute parenchymal inflammatory processes like crescentic glomerulonephritis or acute interstitial nephritis sometimes predisposes individuals to measurable organ swelling. The cortical and medullary pyramids have in this case an anechoic profile. However, the morphological alterations seen via ultrasound in the acute kidney processes are less prominent than those seen in chronic kidney damage. Thus, the diagnostic performance in acute inflammatory renal disease is less effective. Chronic parenchymal diseases, such as chronic interstitial nephritis, glomerulonephritis or nephrosclerosis contribute to a progressive decrease in organ size. A kidney size below 90 mm should be interpreted as pathological. Over the course of the organ decrease, small scarring cortical retractions develop, which give the kidney surface a humped aspect. The renal parenchyma develops a hyperechoic pattern through progressive scarring. The border between parenchyma and pyelon becomes progressively nondescript. A variety of chronic parenchymal diseases can lead to the morphological end stage of a shrunken kidney. Sonographically, it is not possible to differentiate whether small kidneys are the cause or the result of hypertension. A unilateral small kidney as a possible indicator for a hemodynamic relevant renal artery stenosis should always lead to a further evaluation of the renal arteries. Renal cell carcinomas as a rare cause of hypertension are depicted as a well delimitable structure from the surrounding tissue. Usually they can be depicted via ultrasound when they exceed 1 cm. With increasingly size there is an increase in their inhomogeneity, so that it is possible to detect areas of liquefied necrosis for example.

In the screening of secondary forms of hypertension abdominal ultrasound plays also a role in the depiction of the adrenal glands. For this purpose a detailed knowledge of the local anatomy is required. The adrenal glands are located within the retroperitoneum. The left adrenal gland, lacking the acoustic window of the liver and being obscured by air in the stomach, is inherently more difficult to scan than the right adrenal gland. On the right side, the right kidney and the inferior vena cava are landmarks for the examination of adrenal glands, whereas on the left side the aorta, the lower pole of the spleen and the upper pole of the kidney are points of orientation. The right adrenal gland is usually scanned with a right transcostal scan or a subcostal flank scan or oblique subcostal scan. On the left side it is better to use an intercostal flank scan through the spleen. The normal sized adrenal glands are only visible with trained examination techniques and by using high resolution technology, whereas enlarged adrenal glands are detectable in a high percentage of cases. Thirty percent of cases of primary aldosteronism are caused by adrenal adenomas. Seventy percent of cases are caused by adrenal hyperplasia. There are rare cases of adrenal carcinoma and the autosomal dominant condition of glucocorticoid remediable aldosteronism [2]. The micronodular hyperplasia is not possible to be detected via sonography. Adrenal adenomas have a round to oval shape and are uniformly hypoechoic with smooth margins, although some lesions have scalloped borders (polycyclic). Adenomas occasionally have an inhomogeneous appearance. Autopsy statistics indicate that they are quite common (10–20%), but most adenomas (90%) produce no endocrine symptoms, they are silent and too small to be detected by ultrasound. In one study the average size of adenomas was reported to be 1.5 cm, although they may exceed 5 cm in diameter. In a small percentage of patients adenomas are bilateral. Functioning and nonfunctioning adenomas are indistinguishable by their sonographic features [3]. Thus, ultrasound is not a sufficient test in the morphologic diagnosis of Conn syndrome. Upon the detection of a high aldosterone-to-renin ratio and after a confirmation test (e.g. suppression after administration of sodium chloride) the use of a CT or MRT scan is indicated. On the other hand, the detection of a unilateral adrenal mass seen in the ultrasound should be followed by a laboratory evaluation for the evaluation of Conn-Syndrome.

Phaeochromocytoma, a tumor of the adrenal medulla, is a rare secondary cause of hypertension (0.2 – 0.4% of all cases of elevated blood pressure) with an estimated annual incidence of 2 – 8 per million population.[4]. It can be inherited or acquired. Hypertension occurs in about 70% of all cases of phaeochromocytoma, being stable or paroxysmal in approximately equal proportions. The diagnosis is based on establishing an increase in plasma or urinary catecholamines or their metabolites (e.g. (nor-) metanephrines). Following the appearance of clinical symptoms (hypertension and tachycardia caused by increased catecholamine secretion), pheochromocytoma can be detected in 80-90% of cases via abdominal ultrasound. Most pheochromocytomas are already several centimeters in diameter when diagnosed. They have smooth margins, a round shape, and an inhomogeneous or complex echo structure. Hypoechoic liquid components may also be observed. A spectrum of appearances is possible. Pheochromocytomas are bilateral in approximately 10% of cases and extra-adrenal in 10–20%. The organ of Zuckerkandl should be looked for at the level of the origin of the inferior mesenteric artery, anterior to the aorta. Other extra-adrenal sites are the renal hilum, bladder wall, and thorax. Pheochromocytoma is occasionally seen posterior to the renal vein in transverse scans. Rarely, pheochromocytoma is diagnosed in the setting of multiple endocrine neoplasia (MEN). About 2% to 5% of pheochromocytomas are malignant. In recent years endosopic sonography is being used to obtain an adrenal gland biopsy [5-7].

Abdominal ultrasound is also being used in the evaluation of hypertension induced end-organ damage. Vascular end-organ damage may be visualized as atherosclerotic as well as aneurysmatic wall alterations, e.g. of the aorta. In the elderly (> 65 years) approximately 60% of the patients with hypertension have an isolated systolic hypertension. This is a result of the diminished elasticity of the large arterial vessels. Ultrasound can indicate a morphological correlate in form of a manifest aortosclerosis. Besides vascular end-organ damage abdominal ultrasound detects renal end organ damage. The correlate of hypertensive end-organ damage of the kidney is (benign) nephrosclerosis. The sonographic features include a reduced size, hyperechoic parenchyma, indefinite margin of parenchyma and pyelon, and scarring cortical retractions. As stated above, this unspecific sonographic appearance does unfortunately not allow a differentiation between cause and result of hypertension.

3. Echocardiography

Hypertension is one of the most important risk factors for heart failure with increasing risk in all age groups. The lifetime risk for developing heart failure is doubled for subjects with blood pressure > 160/100mm Hg compared to those with blood pressure < 140/90 mm Hg [8]. Systolic and diastolic heart failure are both associated with hypertension. There are several mechanisms, alone or in combination, leading to development of heart failure in the presence of hypertension: left ventricular hypertrophy (LVH), chamber remodeling, hemodynamic load and coronary microvascular disease with impaired coronary hemodynamics. To assess subclinical organ damage, such as ventricular hypertrophy, echocardiography is more sensitive than electrocardiography [9], which is a routine examination in all subjects with high blood pressure. However, the ESC/ESH guidelines suggest that in patients with low and intermediate cardiovascular risk an echocardiography should be performed for better global cardiovascular risk stratification which may implicate the appropriate pharmacological treatment [10]. The role of echocardiography is not limited to identification of (sub-) clinical organ damage in the pre-treatment phase. Since changes of the left ventricular hypertrophy in response to treatment are associated to cardiovascular fatal and non-fatal events [11], echocardiography can also be used to monitor treatment's success and re-assess overall risk.

Left ventricular hypertrophy is the first step toward the development of hypertensive heart disease. The echocardiographic evaluation of LVH includes measurements of the interventricular septum, left ventricular posterior wall thickness and end-diastolic diameter. Upon these parameters obtained by M-Mode at the end of diastole (under two-dimensional control), the left ventricular mass is calculated according to the proposed formula [12]. Since LV mass is depended on gender and obesity, the thresholds for presence of LVH mass are indexed to body surface area and estimated for men (above $125g/m^2$) and for women (above $110g/m^2$) [10]. The adaptation of the left ventricle to hypertension is heterogenic and can be classified in three geometric patterns based on the LV mass and on the index of relative wall thickness (LV wall thickness / chamber radius). An increased ratio ≥ 0.42 combined with increased mass is referred to as concentric hypertrophy. The term eccentric hypertrophy refers to subjects with normal wall to radius ratio (< 0.42) but increased LV mass. The last pattern, the concentric remodeling, refers to subjects with normal ventricular mass but increased ratio (≥ 0.42). All three types of chamber remodeling in response to hypertension are related to increased cardiovascular risk. Interestingly, the incidence of cardiovascular events correlates with changes in geometric adaptation, independent of changes of the LV mass. The development or the persistence of a concentric geometry during treatment has been found to be associated with a greater incidence of cardiovascular events [13]. In the Losartan Intervention For Endpoint reduction in hypertension (LIFE) study [11] a regression of the left ventricular mass of about $25g/m^2$ was associated with a 20% reduction in the incidence of the primary endpoint (cardiovascular mortality, myocardial infarction, stroke). Recent data have furthermore reinforced the predictive value of echocardiography in hypertensive patients. 35.000 normotensive and hypertensive participants with normal left ventricular ejection fraction were studied retrospectively. An abnormal left ventricular geometric pattern was found in 46% of the patients (35% with left ventricular concentric remodeling and 11% with LVH) and was associated with a double-risk of all-cause mortality compared to the patients with normal left ventricular geometry [14]. A prospective trial showed that hypertensive patients with echocardiographic LVH had significantly higher all-cause mortality and cardiovascular events [15]. Beyond the lower incidence of cardiovascular events, including sudden death, in patients with regression of echocardiographic left ventricular hypertrophy or a delayed increase in left ventricular mass [11], treatment-induced changes of left atrium dimension and ventricular geometry are also correlated with cardiovascular event rates [16, 17].

Even before evidence of left ventricular hypertrophy is present and before hypertension in young normotensive male offspring of hypertensive parents has developed, diastolic dysfunction may develop as an early end organ damage due to hypertension [18]. Patients with diastolic heart failure (also referred as heart failure with preserved ejection fraction) show similar long term impairments as patients with systolic heart failure [19]. The importance of an early recognition of diastolic dysfunction is imperative. Arterial hypertension with or without hypertrophy is the main cause of diastolic dysfunction, namely the inability of the heart to adequately fill with blood during diastole. There are several factors which lead to diastolic dysfunction in hypertension by impeding the active or passive phases of diastole. Of these, contractile alterations in myocytes, structural ventricular hypertrophy, extracellular and perivascular fibrosis, and myocardial ischemia are most often implicated. The European Society of Cardiology has recognized diastolic dysfunction diagnosed by echocardiography as criterion for the diagnosis of diastolic heart failure [20]. There are a number of specific echocardiographic indicators of diastolic dysfunction obtained during the examination. The major four parameters include transmitral Doppler inflow velocity patterns, pulmonary venous Doppler flow patterns, tissue Doppler velocities and color M-mode flow propagation velocity (Vp). Transmitral Doppler flow is acquired by placing a pulsed wave (PW) sample volume at the level of the tips of the mitral leaflets in the apical four-chamber view. Normally, the ventricular inflow consists of an early (E) and a late filling peak (A). Respectively, the early filling peak velocity (E) and the late (atrial) peak velocity (A) should be recorded. In normal young individuals, more forward flow occurs during the early diastole largely due to the rapid decline in left ventricular pressure during the isovolumetric relaxation time (IVRT). Consequently, the E/A ratio is > 1 correlating with a normal relaxation. An E/A ratio < 1 together with prolonged IVRT and deceleration time (DT, rapid decline of the E) indicate an abnormal relaxation. By considering these three parameters two more patterns of impaired diastolic function are known: the "pseudonormal" pattern which turns to an impaired relaxation pattern when a Valsalva maneuver is performed and the restrictive pattern. The last one, occurring mostly in patients with restrictive cardiomyopathies (e.g., infiltrative sarcoidosis, endomyocardial fibrosis) and dilated cardiomyopathies with poor systolic function which is associated with increased mortality [21]. Unfortunately, mitral flow is influenced not only by the diastolic properties of the LV but also by other factors, including preload, afterload, heart rate and the presence of arrhythmias. Another indicator, the pulmonary venous flow can be used to assess diastolic function but it is also limited in case of mitral valve disease, heart block and tachycardia. A more precise assessment of the diastolic function can be made by using the tissue Doppler imaging (TDI). This enables the measurement of frequency Doppler shifts caused by myocardial motion as the mitral annulus recoils back toward the base in early (e') and late (a') diastole. The peak waves (e′ and a′) are obtained in analogy to those recorded by the mitral flow. TDI enables, depending of the placement of the sample volume, assessment of global or regional diastolic function. In patients with hypertension and hypertrophy, diastolic dysfunction is more evident at the basal septal segments [22]. The E/e' ratio (with e' assessed at a lateral segment) has been identified as the best parameter for diagnosis of diastolic heart failure [23]. An E/e' ratio below 8 is associated with normal filling pressures and a ratio > 12 to 15 is associated with elevated filling pressures. For values between 8 and 12 additional echocardiographic parameters (e.g., use of Valsalva with transmitral Doppler, pulmonary venous flow) are recommended to correctly classify diastolic function. By using the Doppler color M-mode another index of diastolic dysfunction, the propagation velocity of early diastolic flow (Vp) into the ventricle has been proposed. This index seems to be independent of the load conditions and can be useful to unmask diastolic dysfunction in hypertensive patients with pseudonormal mitral flow. However, in patients with normal left ventricular function the Vp may be normal despite an impaired left ventricular relaxation indicating a major limitation of the index. Beside diastolic dysfunction, an enlarged left atrium was found in patients with hypertension and preserved ejection fraction and is associated with elevated filling pressures of the left ventricle leading to clinical heart failure [24].

As described earlier, echocardiography assesses two main features of the hypertensive heart disease, left ventricular hypertrophy and diastolic dysfunction. Systolic dysfunction occurring in the presence or not of the aforementioned changes is assessed in the clinical practice by echocardiography. Assessment of the ejection fraction can be made visually, it requires however a high level of expertise and is limited by subjectivity. Quantified, objective measurements of the LV systolic function have become standard practice in echocardiography. One parameters of the systolic function is fractional shortening obtained from M-Mode tracings in the parasternal long axis (method according to Teichmann). Though it is a simple and quick method, it is limited by the fact that it provides information about contractility along a single line. If regional wall motion abnormalities occur (e.g. in the presence of coronary artery disease) the severity of the dysfunction may be under - or overestimated, depending if the region of an abnormal wall motion is interrogated or not. As long as this method is only valid in symmetrically contracting hearts, it is inappropriate for the remodeled ventricles of patients with heart failure. The European and American guidelines recommended the biplane method of discs (modified Simpson's rule) as the echocardiographic method of choice for volume measurements and estimation of ejection fraction [25, 26]. The principle underlying this method is that the total LV volume is calculated from the summation of a stack of elliptical discs. The height of each disc is calculated as a fraction of the LV long axis based on the longer of the two lengths from the two and four-chamber views. The cross-sectional area of the disk is based on the two diameters obtained from the two- and four-chamber views. The method can also be used with one single plane, when two orthogonal views are not available. In this case, the presence of any extensive wall motion abnormalities may limit the results [25]. Practically, the endocardial borders in the apical 4- and 2-chamber views in end-diastole and end-systole are traced manually or automatically. The end-diastolic and end-systolic volumes (EDV, ESV) are calculated and the ejection fraction is estimated as follows: Ejection fraction = (EDV – ESV) / EDV. The reference values for the ejection fraction do not differ between men und women. An EF > 55% indicates a normal systolic function. An EF between 45-54% suggests a mildly abnormal function and an EF between 30-44% a moderately abnormal systolic function. A severely abnormal left ventricular function is indicated by an EF < 30%. This 2-D approach to assess EF is based on geometric assumptions, which are invalid in a nonsymmetrical contracting, remodeled ventricle. Over the last decade, several three-dimensional (3-D) echocardiographic techniques became available to measure LV volumes and mass. 3-D echocardiography does not rely on geometric assumptions for volume/mass calculations and is not subject to plane positioning errors, which can lead to chamber foreshortening. Compared to the gold-standard for assessment of left ventricular volumes and EF, the cardiac magnetic resonance, 3-D echocardiography showed significantly better agreement (smaller bias), lower scatter and lower intra- and inter-observer variability than 2-D echocardiography [27, 28]. Furthermore, 3-D echocardiography is also used in the assessment of diastolic function, as it is independent of load conditions.

In summary, echocardiography is a necessary diagnostic tool for risk stratification of patients with hypertension before treatment but also for follow-up assessment of end-organ damages during treatment. In 25-30% of hypertensive patients with low or moderate cardiovascular risk (based on risk factor evaluation and ECG), an increase of the LV mass may be identified by echocardiography leading to higher risk stratification and changes of therapeutic strategy [29, 30].

4. Doppler ultrasound of renal arteries

Renovascular hypertension is the second most common cause of secondary hypertension in approximately 2% of adult patients who present with blood pressure elevation when assessed in specialized centres [31]. This is caused by one or more stenoses of the extrarenal arteries, which in the elderly population have frequently an atherosclerotic nature. Fibromuscular dysplasia accounts for up to 25% of total cases and is the most common variety in young adults. Unfortunately there is not any optimal screening test available for the time. A screening test should have a high sensitivity in order to keep the false negative results in the lowest possible level. The Doppler ultrasound of renal arteries allows an analysis of the renal perfusion. According to various studies the sensitivity and specificity of Doppler ultrasound in the diagnosis of renal artery stenosis lies approximately at 90% [32, 33]. Due to the fact that renovascular hypertension in individuals with mild and medium hypertension has a prevalence below 1%, an unselective examination of all individuals with hypertension would lead to a high rate of false positive results. That would result to a high rate of unnecessary angiographies. On the other hand in a preselected population of hypertensives with clinical implications of increased probability of renal artery stenosis the Doppler ultrasound of the renal arteries is a very appropriate screening examination, due to the fact that the prevalence of renovascular hypertension in acute, severe and resistant hypertension is significantly higher (10-45%). In other words, the use of Doppler ultrasound as a diagnostic tool in a selected population, has a significantly higher positive predictive value with a still acceptable negative predictive value.

Clinical signs for a renovascular hypertension include the following:

- Hypertension in individuals younger than 30 years of age
- A unilateral small kidney or a difference in renal size more than 1.5cm
- Generalized atherosclerosis
- Abdominal bruit with lateralization,
- Resistant hypertension, defined as hypertension refractory to treatment with at least three antihypertensive drugs (including a diuretic agent)
- An elevation of the serum creatinine level > 30% under the treatment with an ACE inhibitor or an AT1-receptor antagonist

It should be mentioned, that a difference of more than 1.5 cm in length between the two kidneys, which is usually considered as being diagnostic for renal artery stenosis is only found in 60 – 70% of the patients with renovascular hypertension [34].

The examination itself can be limited by factors such as bowel gas, obesity, cooperation of the patient and from the fact that it is a highly operator dependent examination. The atherosclerotic induced renal artery stenosis is easily detectable, because it usually involves the ostium and the proximal 1/3 of the renal artery. On the other hand fibromuscular dysplasia involves the distal 2/3 of renal artery and their segmental branches and is thus difficult to depict. With

http://dx.doi.org/10.5772/56171

today's ultrasound technology it is possible to visualize approximately 88% of all main and accessory renal arteries [35]. In every renal artery angle corrected flow velocity measurements should be performed in at least 5 points. A velocity of 60-100cm/s is considered as normal, whereas a 70% stenosis leads to velocities of at least 180-200cm/s. Stenoses proximal to the ostium are easily obtainable with an epigastric transverse scan and distal stenoses or stenoses of segmental branches are better seen with a longitudinal flank scan (lateral position).

Additional intrarenal scanning permits the diagnosis of renal artery stenosis without direct imaging of the main renal artery. In 1994, Schwerk *et al.* introduced the Resistive Index (RI) obtained in the interlobar arteries as a reliable indirect parameter for detecting renal artery stenosis. The RI is a ratio of peak systolic and end diastolic velocity, derived from the Doppler spectrum of any vessel. The authors calculated the side-to-side difference of intrarenal RI > 5% with the lower RI in the post-stenotic kidney. Sensitivity and specificity were 100% and 94%, respectively, for moderate and severe RAS [36]. In the meantime, intrarenal RI has been frequently evaluated for different nephrological issues [37, 38]. In a single prospective study a high intrarenal RI was found to be negatively correlated with the outcome of intervention in patients with atherosclerotic renal artery stenosis [39]. A high RI (RI ≥ 80) was felt to reflect advanced renal damage, which would explain the interventional treatment failure. Radermacher et al. [39] investigated the efficacy of angioplasty of a renal artery stenosis in dependence of the RI. They concluded that an increased renal resistance index > 0.8 is associated with a poor prognosis despite correction of the stenosis. To date, the clinical impacts of these findings are discussed controversially.

5. Ultrasound of carotid arteries

The carotid wall thickening is an early marker of atherosclerosis and subclinical organ damage. It precedes the evolution of arteriosclerotic plaques. Ultrasound of the carotid arteries constitutes a very good opportunity to evaluate hypertension-induced vascular end organ damage. Several cardiovascular risk factors including male sex, ageing, elevated blood pressure, diabetes, smoking and obesity are positively associated with increased carotid intima-media thickness (IMT) in observational and epidemiological studies. Above these factors, high systolic blood pressures have the greatest effect on IMT [40]. An IMT > 0.9 mm in the common carotid artery is generally seen as abnormal; however there is a continuous relationship between IMT and cardiovascular events. An intima-media thickness (IMT) > 0.9 mm or the presence of a carotid plaque predict the occurrence of stroke and myocardial infarction [2, 41]. Particularly, in a meta-analysis of data from 8 studies in general populations, including about 37,000 subjects who were followed up for a mean of 5.5 years, the risk for a myocardial infarction increases by 10-15% and the stroke risk by 13-18% for every 0.1 mm increase of the IMT [42]. For the assessment of CVD risk, the carotid artery wall, rather than the degree of luminal narrowing, is examined to identify areas of increased thickness and non-occlusive atherosclerotic plaque, which represent early stages of arterial injury and atherosclerosis. Furthermore, the detection of early signs of vascular damage has to include ultrasound not only of the common carotid arteries, but of bifurcations and/or internal carotids where atherosclerosis progresses more rapidly and plaques are more frequent [43]. Ultrasound imaging of the far wall of the carotid artery produces two echogenic lines, which correspond to the lumen-intima interface and the media-adventitia interface. The current ultrasound technology enables in the clinical practice the combined measurement of the thickness of the intimal and medial layers of the arterial wall which constitute the IMT. Carotid plaque is defined as the presence of focal wall thickening that is at least 50% greater than that of the surrounding vessel wall or as a focal region with IMT greater than 1.5 mm that protrudes into the lumen. Both near and far walls can be used for assessment of the IMT. However, IMT of the near wall is less accurate because the ultrasound beam is traveling from more to less echogenic layers at the adventitia-media and intima-lumen interfaces of the near wall [44]. Histological data suggest an underestimation of the IMT around 20% when the near wall is used [45]. A linear-array transducer operating at a frequency of at least 7 MHz [44]. Three methods most frequently used to measure the IMT by using B –Mode are the following: 1. Averaging the maximum IMT of the four far walls of the carotid bifurcations and of the distal common carotid arteries. 2. Assessing the mean maximum thickness (M max) of up to 12 different sites (right and left, near and far walls, distal common, bifurcation, and proximal internal carotid). 3. The maximum measured IMT of a single measurement is taken into account. The last method provides more reproducible results when IMT measurement is restricted to the far wall of the distal segment of the common carotid artery, providing only a 3% of relative difference between two successive measurements [46]. Analysis may be performed by manual cursor placement or by automated computerized edge detection. As we mentioned above, B-mode imaging is preferred over M-mode imaging. M-mode, in spite of a superior temporal resolution, provides measurement of one single point of thickness, rather than a segmental value as it is enabled by B-mode. However, carotid wall thickening is not uniform and a singe point measurement may not represent accurately the arterial status and is less reproducible for follow-up measurements. A novel noninvasive echo-tracking system measuring the IMT and other mechanical properties of the carotid wall has been proposed [47]. This method enables an additional evaluation of the carotid plaque stability and composition.

The normal IMT values are influenced by age and sex and IMT normal values may be defined in terms of statistical distribution within a healthy population. IMT values greater than the 75th percentile are considered high and indicate an increased cardiovascular risk. Values in the 25th to 75th percentile are considered average and indicative of unchanged CVD risk. Values less than or equal to 25th percentile are associated with a low CVD risk [44]. However, available data indicate that IMT > 0.9 mm represents a risk of myocardial infarction and/or cerebrovascular disease and in the clinical practice this cut-off value may better defined in terms of increased risk [48]. Recent data have further strengthened the relationship of carotid IMT and plaques with cardiovascular events. A new report from the European Lacidipine Study on Atherosclerosis (ELSA) trial suggests that baseline carotid IMT predicts cardiovascular events independent of blood pressure and this occurs both for the IMT value at the carotid bifurcations and for the IMT value at the level of the common carotid artery [49]. The adverse prognostic significance of carotid plaques has also been reported in patients with high normal blood pressure prospectively followed for about 13 years [50]. In the Risk Intervention Study (RIS) study patients with severe essential hypertension and high cardiovascular risk had a significantly higher prevalence of atherosclerotic lesions compared to control subjects [51]. Assessment of IMT plays an important role in the risk stratification. Interestingly, about 30% of hypertensive subjects classified as at low or moderate added risk without ultrasound for carotid artery thickening or plaque were placed in the high added risk group after detecting of vascular damages [29].

The predictive value of the carotid ultrasound and its role in risk stratification has been demonstrated in a lot of trials as aforementioned. Whether a decrease of IMT progression is associated with a reduction of cardiovascular events and an improvement in prognosis remains at the time elusive. Therapeutic double blind trials have shown that antihypertensive drugs may have a more or less marked effect on carotid IMT progression. A recent meta-analysis of 22 randomized controlled trials has evaluated the effects of an antihypertensive drug versus placebo or another antihypertensive agent of a different class on carotid intima-media thickness. The results have shown that compared with no treatment, diuretics/± beta-blockers, ACE inhibitors and calcium antagonists attenuate the rate of progression of carotid intima-media thickening, in some trials even in the absence of any significant reduction of the blood pressure [52]. In patients with hypertension and hypercholesterolemia the administration of pravastatin prevents the progression of carotid intima-media thickness [53]. In the ELSA trial the treatment-induced changes of the IMT did not predict cardiovascular events as was the case by the baseline values. However, these results are not conclusive due to the smallness of the IMT changes and the large individual differences in baseline IMT [49].

Beyond the identification of subclinical organ damage of the carotid arteries, ultrasound is a useful tool for identification of carotid stenoses in progressive atherosclerosis. High blood pressure is a major risk factor for stroke with a correlation between elevated BP and occurrence of stroke. This correlation holds over a wide BP range, from systolic levels as low as 115 mm/Hg and diastolic levels as low as 70 mm/Hg [54], with systolic BP having a stronger association with higher stroke risk. Elevated BP is positively associated with both ischemic and hemorrhagic stroke, with a higher association appearing in hemorrhagic stroke and secondary prevention [56]. Large vessel disease of the extracranial arteries accounts for half of the ischemic strokes.

Doppler sonography is the most common imaging study performed for the diagnosis of carotid disease. It is part of the imaging tests taking place early after a transient ischemic attack (TIA) or stroke in order to identify patients with tight symptomatic arterial stenosis who could benefit from endarterectomy or angioplasty. Carotid Doppler-studies are fast, non-invasive and easily applicable however provide limited information, require skilled operators and are investigator-dependent. Doppler ultrasound has a similar specificity and sensitivity for carotid artery stenosis with computed tomography angiography (CTA) but both are inferior to contrast-magnetic resonance angiography (MRA) [57]. For asymptomatic patients with hypertension, assessment for carotid artery stenosis is also useful as part of risk stratification and is recommended for patients with two or more risk factors for atherosclerosis. Evidence of an internal carotid artery stenosis (ICA) supports recommendation of antiplatelet therapy and more strict control of risk factors to prevent stroke [58].

The first step of a carotid ultrasound test is to identify plaques via B-mode as referred above. Addition of color Doppler enables identification of origin and course of the internal carotid artery and a differentiation between severe stenosis and occlusion. Stenotic areas are identified in the presence of the "aliasing" phenomenon occurring due to high velocities in the center of the stenotic lumen and post-stenotic flow disturbances. Flow velocities in the spectral analysis are the main parameters used for evaluating the severity of carotid stenosis. Flow velocity must be sampled through the whole area of presumed stenosis until the distal end of the plaque is seen to ensure that the site of the highest velocity has been detected. Compared to angiographic data, a wide range of flow velocities was recorded for any given degree of angiographic stenosis so that the sensitivity and specificity of the method may vary [59]. A better correlation to angiographic determined stenoses is achieved by assessing the peak systolic velocity in the internal carotid artery and the ratio of the peak systolic velocity in the internal carotid artery to that in the ipsilateral common carotid artery as proposed by the current guidelines [60]. Based on Doppler sonography, carotid stenoses are classified into two grades: Grade 1- with the rate of stenosis measuring between 50% to 69% and Grade 2 measuring 70-99%, which also represents a severe non-occlusive disease. In equivocal cases, further imaging methods may be additionally used. In Table 1 the sonographic criteria for grading of carotid artery stenosis are summarized.

An ultrasound examination for detection of carotid stenoses and plaques and evaluation of the intima-media thickness should be performed in hypertensive patients with concomitant risk factors such as smoking, dyslipidemia, diabetes, obesity and family history of cardiovascular disease. The results can be useful for re-assessing CVD risk in some asymptomatic patients and consequently re-assessing therapeutic strategies. For accurate results, strict attention to quality control in image acquisition, measurement and interpretation are necessary.

Grade of Stenosis	Peak systolic velocity and visible criteria
no stenosis	< 125 cm/s and no visible plaque or IMT
< 50%	< 125cm/s with visible plaque or IMT
50-69%	125 – 230 cm/s with visible plaque
> 70% to near occlusion	> 230cm/s with visible plaque and lumen narrowing
100%	No detectable patent lumen and flow is seen

Table 1. Grading of internal carotid artery stenosis upon Doppler velocities and B-mode

6. Flow mediated dilation

Endothelial function is linked to cardiovascular risk factors and provides prognostic information for cardiovascular diseases [61]. Endothelial dysfunction is regarded as the initial step of atherosclerosis and therefore as the earliest detectable manifestation of vascular end-organ damage. It can be assessed using several methods, with flow-mediated dilation (FMD) being currently the gold-standard in non-invasive evaluation of endothelial dysfunction. In this ultrasound-based method brachial artery diameter is measured before and after an increase in shear stress that is induced by reactive hyperemia. When a sphygmomanometer cuff placed on the forearm or upper-arm and is inflated at 50 mm/Hg above systolic pressure, arterial inflow is occluded causing a local ischemia and dilation of downstream arteries. Cuff deflation induces a high-flow state through the brachial artery (reactive hyperemia) to accommodate the dilated resistance vessels. The increased shear stress leads to endothelium dependent dilation of the brachial artery. FMD occurs predominantly as a result of local endothelial release of nitric oxide. Figure 1 shows the B-mode and Doppler flow images of the brachial artery of a patient with hypertension at baseline and after deflation of the cuff (hyperemia). The FMD was calculated by the equation: FMD = (diameter hyperemia – diameter baseline) * 100 / diameter baseline. A value of 8.1% suggesting a near normal value (>8%) was found.

By using invasive and non-invasive methods impaired endothelial function has been found in uncomplicated hypertensive patients [62, 63]. In one prospective trial a reduction of blood pressure in response to antihypertensive treatment leads to improvement of the FMD suggesting a beneficial effect of antihypertensive treatment on endothelial function [64]. Several other large trials have found relationships between endothelial dysfunction assessed by FMD and prognostic markers of cardiovascular disease and atherosclerosis [65, 66]. Although the FMD test has opened a new field in the clinical research of conduit artery endothelial biology, some practical challenges of this technique have prevented its broad use in daily clinical practice so far. The most important of these are the need for highly trained operators, the time-consuming analysis of results and the care required to minimize environmental or physiological influences such as eating, caffeine ingestion and variations of temperature [67].

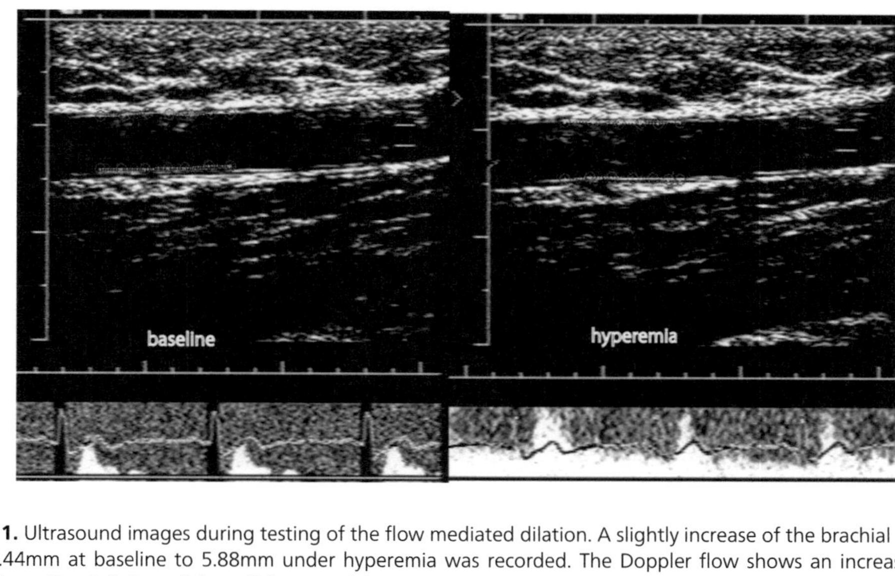

Figure 1. Ultrasound images during testing of the flow mediated dilation. A slightly increase of the brachial diameter from 5.44mm at baseline to 5.88mm under hyperemia was recorded. The Doppler flow shows an increase of the blood flow after deflation of the cuff (hyperemia).

7. Conclusions

In summary, sonography is essential in the workup of a hypertensive patient. Abdominal sonography should be performed in the evaluation of hypertension. The last European guidelines have emphasized that treatment-induced changes of organ damage affect the incidence of cardiovascular events, thereby recommending performance of organ damage examinations including sonography during treatment. When a search for secondary hypertension is indicated, abdominal sonography and Doppler ultrasound of the renal arteries are also recommended. Table 2 summarizes the use of ultrasound in the evaluation of hypertension.

Ultrasound examination	Use in diagnostic workup of hypertension
Abdominal ultrasound	Identification of subclinical and end-organ damage (recommended) • Aortosclerosis • Aortic aneurysm • Nephrosclerosis Screening for secondary causes of hypertension • Renal parenchymal disease • Renal vascular disease • Adrenal adenomas • Phaeochromocytoma
Echocardiography	Identification of subclinical and end organ damage (recommended) • Left ventricular hypertrophy (LVH) • Systolic and diastolic dysfunction • Left atrium dimension and geomertry
Doppler ultrasound of the renal arteries	Screening for secondary causes of hypertension • Renovascular hypertension
Ultrasound of the carotid arteries	Identification of subclinical and end-organ damage (recommended) • Intima – media thickness (IMT) • Carotid plaques • Carotid artery stenosis
Assessment of flow-mediated dilation of brachial artery	Identification of subclinical organ damage (not in clinical use) • Endothelial dysfunction

Table 2. Ultrasound examinations in hypertension

In summary, sonography is essential in the workup of a hypertensive patient. Abdominal sonography should be performed in every newly diagnosed case of hypertension. Performance of further ultrasound techniques depends on age, concomitant diseases, symptoms, and overall cardiovascular risk. Table 2 summarizes the use of ultrasound in the evaluation of hypertension.

Author details

Nikolaos Pagonas, Stergios Vlatsas and Timm H. Westhoff

*Address all correspondence to: timm.westhoff@charite.de

Charité – Campus Benjamin Franklin, Dept. of Nephrology, Berlin, Germany

References

[1] Campos C SJ, Rodicio JL. Campos C, Segura J, Rodicio JL.. Investigations in secondary hypertension: renal disease. Hypertension. 2001:119-26.

[2] Hodis HN, Mack WJ, LaBree L, Selzer RH, Liu CR, Liu CH et al. The role of carotid arterial intima-media thickness in predicting clinical coronary events. Ann Intern Med. 1998;128(4):262-9.

[3] Rezneck RH. AP. Imaging in endocrinology. The adrenal glands.. Clin Endocrinol (Oxf). 1994;40(5):561-76.

[4] Reisch N, Peczkowska M, Januszewicz A and Neumann HP. Pheochromocytoma: presentation, diagnosis and treatment. Journal of hypertension. 2006;24(12):2331-9.

[5] Burton S. RP. Adrenal Glands. Magnetic Resonanc Imaging. 1999.

[6] Goldstein RE ONJ, Jr., Holcomb GW. Clinical experience over 48 years with pheochromocytoma. Ann Surg. 1999;229(6):755-64.

[7] Schwerk WB, Gorg C, Gorg K and Restrepo IK. Adrenal pheochromocytomas: a broad spectrum of sonographic presentation. Journal of ultrasound in medicine: official journal of the American Institute of Ultrasound in Medicine. 1994;13(7):517-21.

[8] Lloyd-Jones DM, Larson MG, Leip EP, Beiser A, D'Agostino RB, Kannel WB et al. Lifetime risk for developing congestive heart failure: the Framingham Heart Study. Circulation. 2002;106(24):3068-72.

[9] Reichek N and Devereux RB. Left ventricular hypertrophy: relationship of anatomic, echocardiographic and electrocardiographic findings. Circulation. 1981;63(6):1391-8.

[10] Mancia G, De Backer G, Dominiczak A, Cifkova R, Fagard R, Germano G et al. [ESH/ESC 2007 Guidelines for the management of arterial hypertension]. Rev Esp Cardiol. 2007;60(9):968 e1-94.

[11] Devereux RB, Wachtell K, Gerdts E, Boman K, Nieminen MS, Papademetriou V et al. Prognostic significance of left ventricular mass change during treatment of hypertension. Jama. 2004;292(19):2350-6.

[12] Devereux RB, Alonso DR, Lutas EM, Gottlieb GJ, Campo E, Sachs I et al. Echocardiographic assessment of left ventricular hypertrophy: comparison to necropsy findings. Am J Cardiol. 1986;57(6):450-8.

[13] Muiesan ML, Salvetti M, Monteduro C, Bonzi B, Paini A, Viola S et al. Left ventricular concentric geometry during treatment adversely affects cardiovascular prognosis in hypertensive patients. Hypertension. 2004;43(4):731-8.

[14] Milani RV, Lavie CJ, Mehra MR, Ventura HO, Kurtz JD and Messerli FH. Left ventricular geometry and survival in patients with normal left ventricular ejection fraction. Am J Cardiol. 2006;97(7):959-63.

[15] Tsioufis C, Vezali E, Tsiachris D, Dimitriadis K, Taxiarchou E, Chatzis D et al. Left ventricular hypertrophy versus chronic kidney disease as predictors of cardiovascular events in hypertension: a Greek 6-year-follow-up study. J Hypertens. 2009;27(4): 744-52.

[16] Gerdts E, Wachtell K, Omvik P, Otterstad JE, Oikarinen L, Boman K et al. Left atrial size and risk of major cardiovascular events during antihypertensive treatment: losartan intervention for endpoint reduction in hypertension trial. Hypertension. 2007;49(2):311-6.

[17] Gerdts E, Cramariuc D, de Simone G, Wachtell K, Dahlof B and Devereux RB. Impact of left ventricular geometry on prognosis in hypertensive patients with left ventricular hypertrophy (the LIFE study). Eur J Echocardiogr. 2008;9(6):809-15.

[18] Aeschbacher BC, Hutter D, Fuhrer J, Weidmann P, Delacretaz E and Allemann Y. Diastolic dysfunction precedes myocardial hypertrophy in the development of hypertension. Am J Hypertens. 2001;14(2):106-13.

[19] Gotsman I, Zwas D, Lotan C and Keren A. Heart failure and preserved left ventricular function: long term clinical outcome. PLoS One. 2012;7(7):e41022.

[20] Paulus WJ, Tschope C, Sanderson JE, Rusconi C, Flachskampf FA, Rademakers FE et al. How to diagnose diastolic heart failure: a consensus statement on the diagnosis of heart failure with normal left ventricular ejection fraction by the Heart Failure and Echocardiography Associations of the European Society of Cardiology. Eur Heart J. 2007;28(20):2539-50.

[21] Moller JE, Sondergaard E, Poulsen SH and Egstrup K. Pseudonormal and restrictive filling patterns predict left ventricular dilation and cardiac death after a first myocardial infarction: a serial color M-mode Doppler echocardiographic study. J Am Coll Cardiol. 2000;36(6):1841-6.

[22] Galderisi M, Caso P, Severino S, Petrocelli A, De Simone L, Izzo A et al. Myocardial diastolic impairment caused by left ventricular hypertrophy involves basal septum more than other walls: analysis by pulsed Doppler tissue imaging. J Hypertens. 1999;17(5):685-93.

[23] Kasner M, Westermann D, Steendijk P, Gaub R, Wilkenshoff U, Weitmann K et al. Utility of Doppler echocardiography and tissue Doppler imaging in the estimation of diastolic function in heart failure with normal ejection fraction: a comparative Doppler-conductance catheterization study. Circulation. 2007;116(6):637-47.

[24] Melenovsky V, Borlaug BA, Rosen B, Hay I, Ferruci L, Morell CH et al. Cardiovascular features of heart failure with preserved ejection fraction versus nonfailing hypertensive left ventricular hypertrophy in the urban Baltimore community: the role of atrial remodeling/dysfunction. J Am Coll Cardiol. 2007;49(2):198-207.

[25] Lang RM, Bierig M, Devereux RB, Flachskampf FA, Foster E, Pellikka PA et al. Recommendations for chamber quantification. Eur J Echocardiogr. 2006;7(2):79-108.

[26] Lang RM, Bierig M, Devereux RB, Flachskampf FA, Foster E, Pellikka PA et al. Recommendations for chamber quantification: a report from the American Society of Echocardiography's Guidelines and Standards Committee and the Chamber Quantification Writing Group, developed in conjunction with the European Association of Echocardiography, a branch of the European Society of Cardiology. J Am Soc Echocardiogr. 2005;18(12):1440-63.

[27] Gopal AS, Schnellbaecher MJ, Shen Z, Boxt LM, Katz J and King DL. Freehand three-dimensional echocardiography for determination of left ventricular volume and mass in patients with abnormal ventricles: comparison with magnetic resonance imaging. J Am Soc Echocardiogr. 1997;10(8):853-61.

[28] Buck T, Hunold P, Wentz KU, Tkalec W, Nesser HJ and Erbel R. Tomographic three-dimensional echocardiographic determination of chamber size and systolic function in patients with left ventricular aneurysm: comparison to magnetic resonance imaging, cineventriculography, and two-dimensional echocardiography. Circulation. 1997;96(12):4286-97.

[29] Cuspidi C, Ambrosioni E, Mancia G, Pessina AC, Trimarco B and Zanchetti A. Role of echocardiography and carotid ultrasonography in stratifying risk in patients with essential hypertension: the Assessment of Prognostic Risk Observational Survey. J Hypertens. 2002;20(7):1307-14.

[30] Schillaci G, De Simone G, Reboldi G, Porcellati C, Devereux RB and Verdecchia P. Change in cardiovascular risk profile by echocardiography in low- or medium-risk hypertension. J Hypertens. 2002;20(8):1519-25.

[31] Elliott W. Secondary hypertension: renovascular hypertension. Hypertension: a Companion to Braunwald's Heart Disease. 2007:93-105.

[32] Radermacher J, Chavan A, Schaffer J, Stoess B, Vitzthum A, Kliem V et al. Detection of significant renal artery stenosis with color Doppler sonography: combining extrarenal and intrarenal approaches to minimize technical failure. Clinical nephrology. 2000;53(5):333-43.

[33] Simoni C, Balestra G, Bandini A and Rusticali F. [Doppler ultrasound in the diagnosis of renal artery stenosis in hypertensive patients: a prospective study]. Giornale italiano di cardiologia. 1991;21(3):249-55.

[34] Safian RD and Textor SC. Renal-artery stenosis. N Engl J Med. 2001;344(6):431-42.

[35] Radermacher J and Brunkhorst R. Diagnosis and treatment of renovascular stenosis--a cost-benefit analysis. Nephrology, dialysis, transplantation: official publication of the European Dialysis and Transplant Association - European Renal Association. 1998;13(11):2761-7.

[36] Schwerk WB, Restrepo IK, Stellwaag M, Klose KJ and Schade-Brittinger C. Renal artery stenosis: grading with image-directed Doppler US evaluation of renal resistive index. Radiology. 1994;190(3):785-90.

[37] Krumme B. Renal Doppler sonography--update in clinical nephrology. Nephron. Clinical practice. 2006;103(2):c24-8.

[38] Pearce JD, Edwards MS, Craven TE, English WP, Mondi MM, Reavis SW et al. Renal duplex parameters, blood pressure, and renal function in elderly people. American journal of kidney diseases: the official journal of the National Kidney Foundation. 2005;45(5):842-50.

[39] Radermacher J, Chavan A, Bleck J, Vitzthum A, Stoess B, Gebel MJ et al. Use of Doppler ultrasonography to predict the outcome of therapy for renal-artery stenosis. N Engl J Med. 2001;344(6):410-7.

[40] Zanchetti A, Bond MG, Hennig M, Neiss A, Mancia G, Dal Palu C et al. Calcium antagonist lacidipine slows down progression of asymptomatic carotid atherosclerosis: principal results of the European Lacidipine Study on Atherosclerosis (ELSA), a randomized, double-blind, long-term trial. Circulation. 2002;106(19):2422-7.

[41] Bots ML, Hoes AW, Koudstaal PJ, Hofman A and Grobbee DE. Common carotid intima-media thickness and risk of stroke and myocardial infarction: the Rotterdam Study. Circulation. 1997;96(5):1432-7.

[42] Lorenz MW, Markus HS, Bots ML, Rosvall M and Sitzer M. Prediction of clinical cardiovascular events with carotid intima-media thickness: a systematic review and meta-analysis. Circulation. 2007;115(4):459-67.

[43] Mansia G, De Backer G, Dominiczak A, Cifkova R, Fagard R, Germano G et al. 2007 ESH-ESC Guidelines for the management of arterial hypertension: the task force for the management of arterial hypertension of the European Society of Hypertension (ESH) and of the European Society of Cardiology (ESC). Blood Press. 2007;16(3): 135-232.

[44] Stein JH, Korcarz CE, Hurst RT, Lonn E, Kendall CB, Mohler ER et al. Use of carotid ultrasound to identify subclinical vascular disease and evaluate cardiovascular disease risk: a consensus statement from the American Society of Echocardiography

Carotid Intima-Media Thickness Task Force. Endorsed by the Society for Vascular Medicine. J Am Soc Echocardiogr. 2008;21(2):93-111; quiz 89-90.

[45] Wong M, Edelstein J, Wollman J and Bond MG. Ultrasonic-pathological comparison of the human arterial wall. Verification of intima-media thickness. Arterioscler Thromb. 1993;13(4):482-6.

[46] Touboul PJ, Hennerici MG, Meairs S, Adams H, Amarenco P, Bornstein N et al. Mannheim carotid intima-media thickness consensus (2004-2006). An update on behalf of the Advisory Board of the 3rd and 4th Watching the Risk Symposium, 13th and 15th European Stroke Conferences, Mannheim, Germany, 2004, and Brussels, Belgium, 2006. Cerebrovasc Dis. 2007;23(1):75-80.

[47] Paini A, Boutouyrie P, Calvet D, Zidi M, Agabiti-Rosei E and Laurent S. Multiaxial mechanical characteristics of carotid plaque: analysis by multiarray echotracking system. Stroke. 2007;38(1):117-23.

[48] EA Rosei MM. Assessment of preclinical target organ damage in hypertension: carotid intima-media thickness and plaque. European Society of Hypertension Schientific Newsletter. 2011pp. 19-20.

[49] Zanchetti A, Hennig M, Hollweck R, Bond G, Tang R, Cuspidi C et al. Baseline values but not treatment-induced changes in carotid intima-media thickness predict incident cardiovascular events in treated hypertensive patients: findings in the European Lacidipine Study on Atherosclerosis (ELSA). Circulation. 2009;120(12): 1084-90.

[50] Sehestedt T, Jeppesen J, Hansen TW, Rasmussen S, Wachtell K, Ibsen H et al. Which markers of subclinical organ damage to measure in individuals with high normal blood pressure? J Hypertens. 2009;27(6):1165-71.

[51] Salonen JT and Salonen R. Ultrasonographically assessed carotid morphology and the risk of coronary heart disease. Arterioscler Thromb. 1991;11(5):1245-9.

[52] Werner GS, Fritzenwanger M, Prochnau D, Schwarz G, Ferrari M, Aarnoudse W et al. Determinants of coronary steal in chronic total coronary occlusions donor artery, collateral, and microvascular resistance. J Am Coll Cardiol. 2006;48(1):51-8.

[53] Zanchetti A, Crepaldi G, Bond MG, Gallus G, Veglia F, Mancia G et al. Different effects of antihypertensive regimens based on fosinopril or hydrochlorothiazide with or without lipid lowering by pravastatin on progression of asymptomatic carotid atherosclerosis: principal results of PHYLLIS--a randomized double-blind trial. Stroke. 2004;35(12):2807-12.

[54] Chalmers J, Todd A, Chapman N, Beilin L, Davis S, Donnan G et al. International Society of Hypertension (ISH): statement on blood pressure lowering and stroke prevention. J Hypertens. 2003;21(4):651-63.

[55] Collins R, Peto R, MacMahon S, Hebert P, Fiebach NH, Eberlein KA et al. Blood pressure, stroke, and coronary heart disease. Part 2, Short-term reductions in blood pres-

sure: overview of randomised drug trials in their epidemiological context. Lancet. 1990;335(8693):827-38.

[56] Rodgers A, MacMahon S, Gamble G, Slattery J, Sandercock P and Warlow C. Blood pressure and risk of stroke in patients with cerebrovascular disease. The United Kingdom Transient Ischaemic Attack Collaborative Group. Bmj. 1996;313(7050):147.

[57] Wardlaw JM, Chappell FM, Best JJ, Wartolowska K and Berry E. Non-invasive imaging compared with intra-arterial angiography in the diagnosis of symptomatic carotid stenosis: a meta-analysis. Lancet. 2006;367(9521):1503-12.

[58] Guidelines for management of ischaemic stroke and transient ischaemic attack 2008. Cerebrovasc Dis. 2008;25(5):457-507.

[59] Grant EG, Duerinckx AJ, El Saden SM, Melany ML, Hathout GM, Zimmerman PT et al. Ability to use duplex US to quantify internal carotid arterial stenoses: fact or fiction? Radiology. 2000;214(1):247-52.

[60] Brott TG, Halperin JL, Abbara S, Bacharach JM, Barr JD, Bush RL et al. 2011 ASA/ACCF/AHA/AANN/AANS/ACR/ASNR/CNS/SAIP/SCAI/SIR/SNIS/SVM/SVS guideline on the management of patients with extracranial carotid and vertebral artery disease: executive summary. J Neurointerv Surg.3(2):100-30.

[61] Celermajer DS, Sorensen KE, Gooch VM, Spiegelhalter DJ, Miller OI, Sullivan ID et al. Non-invasive detection of endothelial dysfunction in children and adults at risk of atherosclerosis. Lancet. 1992;340(8828):1111-5.

[62] Iiyama K, Nagano M, Yo Y, Nagano N, Kamide K, Higaki J et al. Impaired endothelial function with essential hypertension assessed by ultrasonography. Am Heart J. 1996;132(4):779-82.

[63] Panza JA, Quyyumi AA, Brush JE, Jr. and Epstein SE. Abnormal endothelium-dependent vascular relaxation in patients with essential hypertension. N Engl J Med. 1990;323(1):22-7.

[64] Muiesan ML, Salvetti M, Monteduro C, Rizzoni D, Zulli R, Corbellini C et al. Effect of treatment on flow-dependent vasodilation of the brachial artery in essential hypertension. Hypertension. 1999;33(1 Pt 2):575-80.

[65] Kathiresan S, Gona P, Larson MG, Vita JA, Mitchell GF, Tofler GH et al. Cross-sectional relations of multiple biomarkers from distinct biological pathways to brachial artery endothelial function. Circulation. 2006;113(7):938-45.

[66] Juonala M, Viikari JS, Alfthan G, Marniemi J, Kahonen M, Taittonen L et al. Brachial artery flow-mediated dilation and asymmetrical dimethylarginine in the cardiovascular risk in young Finns study. Circulation. 2007;116(12):1367-73.

[67] Corretti MC, Anderson TJ, Benjamin EJ, Celermajer D, Charbonneau F, Creager MA et al. Guidelines for the ultrasound assessment of endothelial-dependent flow-medi-

ated vasodilation of the brachial artery: a report of the International Brachial Artery Reactivity Task Force. J Am Coll Cardiol. 2002;39(2):257-65.

Chapter 5

Ultrasound-Guided Peripheral Nerve Block Anesthesia with Emphasis on the Interscalene Approach to Brachial Plexus Blockade

James C. Krakowski and Steven L. Orebaugh

Additional information is available at the end of the chapter

http://dx.doi.org/10.5772/56645

1. Introduction

Epidemiologic data has revealed a progressive rise in the aggregate number of patient surgical visits with an increasing number occurring within the ambulatory setting [1]. Accompanying this rise has been a growing need for adequate, efficient patient anesthesia and analgesia [2]. With a significant proportion of procedures involving focal orthopedic interventions of the knee and shoulder, peripheral nerve blockade has become an increasing trend in anesthetic practice while neuraxial blockade use has decreased [2]. The popularity of peripheral nerve blockade may stem from its demonstrated effectiveness with studies showing improved analgesia and recovery during the postoperative period versus opioids [3] or general anesthetic [4]. In this chapter, we will review ultrasonography and its application to a commonly employed peripheral nerve block, namely, the interscalene block.

2. Ultrasound guidance for peripheral nerve blockade

2.1. A brief history

The first published account of ultrasound use with peripheral nerve blockade occurred in 1978 when Doppler sonography assisted blood flow detection during supraclavicular brachial plexus block [5]. Although the initial technology did not allow for direct nerve visualization, this was later rectified in 1994, when advancements in technology allowed the first documented use of ultrasound to visually facilitate supraclavicular brachial plexus block [5]. Since this time, ultrasound use for regional anesthesia has shown increasing popularity, and ultrasound technology has mirrored practitioner demand with machines possessing greater portability, simplicity, and image resolution [5]. Literature regarding the utility of ultrasound for a variety of peripheral nerve blocks continues to emerge.

2.2. Advantages

The rising popularity of ultrasound guidance for peripheral nerve blockade (PNB) stems from numerous described advantages supporting its use [6], [7], [5]. Perhaps the principal benefit of ultrasound resides in the technology's inherent ability to directly visualize peripheral nerves and tissue planes in real-time, allowing for optimal injectate or catheter placement with the ultimate goal of optimizing neural blockade [7]. Today's ultrasound machines are equipped with high-frequency probes capable of imaging the majority of nerves necessary for a wide array of regional blocks, and also their oblique course as they traverse the body [7]. This imaging modality permits the identification of relatively diminutive 2 mm diameter digital nerves [7], as well as differentiation of complex neurovascular nuances as found within the brachial plexus [8]. Additional benefit is conveyed in the ability to reposition one's needle in assessing for adequate local anesthetic spread, fascial plane movement, or lack thereof with intravascular injection [7]. The idea of preemptively scanning patient anatomy for neurovascular variations or abnormalities has been suggested as a means of improving patient safety by preventing block complication [9].

A number of objective evaluations have supported the efficacy of ultrasound guidance during PNB. When compared with performance via peripheral nerve stimulation (PNS), PNB executed using ultrasound guidance has been shown to require less time to perform, possesses more rapid onset and longer duration of anesthesia, and is more likely to be successful (less block failure) [6]. The use of ultrasound rather than PNS has also been shown to decrease the risk of vascular puncture [6], [10], and demonstrate improved quality of sensory block [11]. The use of ultrasonography does not exclude the use of PNS for PNB, and the combination for brachial plexus block was shown to have decreased risk of central nervous system toxicity secondary to local anesthetic versus a PNS-landmark technique [12]. Another study demonstrated high rates of success with axillary brachial plexus block using sonography regardless of concurrent PNS use [13]. Compared with PNS for femoral nerve block, ultrasound guidance also provides a reduction in the minimum effective anesthetic volume (MEAV50) [14], and has allowed reduced dosing for many blocks, with a potential impact on local anesthetic systemic toxicity and therefore patient safety [15]. Lastly, given the steady rise in yearly surgical procedures [1], findings such as decreased time to perform PNB [6], [7] and recent demonstration of cost-effectiveness in clinical practice [5] will likely support the role of ultrasound guidance in regional anesthesia's future.

2.3. Disadvantages

Despite many reported advantages to ultrasound guidance during PNB, several barriers to implementation and training have been described. One such limitation arises from peripheral nerve anatomical variation leading to difficulty in regional pattern recognition [16]. Difficulty to trainees may arise from the necessary knowledge of cross-sectional anatomy, terminology, appropriate local anesthetic spread, as well as an understanding of novel probe operating mechanics and regular needle tip visualization [7], [17], [18]. As a result, images may appear ambiguous to the novice operator [19], and identifying the intricate neurovascular anatomy of a common PNB structure as the brachial plexus may prove formidable [20]. Inexperience leading to inability to recognize common on-screen artifacts stemming from image processing may also skew interpretation [21]. In contrast to a definitive motor response end-point elicited with nerve stimulator, the optimal pattern of local anesthetic deposition and distribution continues to be investigated [22], [18].

Ultrasonography may also prove challenging as a result of current technological limitations. For example, discriminating neuronal tissue and its epineurium from that of connective tissue or tendons may prove difficult due to the similar hyperechoicity, or echotexture [7], [20]. Furthermore, ultrasound imaging has been shown to underrepresent the total number of neuronal fascicles as compared to light microscopy, and the possibility of intraneural injection (a topic of controversy with respect to morbidity) exists [23], [20].

3. The interscalene brachial plexus block

3.1. Block description

Upper extremity peripheral nerve blocks account for the majority of performed regional anesthesia techniques in most anesthesia practices [24]. Of the upper extremity PNBs, the interscalene block (ISB) is the most commonly applied block for patients undergoing shoulder surgery [25], [26], [8], imparting both anesthesia and analgesia with adequate coverage of the shoulder, lateral arm, and lateral forearm [27]. The ISB was first described in 1970 by Winnie, who noted based on anatomic and radiographic imaging that the interscalene space allowed for a novel, percutaneous approach to anesthetizing the proximal brachial plexus [28]. This approach allowed for brachial plexus anesthesia of similar quality to that of thoracic epidural anesthesia [28]. Compared to the previously described axillary and subclavian approaches prior to this time, the ISB was quickly favored for its ease of execution due to readily palpable landmarks in patients with large body habitus, no requirement for unique upper extremity positioning, and ability to readily repeat the block during protracted surgical procedures [28]. Both single-shot and continuous catheter placement have been successfully performed with ISB via landmark-paresthesia, nerve stimulator, or ultrasound-guided technique [8].

3.2. Anatomy

With the exception of the supraclavicular nerves, the brachial plexus is responsible for all motor and sensory innervation to the shoulder area [8]. The brachial plexus is an intricate neuronal network originating as ventral rami from cervical nerve roots, C5-8, and initial thoracic nerve root, T1 [24]. Together, these roots within the neck further subdivide into trunks, divisions, cords, and, ultimately, peripheral branches traveling distally into the upper arm [29]. After exiting the vertebral column, the roots become trunks as they traverse through the apposition of the anterior and middle scalene muscles, or interscalene groove [24]. Beyond the distal first rib, the trunks divide into divisions. At the distal clavicle and latter portion of the axillary artery, the divisions combine to form cords, which further subdivide into terminal branches at the level of the humerus [24].

Winnie described three anatomical spaces comprising the fascial sheath-enveloped area, cradling the neurovasculature of the brachial plexus along its course from the proximal, cervical vertebral bodies distally toward the axilla [28]. These regions included the axillary, subclavian, and interscalene spaces [28]. The interscalene space describes the contiguous area enveloped posteriorly by the fascial sheath covering of the middle scalene muscle and anteriorly by that of the anterior scalene fascia [28]. The interscalene space was noted to be continuous with both the axillary and subclavian spaces, thereby allowing appropriate peripheral nerve blockade introduction at this site [28].

In order to provide effective analgesia for shoulder surgery, one must anesthetize the nerves supplying all of the muscle, ligamentous, and osseous tissues of the shoulder joint and surrounding area [8]. Properly performed interscalene blockade provides anesthesia to the superior and middle trunks of the brachial plexus with C5-7 coverage, while also blocking the supraclavicular nerves arising from C3-4 [26]. The C3-4 blockade of the superficial cervical plexus is both fortunate and necessary as this innervation lies outside of the brachial plexus while supplying cutaneous sensation to the rostral shoulder [24].

3.3. Indications

Since its initial description, the interscalene block has been met with widespread acceptance, demonstrating effective [30], [31], [26], [8] and reliable perioperative analgesia for shoulder surgery [27], [26]. The interscalene block is suitable for a wide array of surgical procedures involving the shoulder with coverage including the shoulder joint, proximal humerus, as well as distal clavicle [8].

ISB offers several advantages afforded by regional anesthesia [8]. ISB may be used as an adjuvant to general anesthesia or as solitary anesthetic technique for shoulder surgery [8]. As a primary anesthetic, ISB may thereby reduce the risk of adverse events associated with general anesthesia, including time to ambulation secondary to impaired motor function, postoperative nausea and vomiting, and prolonged length of stay [4]. ISB also allows for a reduction in opioid analgesics and their consequential ill-effects [27], [8]. Additionally, ISB may prove more cost-effective as solitary anesthetic when compared to general anesthesia [8].

Although ISB has proved well-suited for shoulder surgery, it lacks coverage of C8 and T1 distribution, and so it has not been routinely used for surgeries involving the hand or elbow without supplying additional peripheral nerve block technique [30].

3.4. Landmark and nerve stimulator techniques

Prior to the advent of ultrasound imaging guidance, the primary methods for performing brachial plexus blockade included landmark and peripheral nerve stimulator (PNS) techniques [32], [33]. Both methods of nerve localization involve non-visualization of internal structures, and instead rely on either paresthesias or muscle twitch responses for landmark and PNS, respectively [32]. Originally described by Winnie in 1970, the ISB landmark technique entails localizing the interscalene groove lateral to the cricoid cartilage at approximate C6 level, needle advancement until elicitation of paresthesias along the shoulder and upper arm distribution, and completion with deposition of local anesthetic [28].

After its introduction in performing regional anesthesia, PNS later overcame landmark/ paresthesia technique as the method of choice for performing ISB [6], [34]. A common method for performing PNS guidance involves applying a current, ranging from 0.2 to 0.5 mA, at a frequency of 2 Hz while observing for muscle twitch with needle advancement [35]. Specifically, a contraction of the biceps or triceps may be appreciated, corresponding to cervical nerve stimulation at levels C5-6 and C6-8, respectively, at which point local anesthetic is deposited [35]. Of note, PNS may hold limited effectiveness in diabetic patients complicated by neuropathy, as motor response may not be elicited despite application of a standard stimulus [36]. Despite a theoretical advantage in determining needle tip proximity to neuronal tissue with greater precision using PNS as compared to paresthesia elicitation, both techniques have shown similar efficacy for peripheral nerve blockade [24]. In addition, ultrasound studies have revealed that the 0.2 to 0.5 mA range of current has limitations in predicting the accuracy of needle tip placement [37].

3.5. Ultrasonography for interscalene block

In contrast to prior methods of nerve localization, ultrasound guidance provides visualization of the block needle, neurovascular structures and their anatomical course, and the spread of local anesthetic injectate in real-time [38], [7], [5], [24], [39], [8]. Ultrasound guidance has been implemented both with and without concomitant nerve stimulator for the performance of regional anesthesia [10], although no added benefit has been proven with the addition of PNS [24], [40].

Typical sonoanatomy seen while performing the interscalene block has been described. Application of an ultrasound probe in the vicinity of interscalene groove allows for direct visualization of the C5-7 nerve roots exiting their corresponding intervertebral foramina and subsequently passing between the anterior and middle scalene muscles [20]. One may reliably differentiate the seventh cervical nerve root, as the C7 transverse process possesses no anterior tubercle [24]. Elements of the brachial plexus appear characteristically as a cluster of hypoechoic, or comparably dark, bodies on ultrasound imaging, while surrounding fascial layers appear hyperechoic, or comparably white [20]. Of note, numerous variations of the brachial plexus have been characterized, and these subtle deviations may be appreciated with ultrasonography [24].

Reliable brachial plexus blockade via ISB and ultrasonography has been described using a consistent method [38], [41] (Table 1). Patients undergoing ISB should have routine monitoring and supplemental oxygen in place prior to beginning the PNB, with low dose anxiolytic premedication administered when appropriate. Head positioning away from the intended block site may facilitate probe placement (Figure 1). Antiseptic technique including cleansing solution, drape, transducer dressing, gel, and standard practitioner barriers should be implemented. In order to assist avoidance of initial vascular trauma or injection, the subclavian artery is first visualized in cross-sectional view within the supraclavicular region. Color Doppler mode may assist in identifying additional vasculature surrounding the plexus [9]; [42]. Translation of the transducer probe medially reveals the characteristic hypoechoic cluster of brachial plexus fascicles located between the anterior and middle scalene muscle bellies [38] (Figure 2).

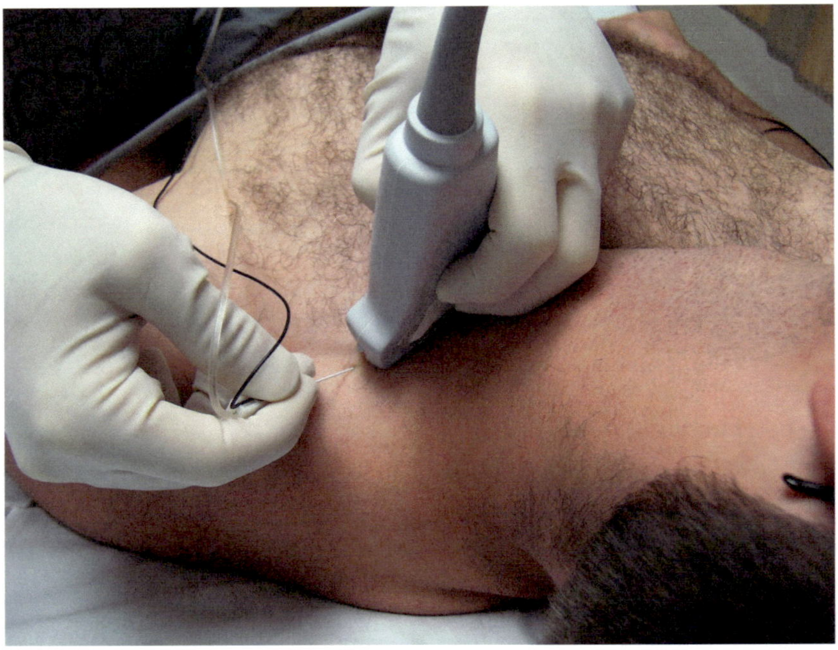

Figure 1. Typical ultrasound probe placement on a patient's neck while performing the interscalene block. Note positioning of the patient's head to the contralateral side of the intended nerve block may facilitate ultrasound probe placement and visualization of brachial plexus anatomy.

Subcutaneous local anesthetic is often administered for patient comfort prior to block needle insertion. Optimally, the entire length of block needle is maintained on-screen during advancement, with particular emphasis on visualizing its tip [7] (Figure 3).

Direct needle tip visualization in relation to neuronal structures allows for repositioning prior to injection while also permitting monitoring of live local anesthetic spread within the interscalene groove [30] (Figure 4). The desired volume of local anesthetic is deposited in 5 cc or less increments following aspiration with each injection [15].

The block needle may be equipped with a PNS for further confirmation of appropriate plexus proximity before deposition of local anesthetic [38]. For example, stimulating with settings of 0.7 to 0.8 mA for 0.1 ms at 2 Hz while approaching the plexus allows for monitoring of desired motor twitch response, which includes contraction of the ipsilateral pectoralis, deltoid, biceps, and triceps muscle groups. These responses indicate adequate proximity to the brachial plexus

http://dx.doi.org/10.5772/56645

1. Apply routine patient monitors and supplemental oxygen
2. Adjust patient bed to comfortable height for block placement
3. Position ultrasound machine with screen readily visible and probe accessible to practitioner
4. Position patient head away from intended block site to facilitate block placement (Figure 1)
5. Provide anxiolytic and/or sedative premedication as necessary
6. Verify patient monitors and vital signs
7. Choose ultrasound probe[1]
8. Prepare ultrasound probe in sterile fashion
9. Prepare patient's skin with antiseptic solution
10. Verify block needle is of appropriate type[2] and primed with selected local anesthetic[3]
11. Verify patient and procedure
12. Verify probe anatomical orientation on patient matches orientation displayed on ultrasound screen
13. Adjust ultrasound machine depth and gain parameters to enhance displayed image
14. Identify subclavian artery at the supraclavicular area
15. Identify brachial plexus lateral/dorsal to subclavian artery
16. Scan with probe to interscalene groove in order to identify optimal local anesthetic injection site (consider ultrasound Doppler function to scan for vessels at chosen injection site)
17. Warn patient of local anesthetic skin infiltration and provide skin wheel
18. Warn patient of needle insertion and insert block needle
19. Visualize block needle tip prior to advancing to desired position within interscalene groove
20. Instruct assistant to provide negative-pressure syringe aspiration to rule out intravascular needle placement
21. Warn patient of possible discomfort and instruct assistant to inject local anesthetic in small (3 – 5 ml) increments (aspirate prior to injecting each aliquot)
22. Assess local anesthetic spread on ultrasound screen for adequacy and reposition block needle if necessary
23. Remove block needle and clean patient's skin at site of insertion
24. Follow-up block adequacy via patient physical exam assessment

[1]Typical ultrasound probe selection for the performance of interscalene block includes a straight, linear array probe due to its higher operating frequencies (5 - 13 MHz), providing increased resolution at the expense of decreased penetration. This probe type facilitates superficial imaging optimal for visualizing the brachial plexus.

[2]Typical block needle selection may include a 22 gauge, beveled needle 5 cm or greater in length. Greater length may allow for superior ultrasound needle visualization due to its ability to provide a less acute angle of approach and thus increased right-angle ultrasound beam reflection.

[3]Local anesthetic choice is typically dependent on desired anesthetic duration. For example, 10 – 12 h of shoulder anesthesia may be elicited when 20 cc of ropivicaine 0.75% is administered via ultrasound-guided interscalene blockade.

Table 1. Routine clinical procedure in performance of the single shot, ultrasound-guided interscalene block

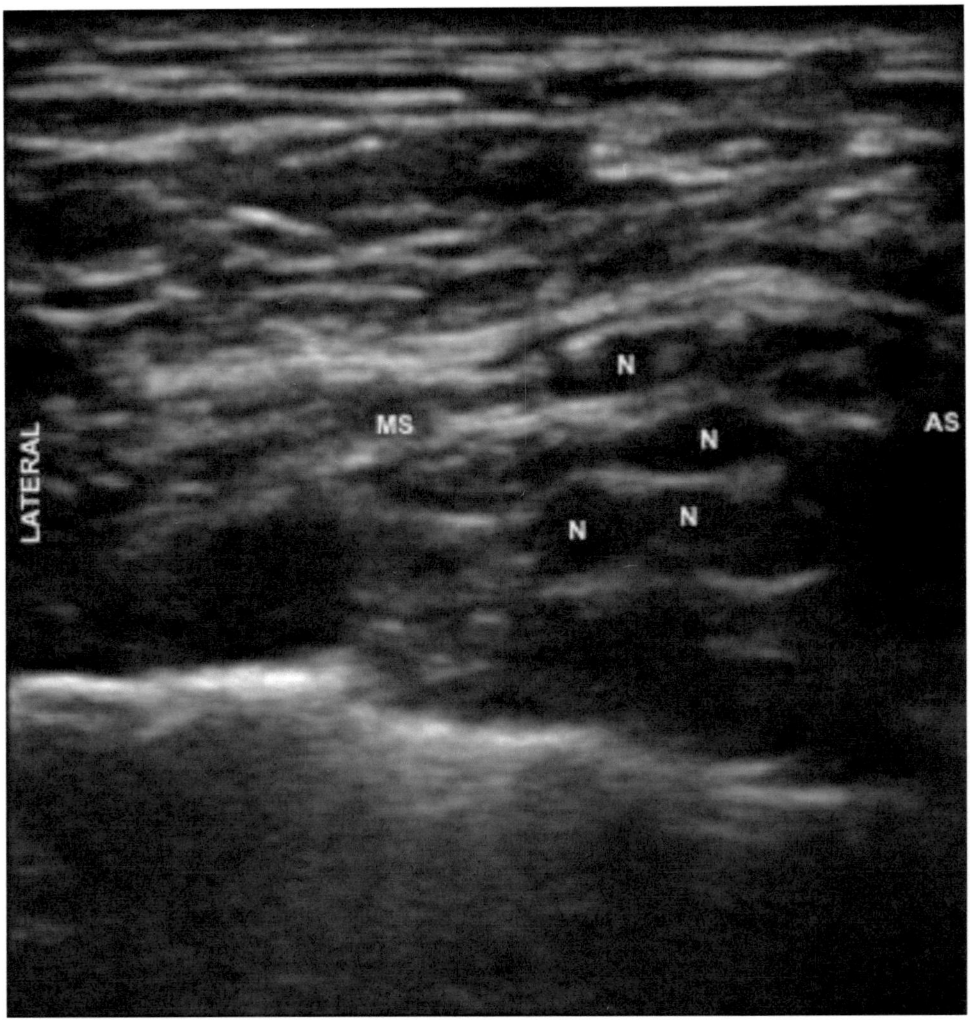

Figure 2. Ultrasound view of the interscalene region demonstrating hypoechoic nerve cross sections of the brachial plexus (N), lying between the middle scalene (MS) and anterior scalene (AS) muscle bellies.

prior to local anesthetic delivery, if consistent with appropriate deposition of local anesthetic solution in the interscalene groove as visualized with real-time ultrasound imaging [41].

Physical examination is used to evaluate for brachial plexus block success. Just as Winnie noted maximal anesthetic effect within 15 min of landmark ISB technique [28], physical examination to assess for appropriate motor and sensory block after ultrasound-guided ISB should be conducted after this timeframe. Examination may include the patient's ability to abduct the arm, assessing deltoid function; flex at the elbow, assessing biceps function; as well as discrimination of pain by prick and temperature by alcohol swab of the shoulder and arm surfaces, or C4 and C5, respectively [38], [30], [41].

http://dx.doi.org/10.5772/56645

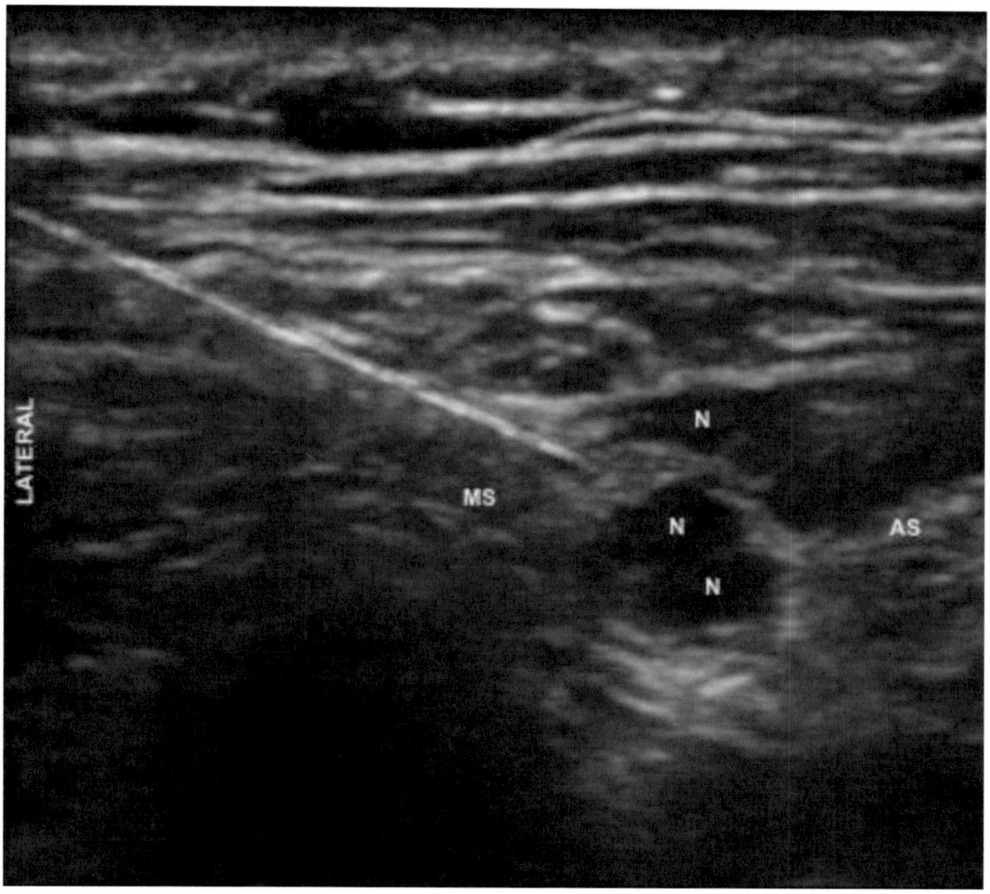

Figure 3. Ultrasound view demonstrating typical lateral approach of a peripheral nerve block needle within the interscale groove. N: nerve cross sections of the brachial plexus; MS: middle scalene muscle belly; AS: anterior scalene muscle belly.

3.6. Efficacy of ultrasound guidance for interscalene block

The successful implementation of ultrasonography for interscalene block has been well-documented with a variety of studies citing its efficacy [6]. Regarding imaging sensitivity, Muhly et al compared ultrasound imaging with cadaveric dissections of ISB anatomy and found that ultrasound was successfully able to detect vasculature branching as well as its course closely bordering nerves of the brachial plexus [42]. Due to individual variation in the neurovasculature surrounding the brachial plexus, one may appreciate the utility of directly visualizing such discrepancies from typical anatomy that might otherwise remain undetected using prior forms of PNB guidance [42].

Several studies have examined the effect of ultrasound with respect to quality of ISB anesthesia. Kapral et al compared performance of ISB using ultrasound versus peripheral nerve stimulation in a randomized trial, finding a significantly greater motor, sensory, and extent of brachial

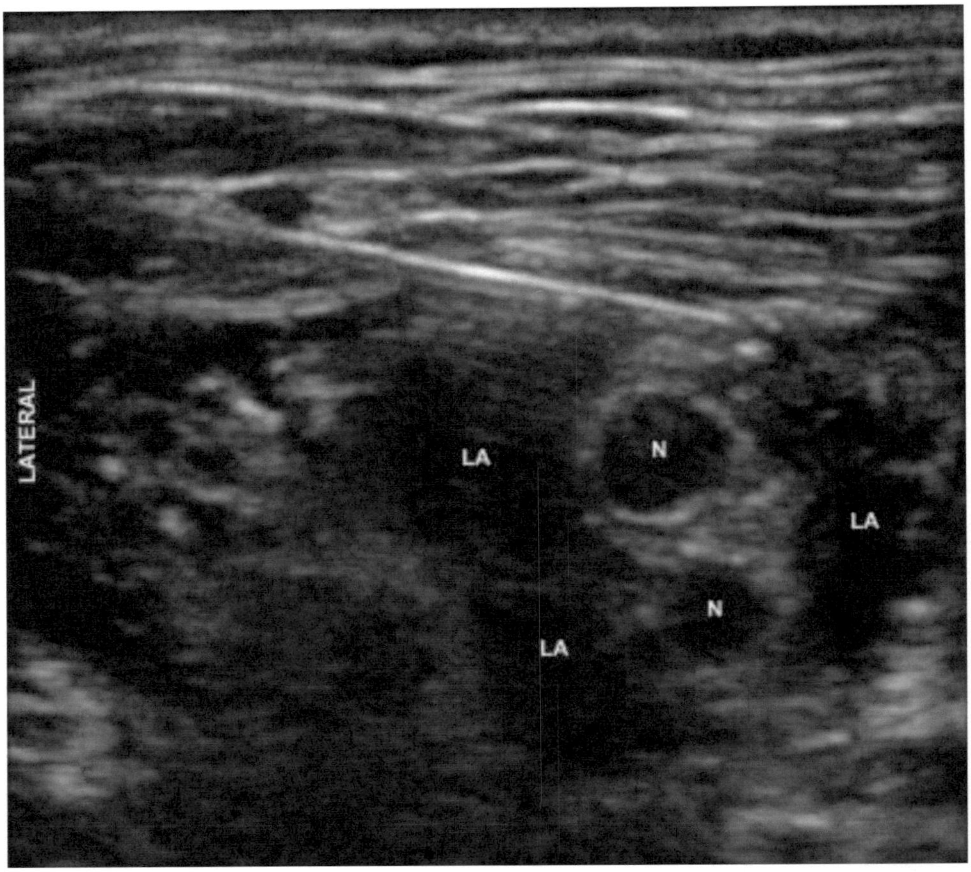

Figure 4. Ultrasound view of areas of local anesthetic (LA) volume deposition surrounding the brachial plexus at the level of the interscalene groove. Note the circumferential enhancement of the brachial plexus nerves (N) after local anesthetic deposition. The peripheral block needle is seen here as a hyperechoic linear structure positioned above the brachial plexus.

plexus blockade while using ultrasound [30]. Similarly, a randomized study by Liu et al, examining ultrasound versus nerve stimulator for ISB in randomized patients, revealed increased motor blockade assessed after five minutes as well as a decreased number of needle attempts for the ultrasound group [25]. McNaught et al also noted decreased needle attempts using ultrasound for ISB, while showing a significant decrease in the minimum effective analgesic volume (MEAV) of local anesthetic, and decreased pain 30 min postoperatively when compared to a nerve stimulator group [27]. When examining ultrasound placement versus nerve stimulator placement of ISB catheters in randomized patients, Fredrickson et al demonstrated greater effectiveness in the ultrasound group, requiring less local anesthetic boluses and tramadol use in addition to fewer needle attempts [43]. Additionally, examination of ISB performance among supervised resident trainees at a large academic center has shown a significant decrease in needle attempts, time required for block completion, and incidence of needle perforation of vasculature [44].

3.7. Revelations with ultrasound and interscalene block

Unexpected findings have been revealed when utilizing ultrasound guidance for interscalene block since the technique's initial application. One such revelation includes the cervical level of block performance. Plante et al carried out a study comparing ultrasound-guided ISB performed at the C5 versus C6 anatomical level in randomized patients undergoing shoulder surgery [39]. This study revealed ISB performed at both levels possessing similar efficacy, however the C6 level resulted in significantly greater block success of the distal brachial plexus, including the ulnar, radial, and medial nerves [39].

Needle proximity and neuronal tissue microanatomy with regard to ISB have also been examined. Spence et al sought to determine the ideal location of local anesthetic deposition for ISB [18]. When comparing needle tip and injection superficial to the brachial plexus sheath versus penetration deep to this plexus covering in randomized patients, both positions showed comparable times to block onset, yet the deeper injection resulted in longer mean block duration [18]. In examining ultrasound-guided needle tip placement relative to the nerve roots of the brachial plexus epineurium in the interscalene groove, using india ink staining in a cadaveric study, it was demonstrated that subepineural injection occurred more often than anticipated despite ultrasound guidance [45].

Although the middle scalene muscle itself was largely thought devoid of neuronal structures, the continued use of ultrasound guidance in performance of the interscalene block has indeed proven useful in both identifying and localizing brachial plexus nerves within this area. In conducting an observational study in 50 adult patients receiving ultrasound-guided, posterior approach interscalene block prior to shoulder surgery, Hanson and Auyong identified the dorsal scapular nerve and/or long thoracic nerve in 90% of these patients (verified with peripheral nerve stimulator twitch monitoring). These nerves were found to occur at a depth approximating the C6 nerve root level and less than 1 cm posterior to the larger brachial plexus with the dorsal scapular nerve identified more commonly than the long thoracic nerve (77% versus 23%, respectively) [46]

Local anesthetic volume and concentration necessary for successful ISB have also been studied. Riazi et al compared the use of 5 ml versus 20 ml ropivicaine 0.5% with ultrasound-guided ISB for randomized patients receiving shoulder surgery [26]. The lower volume group was shown to provide equivalent analgesia to the 20 ml group while resulting in a significant decrease in respiratory complications, including diaphragmatic or phrenic nerve paralysis, declines in oxygen saturation, and reduced function on spirometry testing [26]. A later study by Renes et al examined the minimum effective volume (MEV) of ropivicaine 0.75% necessary to provide successful analgesia for elective shoulder surgery when deposited at the C7 level via ultrasonography [31]. This study revealed the MEV to be 2.9 ml and 3.6 ml for 50% and 95% of patients, respectively [31]. Fredrickson et al compared varying ISB bolus ropivicaine concentrations and volumes for preoperative PNB in randomized patients undergoing shoulder surgery and also receiving postoperative 0.2% ropivicaine infusions [47]. The larger volume, 30 ml of 0.5% ropivicaine demonstrated no significant increase in anesthesia duration as compared to 20 ml of ropivicaine 0.375% [47]. Of note, local anesthetic concentration was shown to be the principle determinant of motor blockade [47].

Goebel et al conducted a randomized trial examining the use of ultrasound-placed ISB catheters in managing postoperative pain for major shoulder surgery [48]. Patient controlled infusions of ropivicaine 0.2% resulted in less concomitant pain medication administration in the first 24 h postoperatively as compared to catheter infusions of normal saline [48].

3.8. Adverse effects with interscalene block

With the performance of interscalene block over the past four decades, notable adverse effects have been established. Perhaps most notable, phrenic nerve (C3-5) paralysis occurs in nearly all patients receiving ISB that may lead to significant decline respiratory function, particularly in patients with underlying pulmonary disease [26], [31]. One ultrasound study found the anatomical separation between the brachial plexus and phrenic nerve lateral to the cricoid cartilage to be as little as 2 mm [49]. Other undesirable effects of regional anesthesia at this site may include blockade of the recurrent laryngeal nerve causing hoarseness, stellate ganglion causing Horner's syndrome, and increased local anesthetic spread rarely causing elements of epidural or spinal quality anesthesia [27]. Inadvertent needle placement during ISB performance may lead to vasculature puncture and direct nerve injury, including reported cases of spinal cord injury [50]. As with other forms of regional anesthesia, systemic local anesthetic toxicity as well as block failure may occur [51]. Failure to anesthetize the distribution of the ulnar nerve is of particular propensity with ISB, as the lower trunk is often spared [24].

3.9. Impact of ultrasound on adverse effects

With the inclusion of ultrasound guidance for interscalene block, several studies have demonstrated an impact on previously reported adverse effects. Renes et al conducted a randomized trial in patients undergoing shoulder surgery, comparing general anesthesia combined with ISB performed with 10 ml ropivacaine deposited via ultrasound versus peripheral nerve stimulator technique [35]. The ultrasound group showed a significantly decreased incidence of diaphragmatic hemiparesis [35]. In addition, the use of ultrasound technique has allowed ISB studies that have revealed decreased incidence of phrenic nerve blockade and respiratory complications based on level of block performance (C7) and reduced volume of local anesthetic [27], [26]. Abrahams et al conducted a systematic review and meta-analysis of randomized trials for a variety of peripheral nerve blocks [6]. When comparing ultrasound guidance versus peripheral nerve stimulation, ultrasound guided blocks were shown to have significantly less risk of vascular puncture [6]. Despite direct visualization when using ultrasound-guidance for PNB, no significant difference in the incidence of neuronal injury or neurologic symptoms postoperatively has been shown [25], [24]. With regard to failure to anesthetize the brachial plexus inferior trunk with ISB, Kapral et al demonstrated improved ulnar nerve and median nerve blockade 30 min post-block when compared to PNS guidance [30].

http://dx.doi.org/10.5772/56645

Perhaps the most important impact of ultrasound guidance during performance of peripheral nerve blockade to date has been related to an increase in patient safety via a decrease in local anesthetic systemic toxicity (LAST). Over a hundred cases of severe toxicity have been described in the medical literature, including some that have resulted in fatality, though the incidence of actual cases are likely much more numerous [15]. Most such cases involve toxicity to the central nervous system, including loss of consciousness, agitation, or, most commonly, seizure. Fifty percent of reported cases showed some evidence of cardiovascular toxicity, for which resuscitation may prove quite challenging [15]. Several studies have recently been published which strongly support the idea that ultrasound imaging has reduced the incidence of serious LAST. Sites, et al, reported over 12,000 cases of ultrasound-guided nerve blocks, with only one case of LAST [52], which compares quite favorably to reports of this complication during the era of nerve stimulator guidance, with rates of 1/1000 to 1/3000. In another large database report from a single site summarizing experience at a single teaching institution, Orebaugh, et al, reported a significant reduction in LAST episodes over a six-year period as the practice transitioned from nerve stimulator to ultrasound guidance-there were no such complications in over 9000 cases in which ultrasound was utilized [53]. Finally, Barrington, et al, reported from a large, multicenter, international database on complications related to peripheral nerve blockade, that the risk of LAST was significantly lowered when ultrasound guidance was utilized (relative risk 0.25-0.31), compared to blocks guided by nerve stimulation alone [54]. These reports have allowed the regional anesthesiologist, using ultrasound guidance, to approach his/her patients with greater certainty, confidence and safety.

4. Conclusions

Peripheral nerve blockade has become an ever-increasing tool in providing analgesia for patients undergoing focal surgical interventions. Advancements in ultrasound guidance for performance of these peripheral nerve blocks have allowed a parallel increase in this technology's utilization. The interscalene approach to brachial plexus blockade is a commonly employed peripheral nerve block that has demonstrated effectiveness in providing perioperative analgesia for patients undergoing shoulder surgery. The use of ultrasound guidance in performing the interscalene block has been shown to be effective in providing postoperative analgesia while decreasing specific respiratory side-effects [26], [27], [35], vascular puncture [6], and local anesthetic toxicity [53] as compared to non-ultrasongraphic, blind techniques. These benefits likely stem from the direct visualization of anatomical structures afforded by ultrasound implementation during block performance. Ultrasound guidance for peripheral nerve blockade remains an exciting advancement in caring for patients during the perioperative period, and this technology will likely continue to become commonplace with an increasing patient population and demonstrated effectiveness.

Author details

James C. Krakowski and Steven L. Orebaugh

Department of Anesthesiology, University of Pittsburgh Medical Center, Pittsburgh, Pennsylvania, USA

References

[1] Cullen KA, Hall MJ, Golosinskiy A. Ambulatory surgery in the United States, 2006. Natl Health Stat Report 2009 Jan 28;(11)(11):1-25.

[2] Memtsoudis SG, Kuo C, Ma Y, Edwards A, Mazumdar M, Liguori G. Changes in anesthesia-related factors in ambulatory knee and shoulder surgery: United States 1996-2006. Reg Anesth Pain Med 2011 Jul-Aug;36(4):327-331.

[3] Hadzic A, Arliss J, Kerimoglu B, Karaca PE, Yufa M, Claudio RE, et al. A comparison of infraclavicular nerve block versus general anesthesia for hand and wrist day-case surgeries. Anesthesiology 2004 Jul;101(1):127-132.

[4] Hadzic A, Williams BA, Karaca PE, Hobeika P, Unis G, Dermksian J, et al. For outpatient rotator cuff surgery, nerve block anesthesia provides superior same-day recovery over general anesthesia. Anesthesiology 2005 May;102(5):1001-1007.

[5] Marhofer P, Harrop-Griffiths W, Kettner SC, Kirchmair L. Fifteen years of ultrasound guidance in regional anaesthesia: part 1. Br J Anaesth 2010 May;104(5):538-547.

[6] Abrahams MS, Aziz MF, Fu RF, Horn JL. Ultrasound guidance compared with electrical neurostimulation for peripheral nerve block: a systematic review and meta-analysis of randomized controlled trials. Br J Anaesth 2009 Mar;102(3):408-417.

[7] Gray AT. Ultrasound-guided regional anesthesia: current state of the art. Anesthesiology 2006 Feb;104(2):368-73, discussion 5A.

[8] Sripada R, Bowens C,Jr. Regional anesthesia procedures for shoulder and upper arm surgery upper extremity update--2005 to present. Int Anesthesiol Clin 2012 Winter; 50(1):26-47.

[9] Manickam BP, Perlas A, Chan VW, Brull R. The role of a preprocedure systematic sonographic survey in ultrasound-guided regional anesthesia. Reg Anesth Pain Med 2008 Nov-Dec;33(6):566-570.

[10] Barrington MJ, Watts SA, Gledhill SR, Thomas RD, Said SA, Snyder GL, et al. Preliminary results of the Australasian Regional Anaesthesia Collaboration: a prospective audit of more than 7000 peripheral nerve and plexus blocks for neurologic and other complications. Reg Anesth Pain Med 2009 Nov-Dec;34(6):534-541.

[11] Marhofer P, Schrogendorfer K, Koinig H, Kapral S, Weinstabl C, Mayer N. Ultrasonographic guidance improves sensory block and onset time of three-in-one blocks. Anesth Analg 1997 Oct;85(4):854-857.

[12] Orebaugh SL, Williams BA, Vallejo M, Kentor ML. Adverse outcomes associated with stimulator-based peripheral nerve blocks with versus without ultrasound visualization. Reg Anesth Pain Med 2009 May-Jun;34(3):251-255.

[13] Swenson JD, Bay N, Loose E, Bankhead B, Davis J, Beals TC, et al. Outpatient management of continuous peripheral nerve catheters placed using ultrasound guidance: an experience in 620 patients. Anesth Analg 2006 Dec;103(6):1436-1443.

[14] Casati A, Baciarello M, Di Cianni S, Danelli G, De Marco G, Leone S, et al. Effects of ultrasound guidance on the minimum effective anaesthetic volume required to block the femoral nerve. Br J Anaesth 2007 Jun;98(6):823-827.

[15] Neal JM, Bernards CM, Butterworth JF,4th, Di Gregorio G, Drasner K, Hejtmanek MR, et al. ASRA practice advisory on local anesthetic systemic toxicity. Reg Anesth Pain Med 2010 Mar-Apr;35(2):152-161.

[16] Orebaugh SL, Pennington S. Variant location of the musculocutaneous nerve during axillary nerve block. J Clin Anesth 2006 Nov;18(7):541-544.

[17] Sites BD, Spence BC, Gallagher JD, Wiley CW, Bertrand ML, Blike GT. Characterizing novice behavior associated with learning ultrasound-guided peripheral regional anesthesia. Reg Anesth Pain Med 2007 Mar-Apr;32(2):107-115.

[18] Spence BC, Beach ML, Gallagher JD, Sites BD. Ultrasound-guided interscalene blocks: understanding where to inject the local anaesthetic. Anaesthesia 2011 Jun;66(6): 509-514.

[19] Sites BD, Beach ML, Spence BC, Wiley CW, Shiffrin J, Hartman GS, et al. Ultrasound guidance improves the success rate of a perivascular axillary plexus block. Acta Anaesthesiol Scand 2006 Jul;50(6):678-684.

[20] Van Geffen GJ, Moayeri N, Bruhn J, Scheffer GJ, Chan VW, Groen GJ. Correlation between ultrasound imaging, cross-sectional anatomy, and histology of the brachial plexus: a review. Reg Anesth Pain Med 2009 Sep-Oct;34(5):490-497.

[21] Antonakakis JG, Sites B. The 5 most common ultrasound artifacts encountered during ultrasound-guided regional anesthesia. Int Anesthesiol Clin 2011 Fall;49(4):52-66.

[22] Brull R, Macfarlane AJ, Parrington SJ, Koshkin A, Chan VW. Is circumferential injection advantageous for ultrasound-guided popliteal sciatic nerve block?: A proof-of-concept study. Reg Anesth Pain Med 2011 May-Jun;36(3):266-270.

[23] Silvestri E, Martinoli C, Derchi LE, Bertolotto M, Chiaramondia M, Rosenberg I. Echotexture of peripheral nerves: correlation between US and histologic findings and criteria to differentiate tendons. Radiology 1995 Oct;197(1):291-296.

[24] Neal JM, Gerancher JC, Hebl JR, Ilfeld BM, McCartney CJ, Franco CD, et al. Upper extremity regional anesthesia: essentials of our current understanding, 2008. Reg Anesth Pain Med 2009 Mar-Apr;34(2):134-170.

[25] Liu SS, Zayas VM, Gordon MA, Beathe JC, Maalouf DB, Paroli L, et al. A prospective, randomized, controlled trial comparing ultrasound versus nerve stimulator guidance for interscalene block for ambulatory shoulder surgery for postoperative neurological symptoms. Anesth Analg 2009 Jul;109(1):265-271.

[26] Riazi S, Carmichael N, Awad I, Holtby RM, McCartney CJ. Effect of local anaesthetic volume (20 vs 5 ml) on the efficacy and respiratory consequences of ultrasound-guided interscalene brachial plexus block. Br J Anaesth 2008 Oct;101(4):549-556.

[27] McNaught A, Shastri U, Carmichael N, Awad IT, Columb M, Cheung J, et al. Ultrasound reduces the minimum effective local anaesthetic volume compared with peripheral nerve stimulation for interscalene block. Br J Anaesth 2011 Jan;106(1): 124-130.

[28] Winnie AP. Interscalene brachial plexus block. Anesth Analg 1970 May-Jun;49(3): 455-476.

[29] Yang WT, Chui PT, Metreweli C. Anatomy of the normal brachial plexus revealed by sonography and the role of sonographic guidance in anesthesia of the brachial plexus. AJR Am J Roentgenol 1998 Dec;171(6):1631-1636.

[30] Kapral S, Greher M, Huber G, Willschke H, Kettner S, Kdolsky R, et al. Ultrasonographic guidance improves the success rate of interscalene brachial plexus blockade. Reg Anesth Pain Med 2008 May-Jun;33(3):253-258.

[31] Renes SH, van Geffen GJ, Rettig HC, Gielen MJ, Scheffer GJ. Minimum effective volume of local anesthetic for shoulder analgesia by ultrasound-guided block at root C7 with assessment of pulmonary function. Reg Anesth Pain Med 2010 Nov-Dec;35(6):529-534.

[32] Chan VW, Perlas A, Rawson R, Odukoya O. Ultrasound-guided supraclavicular brachial plexus block. Anesth Analg 2003 Nov;97(5):1514-1517.

[33] Perlas A, Chan VW, Simons M. Brachial plexus examination and localization using ultrasound and electrical stimulation: a volunteer study. Anesthesiology 2003 Aug; 99(2):429-435.

[34] Tsui B, Hadzic A. Peripheral nerve stimulators and electrophysiology of nerve stimulation. In: Hadzic A, editor. Textbook of Regional Anesthesia and Acute Pain Management New York: McGraw-Hill; 2007. p. 93-104.

[35] Renes SH, Rettig HC, Gielen MJ, Wilder-Smith OH, van Geffen GJ. Ultrasound-guided low-dose interscalene brachial plexus block reduces the incidence of hemidiaphragmatic paresis. Reg Anesth Pain Med 2009 Sep-Oct;34(5):498-502.

[36] Byrne K, Tsui BC. Practical concepts in nerve stimulation: impedance and other recent advances. Int Anesthesiol Clin 2011 Fall;49(4):81-90.

[37] Bigeleisen PE, Moayeri N, Groen GJ. Extraneural versus intraneural stimulation thresholds during ultrasound-guided supraclavicular block. Anesthesiology 2009 Jun; 110(6):1235-1243.

[38] Chan VW. Applying ultrasound imaging to interscalene brachial plexus block. Reg Anesth Pain Med 2003 Jul-Aug;28(4):340-343.

[39] Plante T, Rontes O, Bloc S, Delbos A. Spread of local anesthetic during an ultrasound-guided interscalene block: does the injection site influence diffusion? Acta Anaesthesiol Scand 2011 Jul;55(6):664-669.

[40] Sites BD, Beach ML, Chinn CD, Redborg KE, Gallagher JD. A comparison of sensory and motor loss after a femoral nerve block conducted with ultrasound versus ultrasound and nerve stimulation. Reg Anesth Pain Med 2009 Sep-Oct;34(5):508-513.

[41] Orebaugh SL, Williams BA, Kentor ML, Bolland MA, Mosier SK, Nowak TP. Interscalene block using ultrasound guidance: impact of experience on resident performance. Acta Anaesthesiol Scand 2009 Nov;53(10):1268-1274.

[42] Muhly WT, Orebaugh SL. Sonoanatomy of the vasculature at the supraclavicular and interscalene regions relevant for brachial plexus block. Acta Anaesthesiol Scand 2011 Nov;55(10):1247-1253.

[43] Fredrickson MJ, Ball CM, Dalgleish AJ. A prospective randomized comparison of ultrasound guidance versus neurostimulation for interscalene catheter placement. Reg Anesth Pain Med 2009 Nov-Dec;34(6):590-594.

[44] Orebaugh SL, Williams BA, Kentor ML. Ultrasound guidance with nerve stimulation reduces the time necessary for resident peripheral nerve blockade. Reg Anesth Pain Med 2007 Sep-Oct;32(5):448-454.

[45] Orebaugh SL, McFadden K, Skorupan H, Bigeleisen PE. Subepineurial injection in ultrasound-guided interscalene needle tip placement. Reg Anesth Pain Med 2010 Sep-Oct;35(5):450-454.

[46] Hanson NA, Auyong DB. Systematic ultrasound identification of the dorsal scapular and long thoracic nerves during interscalene block. Reg Anesth Pain Med. 2013 Jan-Feb;38(1):54-7.

[47] Fredrickson MJ, Smith KR, Wong AC. Importance of volume and concentration for ropivacaine interscalene block in preventing recovery room pain and minimizing motor block after shoulder surgery. Anesthesiology 2010 Jun;112(6):1374-1381.

[48] Goebel S, Stehle J, Schwemmer U, Reppenhagen S, Rath B, Gohlke F. Interscalene brachial plexus block for open-shoulder surgery: a randomized, double-blind, placebo-controlled trial between single-shot anesthesia and patient-controlled catheter system. Arch Orthop Trauma Surg 2010 Apr;130(4):533-540.

[49] Kessler J, Schafhalter-Zoppoth I, Gray AT. An ultrasound study of the phrenic nerve in the posterior cervical triangle: implications for the interscalene brachial plexus block. Reg Anesth Pain Med 2008 Nov-Dec;33(6):545-550.

[50] Benumof JL. Permanent loss of cervical spinal cord function associated with interscalene block performed under general anesthesia. Anesthesiology 2000 Dec;93(6): 1541-1544.

[51] Neal JM, Brull R, Chan VW, Grant SA, Horn JL, Liu SS, et al. The ASRA evidence-based medicine assessment of ultrasound-guided regional anesthesia and pain medicine: Executive summary. Reg Anesth Pain Med 2010 Mar-Apr;35(2 Suppl):S1-9.

[52] Sites BD, Taenzer AH, Herrick MD, Gilloon C, Antonakakis J, Richins J, et al. Incidence of local anesthetic systemic toxicity and postoperative neurologic symptoms associated with 12,668 ultrasound-guided nerve blocks: An analysis from a prospective clinical registry. Reg Anesth Pain Med. 2012 Sep-Oct;37(5):478-82.

[53] Orebaugh SL, Kentor ML, Williams BA. Adverse Outcomes Associated with Nerve Stimulator-Guided and Ultrasound-Guided Peripheral Nerve Blocks by Supervised Trainees: Update of a Single-Site Database. Reg Anesth Pain Med 2012 (in press).

[54] Barrington MJ, Kluger R. Use of ultrasound guidance for peripheral nerve blockade is associated with a reduced incidence of local anesthetic systemic toxicity [abstract]. American Society of Anesthesiologists Annual Meeting. October 16, 2012. BOC12.

Chapter 6

A New Functional Transcranial Doppler Spectroscopy (fTCDS) Study of Cerebral Asymmetry During Neuro-Cognitive Functions in Men and Women

Philip C. Njemanze

Additional information is available at the end of the chapter

http://dx.doi.org/10.5772/54877

1. Introduction

The perception of light underlies the processes of cognitive brain function. However, the characterizations of the neuroadaptational processes that relates to the physical quality of light, particularly those implicated in color processing remains largely unknown. Simultaneous color contrast and color constancy have been identified as the memory processes associated with color processing [1-8]. Simultaneous color contrast is the phenomenon that surrounding colors profoundly influence perceived color [1,9]. The mechanism implicated in simultaneous color contrast has been described as wavelength-differencing, implying the ability to differentiate the dominant wavelength of the color of light [10]. Wavelength-differencing involves wavelength-encoding main effect at subcortical peaks, and energy-encoding effects at cortical peaks [11]. On the other hand, frequency-differencing refers to the ability to differentiate the dominant frequency (the inverse of wavelength) of the color of light, and involves energy-encoding main effect at cortical and subcortical peaks [11, 12]. Genetic studies suggest gender-related differences in color vision in primates. Whereas both trichromatic and dichromatic color vision occurs among female monkeys, males appear exclusively dichromatic [13]. It was proposed that, unlike humans, squirrel monkeys have only a single photopigment locus on the X chromosome [13].

Color constancy relates to the invariance of hue, or perceived color of a surface under variation in the spectral content of illumination [3, 14, 15]. In other words, color constancy refers to the unchanging nature of the perceived color of an object despite considerable variation in the wavelength composition of the light illuminating it [16]. It has been suggested that there may exist a color space comprising chromatic axes (red-green and blue-yellow) and achromatic (black-white) luminance axis [8]. However, the non-invasive physiologic measurements at the neural substrates to characterize the 'color space' in humans has not been feasible until now [17]. The anatomy of the main neural substrates for color processing have been characterized within the visual pathways and extrastriate cortex 'color centres' [18], which lie within the distribution territories of the posterior cerebral arteries (PCAs) [19-21] and middle cerebral arteries (MCAs) [19, 21, 22]. The superior parietal aspects of the optic radiation receive blood mainly from the MCA, whereas the inferior aspects are supplied by the PCAs [23]. The macular cortical region receives blood supply, from both the calcarine artery (a branch of the internal occipital artery of the PCA distribution), and branches of the MCA, which explains macular sparing with PCA occlusion [19]. Therefore, it is possible to characterize the 'color space' in the primary visual cortex and extrastriate areas using measurements of changes in blood flow velocity in the MCAs during color stimulation [22]. In prior studies in our laboratory for microgravity simulations, we applied non-invasive transcranial Doppler measurement of mean flow velocity (MFV) in the MCAs, to examine changes in color space in men during head-down rest, and demonstrated neuroplasticity over 25 hours of recordings [11], or more, if testing was continued. These findings have been related to formation of the phenomena of long term potentiation (LTP) and long-term depression (LTD), implicating role for NMDA receptors [11]. The phenomena of LTP [24] and LTD [25], have been applied to explain potential mechanisms of memory, primarily because they exhibit numerous properties expected of a synaptic associative memory mechanism, such as rapid induction, synapse specificity, associative interactions, persistence, and dependence on correlated synaptic activity. Given these important features, LTP and LTD remains only models of the synaptic and cellular events that may underlie memory formation.

Recently, we demonstrated using functional transcranial Doppler spectroscopy (*f*TCDS) technique, that color processing occurred within cortico-subcortical circuits [11, 12]. It was demonstrated that in men, wavelength-differencing of Yellow/Blue pairs occurred within the right hemisphere by processes of cortical long-term depression (CLTD) and subcortical long-term potentiation (SLTP). On the other hand, in women, frequency-differencing of Blue/Yellow pairs occurred within the left hemisphere by processes of cortical long-term potentiation (CLTP) and subcortical long-term depression (SLTD) [11, 12]. In both genders, there was luminance effect in the left hemisphere, while in men it was along an axis orthogonal to chromatic effect, in women it was along a parallel axis [11, 12]. It therefore, may be possible to describe mechanisms for color memory formation using *f*TCD and *f*TCDS techniques. In the present study, it was hypothesized that, the brain functionally integrates within a three-dimensional physiologic 'color space', luminance effect in the left hemisphere with wavelength-differencing activity in the right hemisphere in men, but with frequency-differencing activity in the left hemisphere in women. This functional integration in color space could be mathematically modeled and could have potential applications in the study of color memory, adaptive neuroplasticity in stroke management and rehabilitation, as well as in neurodegenerative diseases. There has not been any in-depth characterization of the neurophysiological processes involved in wavelength-differencing. However, effort has been made to apply the new modality of *f*TCDS, based on wave propagation theory to identify the neural processes implicated in color processing. It was suggested that, simultaneous color contrast implicated

http://dx.doi.org/10.5772/54877

wavelength-differencing processes in men [11], while in women, the underlying process was characterized as frequency-differencing [12]. This is the first hint that, there may be a gender-related difference in color processing. This is a profound finding that may change our overall understanding of perceptive processes in men and women. It was therefore proposed that, the brain color processing mechanisms integrates within a three-dimensional 'color space', luminance effects in the left hemisphere, and wavelength-differencing effects in the right hemisphere in men, but frequency-differencing effects in the left hemisphere in women [17]. The latter finding led to the conclusion that, color processing followed the same rule of lateralization as other major cognitive functions, such as facial processing [26, 27] and general intelligence [30], which implicated the right hemisphere cognitive style in men, and left hemisphere cognitive style in women.

Furthermore, the functional integration in color space was mathematically modeled. It was shown that, the existence of wavelength-differencing in men and frequency-differencing in women, implemented inverse exponential and logarithmic functions, respectively. These gender-related differences that underlie cerebral asymmetry for color processing, has been hypothesized to be associated with the perception of the dual nature of light as a wave and as particulate energy referred to as quanta [11,12]. The presumed genetic and psychophysiologic effects of the physical qualities of light was the basis for the proposal of the light hypothesis of cerebral asymmetry [12]. The light hypothesis for cerebral asymmetry, posits that, the phenotypic neuroadaptation to environmental physical constraints of light as a wave and as quanta energy led to phenotypic evolution, and genetic variation of X-Y gene pairs that determine hemispheric asymmetry [12]. Hence, the evolutionary trend is towards optimization of perception of the 'whole' environment by functional coupling of the genes for complementarity of both hemispheres within self, and between both genders [12]. More specifically, the basic tenant of the Light Hypothesis for cerebral asymmetry posits that, the right hemisphere is implicated in wavelength-differencing in men and the left hemisphere, in frequency-differencing in women, with an overall gender complementarity in adaptive mechanisms for neuropsychophysiological processes. The latter has been characterized as gender-related cognitive styles designed for coupled perceptual experience of the world around us.

Overall, it has been documented that there is a gender-related difference in facial processing [26]. Facial perception occurred in the cortical region of the right hemisphere in men, but in the left in women. The results are similar to previous observations using transcranial Doppler [27], and agree with those made using electrophysiological techniques [28]. Similar gender-related hemisphere differences have been observed at the amygdale for emotionally related stimuli [29], and for performance-related processing [30-32]. Men showed a right lateralization during object processing, but women showed a right tendency or bilateral activation. The effect of perception of faces has to be examined beyond the use of colors.

One presumption about the effects of color would be that, if the neuronal assemblies processing light information shared analogous topological organization as their blood flow supply, then dark would elicit the least effect, followed by colors and other stimuli on increasing complexity. This type of summation of responses related to stimulus complexity could be presumed as evidence for topological organization of these cortical areas was observed in men [26]. It was demonstrated that, the latter extends from the area implicated in color and object perception to a much greater area involved in facial perception. This agrees with the object form topology hypothesis proposed by Ishai and colleagues [33]. However, the relatedness of object, color and facial perception was process based, and appears to be associated with their common holistic processing strategy in the right hemisphere in men. Moreover, when the same men were presented with disarranged facial Paradigm requiring analytic processing, the left hemisphere was activated. This agrees in principle with the suggestion made by Gauthier that, the extrastriate cortex contains areas that are best suited for different computations, and described as the process-map model [34]. It has been proposed that the models of cognitive processing of colors and faces are not mutually exclusive, and this underscores the fact that color and facial processing do not impose any new constraints on the brain other than those used for other stimuli [26]. It may be suggested that each stimulus was mapped by category into color, face or non-face, and by process into holistic or analytic. Therefore, a unified category-specific process-mapping system was implemented for either right or left cognitive styles [26].

Another profound gender-related difference was related to the responsiveness to the dark condition. Studies in the dark condition were included to measure the effects of non-spectral stimuli, since it is known that, some of these can actually result in the production of color experience [35]. It was observed that, there was a tendency towards right lateralization in women but no lateralization in men in dark condition. The latter finding was difficult to interpret, and similar to observations made in previous studies [20]. These observations led to the suggestion that, scotopic visual information was processed in the right hemisphere in women [20]. However, in women data from spectral density estimates showed accentuation for dark responsiveness at the cortical (C-peaks) over those of light conditions. The latter may be an indication that greater neuronal assemblies were involved in processing scotopic vision in women compared to men. Furthermore, it was proposed that, in women the neuronal assemblies may not have the same orderly topological arrangement as in men; rather the neurons involved in processing cone and rod vision were segregated within the right hemisphere cortical region. Hence, in women the right hemisphere responded to luminance effect and object perception, but showed no category-specific face effect or color processing [12, 17, 26]. The latter arrangement explains the observed right lateralization for non-face Paradigm, but left lateralization for facial Paradigms and colors. In other words, similar to men, women employed the holistic mechanism for processing object stimulus in the right hemisphere, but preferred the analytic mechanism for facial and color perception in the left hemisphere. Therefore, one major observed gender-related difference was that, while men employed a category-specific process-mapping system for facial and color perception in the right hemisphere, women used same in the left hemisphere.

Another gender-related difference that has been consistently observed is the higher MFV in women than men [12, 17, 22, 26, 27, 36]. It is noteworthy that, the side differences appear to be related to cognitive changes rather than anatomic differences [37]. To cancel the effects of these initial variations in MFV, laterality index calculations were used [26, 27, 30]. However, if women differed from men in dark responsiveness, then LI calculations relative to dark would be expected to produce differences due to initial variations. In contrast, this limitation is overcome with Fourier-derived spectral density estimates, which assessed the periodicity during each stimulus condition independently, and lacked the properties of the original MFV signals. The absolute differences in MFV values would not affect the periodicity of the time series hence the Fourier transform would be equally sensitive for both men and women.

The rationale for *f*TCDS has been discussed in detail elsewhere [26]. It has been demonstrated that, when measuring at the main stem of the middle cerebral artery (MCA) the origins of the peaks arise from a peripheral circulation reflection site such as the tip of the fingers, the terminal end of the lenticulostriate subcortical branches of the MCA and the terminal of the cortical branches of the MCA. The peaks designated as **F**- (fundamental or finger), **C**- (cortical), and **S**-(subcortical) peaks occurred at regular frequency intervals of 0.125, 0.25, and 0.375, respectively. These frequencies could be converted to cycles per second (Hz), assuming that the fundamental frequency of cardiac oscillation was the mean heart rate. The fundamental frequency *f* of the first harmonic was determined by the mean heart rate per second of for example, 74 bpm/60 seconds or 1.23 Hz. In other words, the **F**-, **C**-, and **S**-peaks occurred at multiples of the first harmonic, at second and third harmonics, respectively. The distance of the reflection site for **F**-peak could be presumed to emanate from a site at:

$$D_1 1/4\lambda \text{ or } c/4\,f, \text{ or } 6.15\left(ms^{-1}\right)/(4*1.23\text{ Hz}) = 125\text{ cm} \tag{1}$$

where *c* is the assumed wave propagation velocity of the peripheral arterial tree [38]. Considering that there is vascular tortuosity, the estimated distance approximates that from the measurement site in the MCA main stem, to an imaginary site of summed reflections from the aorto-iliac junction [38] and the upper extremities, close to the finger tips when stretched sideways [26]. The **C**-peak occurred at the second harmonic, such that the estimated arterial length (using common carotid $c = 5.5\ ms^{-1}$) [39] was given by:

$$D_2 = 1/8\lambda \text{ or } c/8 *2f, \text{ or } 28\text{ cm; and a frequency } f_2 \text{ of } 2.46\text{ Hz} \tag{2}$$

This length approximates the visible arterial length from the main stem of the MCA, through vascular tortuosity and around the cerebral convexity, to the end vessels at distal cortical sites such as the occipito-temporal junction on carotid angiograms of adults [26]. The **S**-peak occurred at the third harmonic, and may have arisen from an estimated site at:

$$D_3 = 1/16\,\lambda \text{ or } c/16*3f, \text{ or } 9.3\text{ cm; and a frequency } f_3 \text{ of } 3.69\text{ Hz} \tag{3}$$

The latter is about the approximate visible arterial length of the lenticulostriate vessels from the main stem of the MCA on carotid angiograms [40]. Although it is not shown, the fourth harmonic would be expected to arise from the MCA bifurcation in closest proximity to the measurement site in the main stem of the MCA. The pre-bifurcation length from the measurement point would be given by:

$$D_4 = 1/32\ \lambda \text{ or } c/32{*}4f, \text{ or } 3.5 \text{ cm; and a frequency } f_4 \text{ of } 4.92 \text{ Hz} \quad (4)$$

The calculated length approximates that of the segment of MCA main stem just after the carotid bifurcation, where probably the ultrasound sample volume was placed, to the MCA bifurcation or trifurcation, as the case may be. Thus, the latter estimates may approximate actual lengths. However, it has been suggested that the estimated distances may not correlate exactly with known morphometric dimensions of the arterial tree [41]. The *f*TCDS examines spectral density estimates of periodic processes induced during mental tasks, and hence offers a much more comprehensive picture of changes related to effects of a given mental stimulus. The spectral density estimates would be least affected by artifacts that lack periodicity, and filtering would reduce the effect of noise. Despite the outlined advantages of *f*TCDS, there are potential problems with the present studies which are conducted with relatively small sample size, which may create greater influence of outliers. However, statistical analysis did not reveal any extreme outliers in the present data set and exclusion of outliers did not alter the lateralization patterns. The choice of eight men and eight women for each of the two data sets for analysis, with a total of 48 points in each data set was ideal for Fourier analysis.

2. Methodological procedures

2.1. Subjects

The study included 64 (32 men and 32 women) healthy subjects, divided in four groups of comprising each 8 men of mean ± SD age of 24.6 ± 2 years, and 8 women of mean ± SD age of 24 ± 2 years, all were right handed on hand preference questionnaire [42]. All subjects had normal sight and color vision, according to testing of visual acuity by Snellen chart, color vision by Ishihara pseudoisochromatic plates and color recognition [43]. Complete physical and mental examination revealed no abnormalities and routine evaluation of the cardiovascular, neurologic and respiratory systems were unremarkable. All were placed on the usual restrictions for cognitive studies [44]. All subjects gave written informed consent according to the Declaration of Helsinki; and the Institutional Ethics Board approved the study protocol. The experimental procedure including TCD scanning was similar for cognitive studies described in detail elsewhere [17, 22, 26]. In summary, TCD studies were performed using two 2 MHz probes of a bilateral simultaneous TCD instrument (Multi-Dop T, DWL, Singen, Germany), with sample volume placed in the RMCA and LMCA main stems at a depth of 50 mm. The MCAs was chosen for measurements since it supplies about 80% of brain blood flow [45], and thus provides a global characterization of the color space than those from the PCAs. Moreover, complex processing of color occurs in the extrastriate cortex perfused by the MCAs, than in the primary visual cortex perfused by the PCAs. All participants were briefed on the protocol for the entire experiment, and all questions and practice sessions on what was required for the visual paradigms were explained prior to the start of the experimental data acquisition.

2.2. TCD scanning procedure

All *f*TCD procedures were performed using examination techniques previously described for cognitive studies [12, 17, 26, 27, 30, 46, 47, 48]. The *f*TCD scanning was performed using bilateral simultaneous *f*TCD instrument (Multi-Dop T, DWL, Sipplingen, Germany). *f*TCD studies were performed as follows: first, the participant was placed in a supine posture with their head up at 30 degrees (Figure 1).

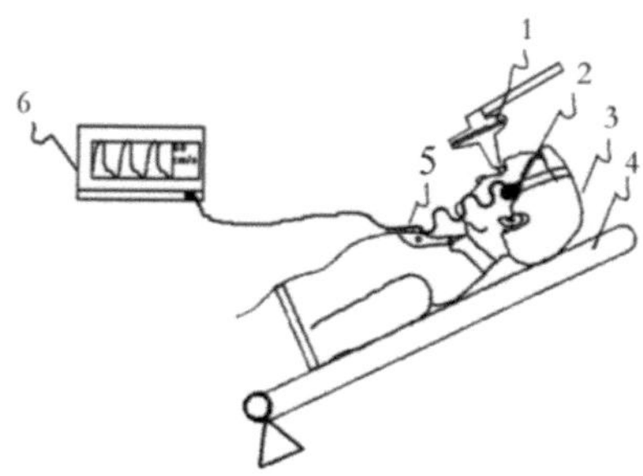

Figure 1. Shows the experimental setup with the subject supine with head-up at 30 degrees looking into the 3D-view-master for color stimulation with two 2MHz transcranial Doppler probes attached bilaterally for simultaneous measurements in both MCAs. (Source modified from Njemanze PC. United States Patent No. 8,152,727 April, 2012).

The Viewmaster *1* is placed in front of the subject where he/she could see clearly through it. The probe holder headgear *2* LAM-RAK (DWL, Sipplingen, Germany) was clamped with a base support the head *3* and on the nasal ridge, while the subject rested supine *4*. Two earplugs were affixed. Two 2-MHz probes connected via transducer cord *5* to the TCD device *6* were affixed in the probe holder and insonation was performed to determine the optimal position for continuous monitoring of both MCA main stems at 50 mm depth from the surface of the probe. The gain and power controls were kept constant for both MCAs in all participants. The headgear was placed comfortably on each participant prior to start of recording. Participants were instructed to remain mute and motionless throughout the short data acquisition time duration. They were informed that their thoughts and subjective feelings would be debriefed after the experimental data acquisition session. All participants were requested to refrain from internal or external verbalization and informed of the deleterious effects that might invalidate the data acquired. Environmental luminance was kept constant for all participants during the study. Effort was made to exclude the effects of environmental noise by sound shielding of the experimental room, and the participant wore earplugs that further reduced environmental noise levels. However, completely sensory deprivation of the participant was avoided. Vital signs were monitored using continuous recording of electrocardiography and respiration. A standard questionnaire was used for monitoring the self-perceived anxiety levels, as measured using state-trait anxiety inventory (STAI) in pre-test and posttest conditions. The STAI has been tested and validated by other investigators [49, 50]. In post-experimental debriefings was focused on what participants were "thinking" during task performance, and any relevance it might have to attention during the data acquisition process. The debriefings were cordial and voluntary to encourage participants to provide full disclosure of their thoughts during the experimental data acquisition, and they were told that, there was no threat of any sanctions regardless of the outcome. Pre-experimental test runs in a different but selected group of participants provided insights into how participants understood the instructions and handled the stimulus used in the present study [22, 27]. The latter was used to modify and simplify the task design for easy comprehension and strict adherence. Baseline vital signs were recorded in full consciousness under normal resting conditions.

2.3. Recordings under dark condition

Measurements in dark condition were considered as light absent condition, as well as including background effects of scotopic vision [20, 51]. It is known that black may evoke a color experience [51]. Recording of a continuous train of velocity waveform envelopes was performed at rest with the participant mute, still, and attention-focused, in a dark visual field within a dark enclosed space with no mental or manual tasks to undertake. Although this had a similar effect to eye closure, but did not require eye muscle contractions and eye ball movements that could elicit motion artifacts. First, dark recording was obtained prior to stimuli administration for 60 seconds, and was used as reference for light stimulation conditions. An observer monitored the subject for movement artifacts, which were marked and removed from recordings.

2.4. Color stimulation recordings

The tasks were designed in our laboratory and the detailed rationale described elsewhere [22]. We have applied these tasks to show consistent and reliable recordings with TCD ultrasonography in prior studies [17, 22]. Briefly, specially adapted 3D-viewing device (Viewmaster, Portland, OR) was painted inside with black paint. The aperture on the right side of the device was closed to light, but the left side aperture was open, to be backlit from white light reflected from a remotely placed light source. In other words, there was left eye monocular vision, with light path from the left visual hemifield reaching the right side of the left eye retina, and crossing at chiasm to project contralaterally to the right visual cortex, while the light path from the right visual hemifield reaching the left side of the left eye retina, project ipsilaterally to the left visual cortex. The rationale for this design, relates to the fact that, in primates including humans, there is virtually total binocular vision; the left half of each retina project to the left visual cortex and the right half of each retina project to the right visual cortex. This means that the right visual cortex receives all its input from the left visual field and the left visual cortex receives all its inputs from the right visual field [52]. Color processing cells, receiving inputs from only one eye are grouped together within the same area of the striate cortex, extending from the upper to the lower cortical layers, and are referred to as ocular dominance columns (blobs) [15, 53, 54]. While those receiving inputs from both eyes are called hypercolumn [53, 55]. During binocular vision, there is binocular interaction due to stereopsis, the perception of depth [15]. Therefore, it is inappropriate to mix the inputs, from both retinas in a single neuron, before the information of color vision has been extracted [15]. The reflection from a light source was used, and projected onto a white surface flat screen, placed 125 cm from the lamp. The screen was positioned 80 cm from the nose ridge of the subject. The light source was a tungsten

http://dx.doi.org/10.5772/54877

coil filament, of a general service lamp ran at a constant 24 V and 200 W, with a color temperature of about 2980 K and approximately 20 lumens/watt. Color stimulation was performed using optical homogenous filters placed on the reel of the Viewmaster, in the light path. Kodak Wratten filters: Deep Blue (No. 47B) with short dominant wavelength (l) of $S\lambda$= 452.7 nm; and Deep Yellow (No. 12) with medium dominant wavelength (l) of $M\lambda$ = 510.7 nm were used. The Kodak manufacturer's manual for Wratten Filters provides the excitation purity and luminous transmittance for each filter [56]. During color stimulation the condition was identical to that of baseline, except for use of slides that were Blue, and Yellow, respectively. White light stimulation was considered as measurements with the left aperture on the reel open to white light reflected from the remote light source.

2.5. Facial stimulation recordings

Figure 2 shows that object and facial paradigms used in the present study.

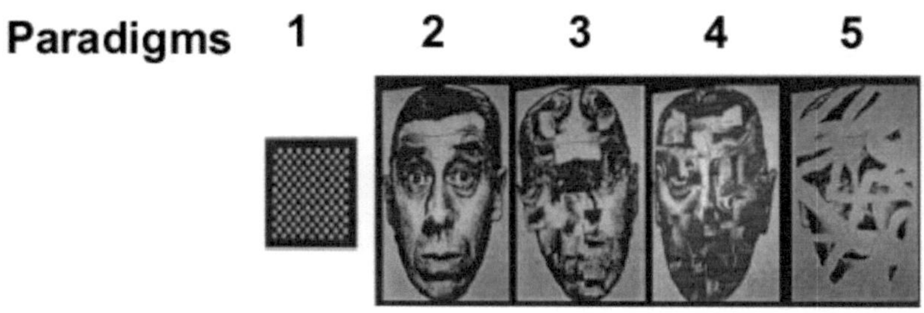

Figure 2. Shows object (Paradigm 1) and facial stimuli (Paradigms 2-5). (Source: Njemanze PC. Aviat Space Environ Med, 2004, 75:800-805).

Paradigm 1: *Object perception* - Checkerboard square paradigm. The paradigm comprised black and white chequered square of alternating black and white square dots. This was a nonverbal passive viewing task of an object foveally presented from a slide projector onto a screen placed in front of the participant, which was inclined at 30 degrees from the horizontal plane at a distance of 80 cm from the nasal ridge. During the presentation, a continuous train of velocity waveform envelopes was recorded with the participant mute, still, with fixed gaze, and attention focused on the object. There were no mental or manual tasks to perform while viewing the object. MFV measurements were made for 60 seconds.

Paradigm 2: *Face encoding task* - whole neutral face. A novel whole male face expressing a neutral emotion was presented. The participant was instructed to commit the face to memory and told that their memory would be tested later. During the presentation, MFV was recorded for 60 seconds while the participant viewed the face.

Paradigm 3: *Facial elements sorting task* – of disarranged face. This facial task comprised sorting elements of a disarranged face. Participants were instructed to sort the elements of the face and arrange them into a whole face, one element at a time, for 60 seconds. The task required a sophisticated perceptual mechanism capable of extraction of components of a face; analysis of their width and height, distances between these elements, angles, contours, illumination, expression, hairline, hair style and so on; and constantly spatially fitting the puzzle by matching each element with that stored in memory and then proceeding to form the picture of the whole face. The task implies that, far more iterations were required to accomplish the recognition task. The rationale is based on the fact that, facial processing comprises several stages [57, 58]. However, on presentation of a face, this multi-stage processing occurs almost simultaneously [59]. The task design was an attempt to break down the processes into several iterative steps, and to exclude verbalizable features that may cause extraneous compounding effects [27]. The MFV was recorded for 60 seconds during the performance of the task.

Paradigm 4. *Facial recognition task:* This facial recognition task comprised disarranged facial elements with a part of the face left in place as a clue. Subjects were asked to recognize the face. The clues left in place were intended to introduce some measure of "automaticity" in the recognition process. In other words, the clue reduced the number of iterations required to accomplish the task.

Paradigm 5. *Facial recognition task:* This facial recognition task comprised a degraded face with missing elements of a greater level of complexity than that of Paradigm 4, but the contour and some elements were preserved in place to aid the subject to recognize the face using a 'fill-in effect' of the missing parts.

The exclusion in the task design of performance ratings by any observer and any competitive indices was done to minimize any role of anxiety. Furthermore, positively and negatively valenced pictures, culturally familiar faces, as well as female faces, were also not used in the present study. Pretest runs suggested that, the latter factors could cause emotional activation both subliminally and supraliminally, with compounding effects on autonomic responses [60]. The design rationale for this pedigree of paradigms have been described in detail elsewhere [27]. Participants were later debriefed on the sequence of task execution and the climax attained. In post-test debriefings, we focused on "what participants were thinking" at each stage of the task, difficulties, distractions, and any confounding experiences or thoughts. The participants described in detail the sequence and strategy used for each task execution, and how they resolved internal conflicts that arose during task performance. Their self-rating of performance on a 4-point scale (from poor to best performance) was also assessed relative to self-attained target performance for the same task during pretest runs. An observer monitored motion artifacts such as eye movements and voluntary and involuntary movements, who documented time of occurrence on the MFV train for use in later analysis.

2.6. Calculations

Artifacts were marked and removed prior to data analysis. Data averaging comprised 10-second segments of the train of velocity waveform envelopes for the dark task and each of the paradigms, respectively. For baseline and each stimulus, 60 seconds of recording resulted in six MFV values for dark and each task, respectively. These values were used for further calculations. In other words, velocity waveform envelopes for the relevant 60-s intervals were first averaged in 10-s segments, to produce six values for black and each color condition respectively. The resulting values were used for further computations of laterality index (LI′). Cerebral lateralization was assessed using LI′ expressed as:

$$LI' = \frac{(\text{RMCA MFV}_{10\text{-s}} \text{ minus LMCA MFV}_{10\text{-s}})}{(\text{RMCA MFV}_{10\text{-s}} \text{ plus LMCA MFV}_{10\text{-s}})} * 100. \tag{5}$$

The relative value of lateralization (LI), for each 10-s segment for each color, was calculated as the difference between LI′ values measured during the 10-s segment of the color and the corresponding 10-s segment of baseline (onset of baseline corresponds with onset of color within the 60-s segment):

$$LI = LI'\text{color}_{10\text{-s}} \text{ minus } LI'\text{baseline}_{10\text{-s}}. \tag{6}$$

In general, positive LI values suggest right lateralization, while negative LI values suggest left lateralization. Zero LI values showed no lateralization from baseline, or possible bilateral response. LI values calculated for each 10-s segment of the MFV envelope, were used for further analysis.

2.7. Three dimensional color space

In the design of the model for three dimensional color space, it could be presumed that opponency was accomplished across two orthogonal coordinates of blue and yellow, respectively [11]. In men, wavelength-differencing activity was captured by changes in the RMCA MFV for Yellow plotted on the Y-axis, and the RMCA MFV for Blue plotted on the X-axis [11]. In women, frequency-differencing [12] was captured by changes in the LMCA MFV for Yellow plotted on the Y-axis, and the LMCA MFV for Blue plotted on the X-axis. The luminance effect on the LMCA MFV in response to White light with the highest luminous flux, was plotted on the (Z - axis), in both men and women [11]. The reconstruction of the 3D-color space plots was performed using the quadratic function [11], fitted by the procedure that has the general form:

$$Z = a_o + a_1X + a_2Y + a_3X^2 + a_4Y^2 + a_5XY \tag{7}$$

The relationships between observed variables were estimated in 3D-surface plot which offered a flexible tool for approximation. Moreover, the quadratic surface plot does not flex to accommodate local variations in data. When the overall pattern of changes in MFV dataset follows some segment of the quadratic surface, then a good fit could be achieved. The raw data spikes were displayed on the surface, to examine goodness of fit and assess the influence of outliers. The MFV gradient produced color scale sequence ranges, from minimum (green) to maximum (red) of Z-values of luminance effect. The color sequence ranges were used to adjudge the level of luminance effect required for wavelength-differencing activity in men, and frequency-differencing activity, in women, respectively.

2.8. Exponential function model

The 3D-graph was examined to uncover the relationship between luminance effects (Z-axis) and wavelength-differencing on the RMCA MFV for Yellow plotted on the *Y*-axis in men. The observation of an exponential growth suggested that, the data could be fitted to an exponential function model. The LMCA MFV for White light (*Y*-axis) and RMCA MFV for Yellow (X-axis) was fitted to an exponential function of a 2D graph, given the following:

The exponential function with positive base $b > 1$ is the function:

$$y = b^x \tag{8}$$

It is defined for every real number x for any base b.

There are two important things to note:

The y-intercept is at (0, 1). For, $b^0 = 1$.

The negative x-axis is a horizontal asymptote. For, when x is a large negative number e.g. $b^{-10,000}$ - then y is a very small positive number.

2.9. Logarithmic function model

In women, the 3D-graph was examined to uncover the relationship between luminance effects (Z-axis) and frequency-differencing on the LMCA MFV for Blue plotted on the X-axis. The observation of a logarithmic growth suggested that, the data could be fitted to a logarithmic function. The LMCA MFV for White light (*Y*-axis) and LMCA MFV for Blue (*X*-axis) was fitted to a logarithmic function of a 2D graph, given the following:

The logarithmic function with base b is the function:

$$y = \log_b x \tag{9}$$

b is normally a number greater than 1 (although it need only be greater than 0 and not equal to 1). The function is defined for all $x > 0$. The negative y-axis is a vertical asymptote.

2.10. Inverse relations of exponential and logarithmic functions

The inverse of any exponential function is a logarithmic function. For, in any base b:

$$i)\ b^{\log_b x} = x, \tag{10}$$

and

$$ii)\ log_b b^x = x \tag{11}$$

Rule *i*) embodies the definition of a logarithm: $\log_b x$ is the *exponent* to which *b* must be raised to produce *x*.

Now, let:

$$\lambda(x) = b^x \text{ and } f(x) = log_b x \tag{12}$$

Then Rule *i*) is $\Lambda(f(x)) = x$.

And Rule *ii*) is $f(\Lambda(x)) = x$.

These rules satisfy the definition of a pair of inverse functions. Therefore for any base *b*, the functions:

$$\lambda(x) = b^x \text{ and } f(x) = log_b x \tag{13}$$

are inverses. This defines the well established relationship between wavelength (λ) and frequency (*f*), respectively, that is given by: $\lambda = c/f$.

where *c* is the speed of light in a vacuum and remains constant at 3.00×10^8 m/s.

2.11. Fourier analysis

The Fourier transform algorithm was applied using standard software (Time series and forecasting module, Statistica for Macintosh, StatSoft, OK, USA). The most efficient approach for Fourier algorithm requires that, the length of the input series is equal to a power of 2. If this is not the case, additional computations have to be performed. To obtain the required time series, the data were averaged in 10-second segments for one minute duration for each stimulus; yielding 6 data points for each participant and a total of 48 data points for all eight men and women, respectively. Smoothing the periodogram values was accomplished using a weighted moving average transformation. Hamming window was applied as a smoother [61, 62]. The spectral density estimates, derived from single series Fourier analysis, were plotted, and the frequency regions with the highest estimates were marked as peaks.

2.12. Other statistics

All analyses were performed using the software package Statistica (StatSoft, OK, USA). Results were given as mean±SD and plots represented as mean/SE/1.96*SE where applicable. Analysis of LI was recomputed after excluding outliers. Analysis of variance (ANOVA) was applied to spectral density estimates between two minima including the peak (as maxima) to examine the effects of paradigms on cortical and subcortical responses. The stimulus effect was assessed by multivariant analyses of variance (MANOVA) with repeated measures applied to the MFV data set, followed by planned Scheffé contrast that compared stimulus response relative to stimulus-absent Dark condition. Analysis of covariance (ANCOVA) with repeated measures was performed to demonstrate that, the difference found during visual stimulation persists even when the differences in baseline condition were partialled out. When applicable, one-way ANOVA of paired groups was used to assess differences in spectral density estimates between two minima including the peak (as maxima), under different stimulation conditions, for the RMCA and LMCA, respectively. The determination of LUMINANCE effect was derived by comparison of Dark versus Light conditions, and the direction relative to chromatic axis was either opposite (orthogonal axis) or parallel axis. WAVELENGTH-encoding was assessed as present when the effects of longer wavelength color (Yellow) were accentuated over shorter wavelength color (Blue) [11]. Conversely, ENERGY-encoding was present when the effects of higher frequency color (Blue), was accentuated over lower frequency color (Yellow) [11]. WAVELENGTH-differencing implicated WAVELENGTH-encoding main effect at S-peaks, and at least a tendency for ENERGY-encoding at C-peaks [11]. The pre-condition for WAVELENGTH-differencing requires that, a chromatic contrast detector sub-serving one area of chromatic space, excite a chromatic detector of opposite type and/or inhibit a chromatic detector of the same type in neighboring areas of chromatic space [11, 15]. On the other hand, FREQUENCY-differencing involved ENERGY-encoding main effect at C-peaks, and at least a tendency at S-peaks. CLTP process accentuated C-peaks over S-peaks due to prevailing SLTD. Conversely, SLTP process accentuated S-peaks over C-peaks, due to prevailing CLTD. The latter was followed by planned contrasts to examine luminance effect (dark versus Paradigm 1), discrimination of face from non-face or category-specific face effect (Paradigm 1 versus Paradigm 2), and face-processing strategy effect (Paradigm 2 versus Paradigm 3). The Paradigms 4 and 5 were used only in the *f*TCD analysis but not in the further, *f*TCDS analysis. The level of significance was at $p=0.05$.

3. Results

3.1. Gender-related asymmetry during color processing by *f*TCD

The gender-related asymmetry for color processing is shown in Figure 3, that displays the box and whiskers plot of the MFV data obtained for all subjects under all conditions. Overall, MFV for women were higher than that for men. The plot shows the five-number summary (the minimum, first quartile, median, third quartile, and maximum) of the distribution of the observations of the MFV data set, and showed a more symmetric distribution during color stimulations (Blue, Yellow, and Red) in men, compared to greater dispersion in women. Table 1A shows the mean ± SE of MFV for men, and the planned contrast (Scheffé P-value) variation from Dark condition. In men, the RMCA MFV increased significantly in response to Light (2.6%), Blue (4.3%), Yellow (2.5%) and Red (2.8%). While LMCA MFV increased only to Blue (2.6%) stimulation. Table 1B shows the mean ± SE of MFV for women. In women, only Blue stimulation evoked increase in MFV in the RMCA (2.6%) and LMCA (2.2%).

http://dx.doi.org/10.5772/54877

Stimulations	RMCA (cm/s)	Scheffé *P* (cm/s)	LMCA	Scheffé P
Dark	64±1.26	-63.9±1.8		
Light	65.7±1.2	*<0.05*	64.2±1.67	*NS*
Blue	66.8±1.28	*<0.0001*	65.6±1.8	*<0.01*
Yellow	65.6±1.26	*<0.05*	64.4±1.7	*NS*
Red	65.8±1.27	*<0.01*	64.4±1.6	*NS*
A				

Stimulations	RMCA (cm/s)	Scheffé *P* (cm/s)	LMCA	Scheffé P
Dark	81.6±2	-	80.7±1.8	-
Light	82.3±2	*NS*	81.26±1.7	*NS*
Blue	83.8±1.9	*<0.0001*	81.6±1.77	*<0.01*
Yellow	82.57±1.86	*NS*	81.3±1.6	*NS*
Red	82.1±1.9	*NS*	80.7±1.68	*NS*
B				

Table 1. A. Mean±SE and Planned Contrasts of MFV Changes during Visual Stimulations from Dark Baseline in Men; B. Mean±SE and Planned Contrasts of MFV Changes during Visual Stimulations from Dark Baseline in Women

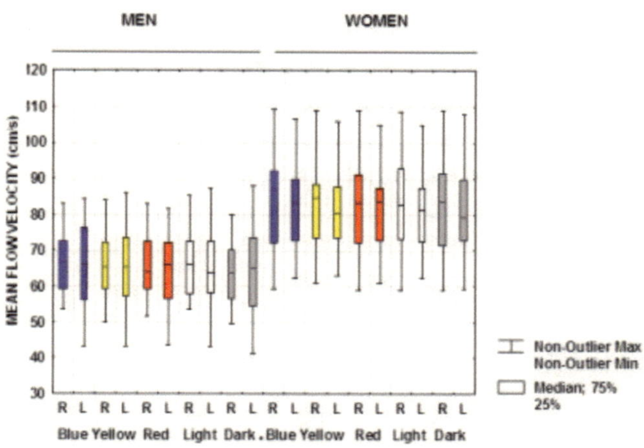

Figure 3. Box and whiskers plots of mean/SE /1.96*SE of MFV (in cm/s) during dark and color stimulation in men and women. (Source modified from: Njemanze PC. Exp Transl Stroke Med 2010, 2:21-27.).

To assess the overall gender-related differences in MFV during color stimulation, a MANOVA test was applied to MFV data set to assess differences between measurements in the RMCA and LMCA in men and women, with a 2 × 5 × 2 design: two levels of GENDER (Men and Women), five levels of STIMULATIONS, (Dark, Light, Blue, Yellow, and Red), and two levels of ARTERY (RMCA and LMCA). The MFV was analyzed as the dependent variable. There was a main effect of GENDER, $F(1,94) = 65.4$, $MSE = 68166$, $p < 0.0001$. There was a main effect of STIMULATIONS, $F(4,376) = 5.6$, $MSE = 111.7$, $P < 0.001$. There was no main effect of ARTERY, P = NS. However, there was STIMULATION × ARTERY interaction, $F(4,376) = 3.3$, $MSE = 5.96$, $P < 0.05$.

The 3D surface quadratic plots of MFV changes in color space are shown in Figures 4(A-B) for men (Figure 4A) and women (Figure 4B), respectively. The male 3D surface quadratic plot (Figure 4A) was 'funnel shaped', indicating overall that, wavelength-differencing activity was narrowed at low luminance effect, but broadened with increasing luminance effect. In men, there was an exponential relationship (Figure 5A) between right hemisphere wavelength-differencing and contralateral left hemisphere luminance effect, as demonstrated in the 2D graph (Figure 5B), showing all subjects within the 95% confidence band. The exponential function model in men (Figure 5B) indicated that brain functional integration of luminance effects and wavelength-differencing activities was maintained within a 'narrow physiologic range' of MFV of 50 to 85 cm/s in the RMCA and LMCA. On the other hand, in women, the 3D-surface quadratic plot was the mirror-image of that observed in men, showing a closed 'cone shape' with a widespread base (Figure 4B). The base of the cone shape suggests that at very low luminance effect on LMCA MFV, frequency-differencing activity occurred over a very wide range. However, with increasing luminance effect, frequency-differencing activity narrowed. In women, there was a logarithmic relationship between ipsilateral left hemisphere frequency-differencing and luminance effect, as demonstrated in the 2D graph of logarithmic function (Figure 5C), showing all subjects but two, within the 95% confidence band. The logarithmic function model in women (Figure 5D) indicates that, brain functional integration of luminance effect and frequency-differencing activities was maintained within a 'narrow physiologic range' of MFV of 60 to 106 cm/s in the LMCA, however, somewhat wider than that for men. In both, men (Figure 5C) and women (Figure 5D), respectively, there appears to be a high level of scatter. However, in men (Figure 5C) it is more disperse than in women (Figure 5D), which may suggest as greater sensitivity to luminance in men (see Figure 4A), than in women (see Figure 4B).

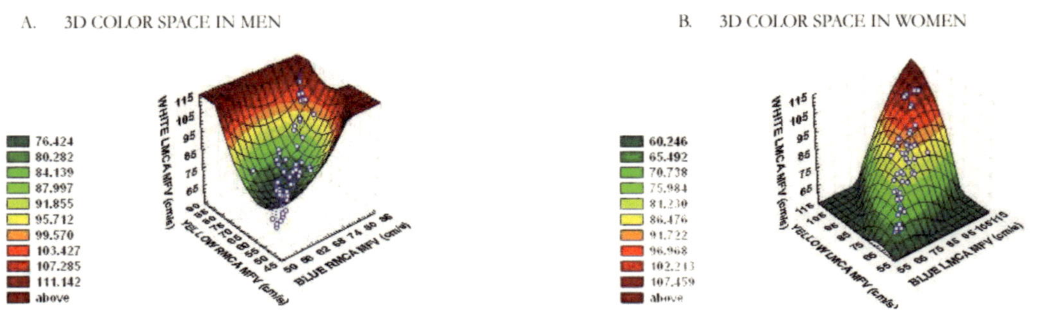

Figure 4. A-B). Shows the 3D surface quadratic plots of MFV changes in color space for men (Figure 4A) and women (Figure 4B), respectively. (Source modified from: Njemanze PC. Exp Transl Stroke Med 2011, 3:1-8.).

http://dx.doi.org/10.5772/54877

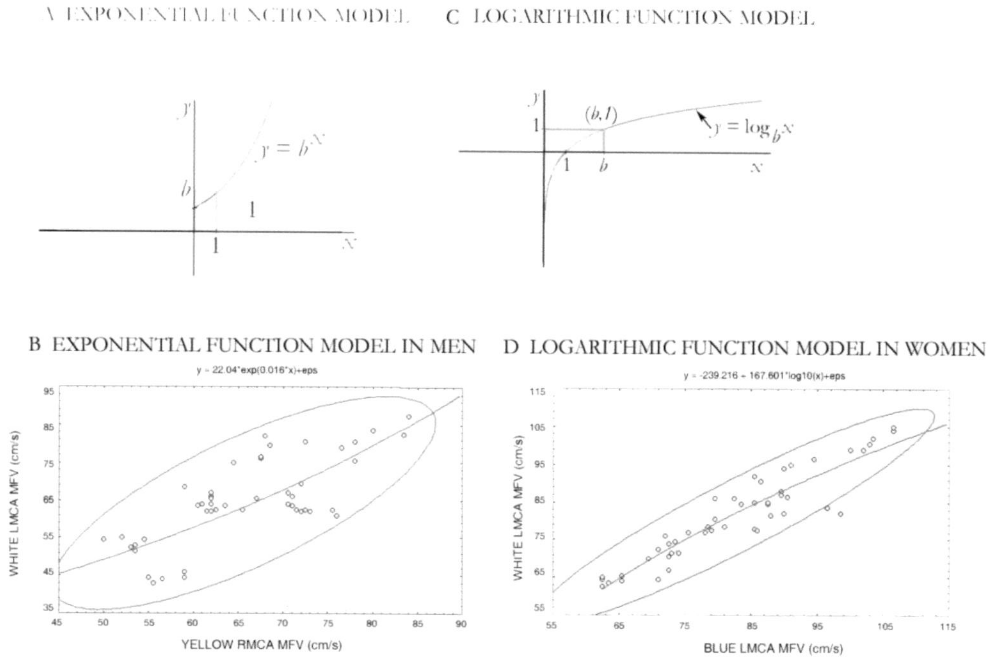

Figure 5. A-D). Shows the exponential function curve used for any base *b* (Figure 5A) that was used for the exponential function model fitted to the data in men (Figure 5B); in contrast, to the logarithmic function curve used for any base *b* (Figure 5C) that was used for the logarithmic function model fitted to the data in women (Figure 5D). All subjects were plotted with the 95% confidence band shown. (Source modified from: Njemanze PC. Exp Transl Stroke Med 2011, 3:1-8.).

3.2. Gender-related asymmetry for color processing by *f*TCDS

Figures 6 (A-D) demonstrates the conventional spectral density plots for each artery during Dark, Light, Blue and Yellow stimulations in men (Figures 6A-B) and women (Figures 6C-D), respectively.

In general, for all stimulations in both men and women there were three peaks designated as fundamental (F-peak), cortical (C-peak), and subcortical (S-peak), which occurred at regular frequency intervals of the first (0.125 Hz), second (0.25 Hz), and third (0.375 Hz) harmonics, respectively. Given the differential MFV response in men and women, the spectral density estimates for men and women were analyzed separately, to uncover changes at cortical and subcortical peaks. A MANOVA with repeated measures was applied to spectral density estimates in a 2 × 5 × 2 design: two levels of REGIONS (Cortical, Subcortical), five levels of STIMULATIONS (Dark, Light, Blue, Yellow and Red) and two levels of ARTERIES (RMCA and LMCA). In men, there was no main effect of REGIONS, p = NS, but there was a tendency for subcortical peaks to be higher than cortical peaks in men. There was a main effect of STIMULATIONS, $F(4,24) = 4.2$, MSE = 11586, $p < 0.01$. There was no main effect of ARTERIES, p = NS. There was a REGIONS × STIMULATIONS interaction, $F(4,24) = 4.8$, MSE = 31945, $p < 0.01$. There was no REGIONS × ARTERIES interaction, p = NS. There was a STIMULATIONS × ARTERIES interaction, $F(4,24) = 4.7$, MSE = 7397, $p < 0.01$. There was a three-way interaction,

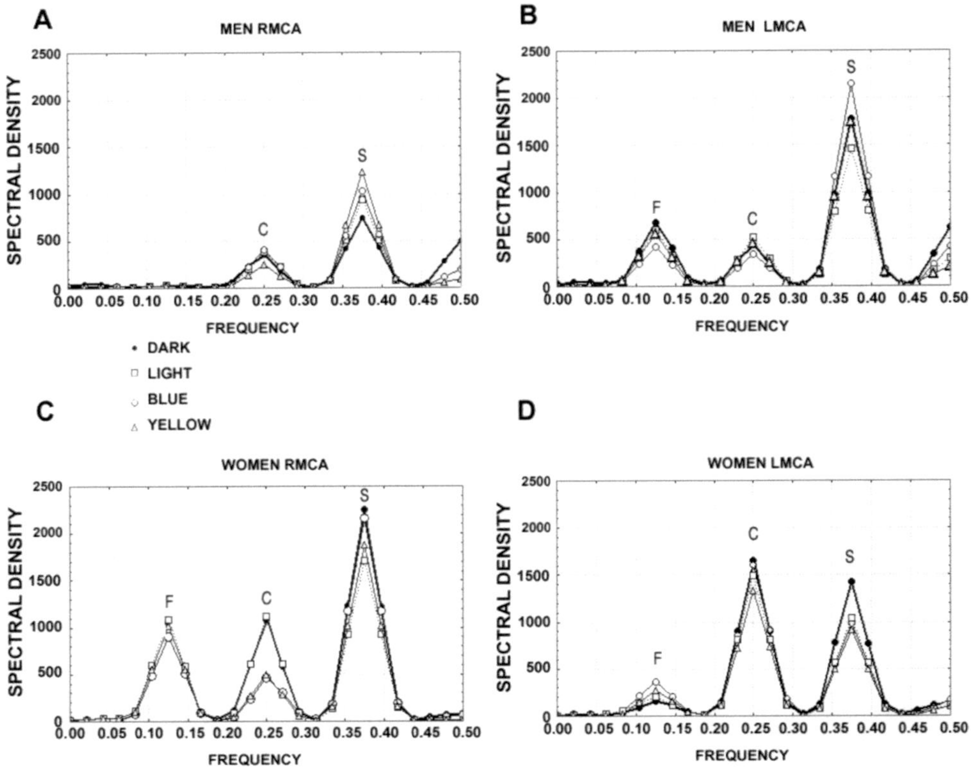

Figure 6. A-D). Shows the plots of spectral density estimates for dark, light and color stimuli (blue, yellow) for the RMCA in men (Figure 6A), for the LMCA in men (Figure 6B); for the RMCA in women (Figure 6C) and LMCA in women (Figure 6D). (Source modified from: Njemanze PC. Exp Transl Stroke Med 2010, 2:21-27.).

REGIONS × STIMULATIONS × ARTERIES, $F(4,24) = 4.76$, MSE = 25392, $p < 0.01$. An analysis of covariance (ANCOVA) with repeated measures was applied to demonstrate that the difference found during color stimulation persists even when the difference due to baseline condition was partialled out. In men, there was significant increase in MFV produced by luminance, hence WAVELENGTH-encoding activity could only be adjudged after partialling out the changes under Dark and Light conditions as changing covariates. Conversely, in women, there was no change in MFV associated with luminance, and hence only baseline Dark condition was used as a covariate.

In men, in the RMCA, at C-peaks, there was a tendency for ENERGY-encoding, $F(1,5) = 5.95$, MSE = 10315, $p = 0.058$. However, at S-peaks, there was a significant main effect of WAVELENGTH-encoding, $F(1,5) = 9.98$, MSE = 1016.8, $p < 0.05$. This may suggest that, there was WAVELENGTH-differencing in the right hemisphere in men. There was no luminance effect in the RMCA territory, p = NS. However, in the LMCA, there was an orthogonal LUMINANCE effect, $F(1,5) = 6.27$, MSE = 6834.6, $p < 0.05$. Figure 6A shows that the RMCA S-peaks were 'topologically' separated, achromatic from chromatic peaks, and between the latter, short wavelength (Blue) from long wavelength (Yellow and Red). There was a reverse tendency at the C-peaks. Overall, in men, wavelength-differencing in the right hemisphere (Figure 6A), and luminance effect in the left hemisphere (Figure 6B), occurred by processes of CLTD and SLTP. In women, in the RMCA, the C-peaks were unremarkable, p = NS. However, at S-peaks, there was some residual tendency for ENERGY-encoding effect, $F(1,6) = 5.65$, $MSE = 31823$, $p = 0.054$, and LUMINANCE sensitivity, $F(1,6) = 5.52$, $MSE = 58620.5$, $p = 0.057$. On the other hand, in the LMCA, a main effect for ENERGY-encoding occurred at C-peaks, $F(1,6) = 6.35$, $MSE = 34730$, $p < 0.05$, as well as at S-peaks, $F(1,6) = 7.5$, $MSE = 2197.7$, $p < 0.05$. This may suggest that in women, FREQUENCY-differencing occurred in the left hemisphere. A parallel LUMINANCE main effect, occurred at C-peaks, $F(1,6) = 6.27$, $MSE = 10461.6$, $p < 0.05$, but showed a tendency at S-peaks, $F(1,6) = 5.5$, $MSE = 58620$, $p = 0.057$. In women, both frequency-differencing and luminance effect responsiveness in the left hemisphere (Figure 6D), occurred by processes of CLTP and SLTD.

3.3. Gender-related asymmetry during facial processing by *f*TCD

The LI for men is displayed in Figure 7A, and for women in Figure 7B, respectively.

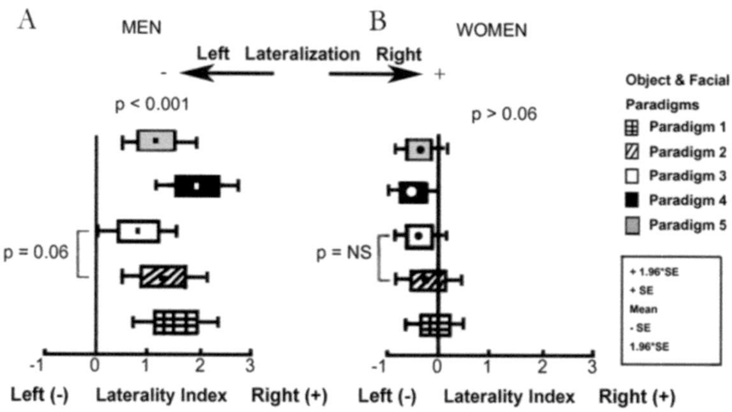

Figure 7. A-B). Shows the box and whiskers plot of mean/SE /1.96*SE of LI during object (Paradigm 1) and facial (Paradigms 2-5) stimulation in men (Figure 7A) and women (Figure 7B).

Overall, men were right lateralized for facial Paradigms 2-5 as well as non-face object Paradigm 1. On the other hand, women were left lateralized for facial Paradigms 2-5, but right lateralized for object Paradigm 1. However, on exclusion of outliers, women showed no lateralization with zero LI value or bilateral activation during object processing. In men, at baseline MFV in dark condition did not differ between RMCA and LMCA. Paradigms 1–5 induced significant variation in MBFV in the RMCA ($p < 0.01$) and LMCA ($p < 0.001$), that resulted in right lateralization for all tasks. There was a marginal difference between Paradigm 2 and Paradigm 3 ($p = 0.06$), due to more pronounced activation in the LMCA ($p < 0.01$) than RMCA ($p = 0.053$) (Figure 7A) during Paradigm 3. Overall, tasks were right lateralized ($p < 0.001$), showing stimulus-specific effect in lateralization. The LI for women is displayed in Figure 7B. At baseline MFV in dark condition was higher in LMCA than R-MCA, and Paradigms 1–5 induced significantly greater attenuation of MFV in the RMCA ($p < 0.05$) than in the L-MCA ($p < 0.001$). As a result, there was left lateralization for all Paradigms 1-5 (Figure 7B). There was no difference between Paradigm 2 and Paradigm 3. In other words, in women, stimulus-specific effects did not yield lateralization of MFV. Given the observed marginal tendencies for changes between Paradigms 1-3, the *f*TCDS analysis was carried out for dark and Paradigms 1-3 effects.

3.4. Gender-related asymmetry during facial processing by *f*TCDS

The spectral density plots for each artery during all study conditions in Figures 8 A-D, in men (Figure 8 A-B) and women (Figure 8 C-D), respectively.

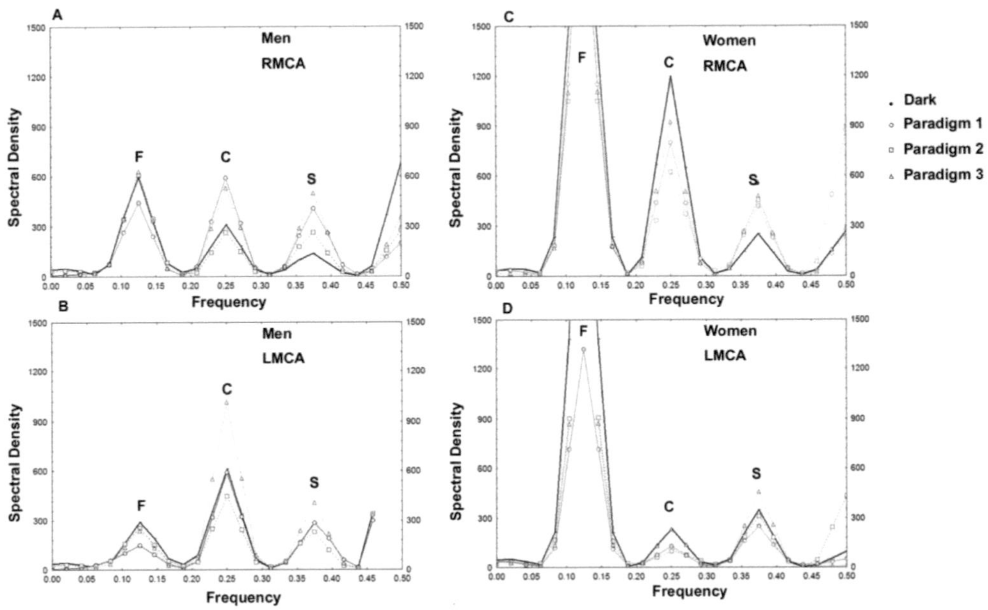

Figure 8. A-D). Shows the plots of spectral density estimates for dark, object (Paradigm 1) and facial (Paradigms 2-3) stimulation for the RMCA in men (Figure 8A), for the LMCA in men (Figure 8B); for the RMCA in women (Figure 8C) and LMCA in women (Figure 8D). (Source modified from: Njemanze PC. Laterality 2007, 12:31-49.).

In general, for all stimulations in both men and women there were three peaks designated as **F**-, **C**-, and **S**-peaks, representing the fundamental, cortical, and subcortical peaks, which occurred at regular frequency intervals of 0.125, 0.25, and 0.375, respectively. The spectral density peaks were analyzed for each gender separately to examine the effect of dark and stimulations at **C**- and **S**-peaks for the RMCA and LMCA, respectively. A one-way ANOVA with repeated measures for all four levels of STIMULATION (Dark, Paradigms 1-3) was used. This was followed by planned contrasts. In men, in the RMCA at C-peaks, there was a main effect of STIMULATION, $F(3, 18) = 4.2$, MSE= 16804.3, $p=0.05$. Planned contrast revealed a category-specific face effect, $p = 0.05$, (Figure 8A). However, at the S-peaks there was only a marginal tendency for luminance effect. In men, in the LMCA at C-peaks, there was a main effect of STIMULATION, $F(3, 18) = 4.4$, MSE = 39947, $p = 0.05$. Planned contrast revealed a facial processing strategy effect, $p = 0.05$, (Figure 8B). However, at S-peaks there was no main effect of STIMULATION. In women, in the RMCA at C-peaks, there was a main effect of STIMULATION, $F(3, 18) = 4.2$, MSE = 38441.9, $p = 0.05$. Planned contrast revealed a luminance effect, $p = 0.05$ (Figure 8C). Similarly, at the S-peaks there was a marginal tendency for luminance effect. In women, in the LMCA at C-peaks, there was a main effect of STIMULATION, $F(3, 18) = 3.2$, MSE = 2791.4, $p = 0.05$. Planned contrast revealed a facial processing strategy effect, $p = 0.05$ (Figure 8D). However, at S-peaks there was no main effect of STIMULATION.

3.5. Confounding effects

The cardiovascular measures that could cause confounding effects were assessed using one-way analysis of variance (ANOVA). In men the heart rate during Paradigm 1 (71.9±10.6 bpm), Paradigm 2 (69.6±11 bpm), and Paradigm 3 (70.5±5 bpm) did not differ from resting baseline (67.5±9 bpm), ($p = 0.05$). Similarly, in women the heart rate during Paradigm 1 (76.9±9.8 bpm), Paradigm 2 (78.9±12 bpm), and Paradigm 3 (79.3±13.8 bpm) did not differ from resting baseline (76.9±9.6 bpm), ($p = 0.05$). In men the respiratory rate during Paradigm 1 (17.3±3.5 per minute), Paradigm 2 (19.9±5.7 per minute), and Paradigm 3 (16.9±3.7 per minute) did not differ from resting baseline (17.9±2.5 per minute), ($p=0.05$). Similarly, in women the respiratory rate during Paradigm 1 (19±4.5 per minute), Paradigm 2 (21±5 per minute), and Paradigm 3 (21±6 per minute) did not differ from resting baseline (19.3±6.4 per minute), ($p > 0.05$). The overall mean heart rate was 74 bpm and respiratory rate was 19 per minute. There was no significant difference between pre-test and post-test blood pressure, ($p > 0.05$). Similarly, there were no significant differences between the stimuli for heart rate, respiratory rate, and anxiety scores ($p > 0.05$). In other words, there were no changes in cardiovascular parameters and anxiety scores during the study. In post-test debriefings, participants described their initial condition as "blank", unaware of subtle emotional state, as they tried to focus attention on the imagery spot within the dark visual field. Women described the paradigms in greater detail than men. For example, on first prompt for description, most men described Paradigm 1 simply as a draught board or chess board, while most women described it as alternating black and white squares within a cube. For execution of Paradigm 3, both men and women reported sorting one part of the face at a time into place before proceeding to the next part, in other words, all followed a step-by-step approach. All rated themselves as not being anxious, and assessed themselves as having good performance, with no difficulty with task execution.

4. Discussion

4.1. Gender-related asymmetry during color processing

Overall, the gender-related differences could be summarized as follows: (1) in men, wavelength-differencing activity was enhanced at high luminance effect, conversely, in women, frequency-differencing activity was enhanced at low luminance effect. (2) In men, luminance effect varied exponentially with wavelength-differencing activity, while in women, luminance effect varied logarithmically with frequency-differencing activity. (3) The physiologic range of MFV in the MCA territories for the relationship between luminance effect and wavelength-differencing activity in men, was narrower than that for frequency-differencing activity in women. The gender-related differences in color processing, which comprised right hemisphere wavelength-differencing in men, but left hemisphere frequency-differencing in women, suggest that, color processing followed the same rule of lateralization as other major cognitive functions, such as facial processing [26, 27] and general intelligence [30], which implicated the right hemisphere cognitive style in men, and left hemisphere cognitive style in women. Prior studies have suggested that, the right hemisphere was implicated in color processing [20, 21, 22] and the left hemisphere in color memory [61, 62]. Functional magnetic resonance studies demonstrated that memory for colors activated the same cortical regions associated with color perception in the left fusiform gyrus [63, 64]. This has led some investigators to suggest that, color memory is a constructive process reflecting the synthesis of features each of which are processed in the different cortical regions [65-67]. The functional integration of color processing and luminance effect could provide a model for the study of the functional integration of color processing and color memory within the color space.

However, the reason for gender-related cerebral asymmetry for color processing remains to be elucidated. It was suggested that, the neuroadaptation to the physical qualities of light as a wave and as quanta energy, pre-conditioned the right hemisphere for wavelength-differencing and left hemisphere for frequency-differencing, respectively. A light hypothesis for cerebral asymmetry was postulated, to infer that, the phenotypic neuroadaptation to the environmental physical constraints of light, led to phenotypic evolution and genetic variation of X-Y gene pairs that determined hemispheric asymmetry [12, 17]. The evolutionary trend is towards optimization of perception of the 'whole' environment by functional coupling of the genes for complementarity of both hemispheres within self, and between both genders [12, 17, 26]. The contralateral hemisphere processing of wavelength-differencing and frequency-differencing was as a result of the inverse relationship between wavelength and frequency. The results further demonstrate that, color processing was organized within cortico-subcortical circuits [11]. It could be presumed that, the neuronal assemblies processing light information as well as their blood flow supply, share analogous topological organization [26]. In men, the distribution of the S-peaks showed that dark elicited the least effect followed by White, Blue, Yellow and Red. This type of summation of responses, with distinction between achromatic and chromatic contrasts along orthogonal axis, on one hand, and between short wavelength and long wavelength on the other, could be presumed to be evidence for stimulus complexity topological organization based on wavelength, in the right hemisphere in men [12, 17, 26]. The latter extends from an area implicated in luminance processing to a much greater area for wavelength-differencing. Similar stimulus complexity topological organization, has been observed in studies involving facial and object stimuli in the right hemisphere in men [26]. In other words, there is a topological organization, based on category-specific stimulus complexity of the functions, located within the ventral temporal cortex of the right hemisphere in men. The latter would be compatible with the findings that thin stripes in V2 contain functional maps where the color of a stimulus is represented by the location of its response activation peak [52, 53]. Conversely, in the left hemisphere in women, at **C**-peaks, frequency-differencing separated the peak for high frequency color (Blue) from low frequency color (Yellow), but was parallel to the luminance axis. Hence, the differentiation was process-mapped only to frequency. Similar process-map model has been proposed for facial processing [26, 34]. It could be suggested that in the left hemisphere in women, there is a category-specific process-mapping system for retrieving color from memory. The latter would be consonant to the proposed distinct map for representation of color in memory [66, 67].

The present work may offer some indication on the neurophysiologic mechanisms underlying vasomotor changes during color processing, which have remained largely unknown until now. The cerebral arteries are innervated by postganglionic nitrergic nerves, originating from the ipsilateral pterygopalatine ganglion, that tonically dilate cerebral arteries in the resting condition [70]. The observed changes in MFV in response to visual stimulations have been related to imbalance between sympathetic vasoconstrictor traffic and vasodilator effects of nitric oxide (NO) [11, 22, 71]. The NO released postsynaptically, diffuses back across the synaptic cleft, to act on the presynaptic terminals, causing increases in presynaptic glutamate release [70, 72], which could account for ipsilateral LTP [11, 72]. Others contend that LTP induced in the visual cortex in animal models is NO dependent [72]. The LTP and LTD recorded non-invasively using *f*TCDS, have shown neuroplasticity during color processing over several hours [11], and hence could be applied to the study of stroke rehabilitation and monitoring of drug effects on N-Methyl- D-aspartate (NMDA) receptors.

Presuming that these mechanisms are present, it could be proposed that in men, wavelength-differencing within the right hemisphere by processes of cortical long-term depression (CLTD) and subcortical long-term potentiation (SLTP) [12, 17], occurred simultaneously with contralateral cortical short-term depression (CSTD) and subcortical short-term potentiation (SSTP) in the left hemisphere, marked by exponential decaying increase in synaptic strength that appears to involve NMDA receptors as well [12, 17, 73, 74], but decays after reaching the asymptotic levels of MFV (Figure 5A-B). Thus, it could be postulated that in men, in the contralateral left hemisphere, memory activation implicated 'exponential expansion' by CSTD and SSTP processes. On the other hand, in women, frequency-differencing within the left hemisphere occurred by processes of cortical long-term potentiation (CLTP) and subcortical long-term depression (SLTD) [11, 12, 17], concurrently, with ipsilateral cortical short-term potentiation (CSTP) and subcortical short-term depression (SSTD) in a selective area of the left hemisphere [11, 12, 17], characterized by logarithmic decaying decrease in synaptic strength that may also involve NMDA receptors, but decays after reaching the asymptotic levels of MFV (Figure 5C). Thus, in women, in the ipsilateral left hemisphere memory activation involved 'logarithmic compression' by CSTP and SSTD processes. Analogous synaptic and cellular activities have been observed in animal experiments [73, 74].

The clinical relevance of the observed profound gender-related differences in cortico-subcortical activation during color stimulation is yet to be fully realized. The plausible implications of the result that, in men, in the right hemisphere, SLTP and CLTD occurred with wavelength-differencing, and conversely, in women in the left hemisphere, CLTP and SLTD occurred with frequency-differencing, is not known. It could be suggested that, there could be a gender-related difference in the effects of brain lesions in men and women. While in men, subcortical lesions of the right hemisphere may be associated with severe color deficits because of impaired SLTP processes for wavelength-differencing, in women, cortical lesions of the left hemisphere could result in more severe deficits due to inability to form CLTP processes for frequency-differencing. The onset of memory deficits may be characterized by loss of the capability to perform 'exponential expansion' in the memory area of the left hemisphere in men, or 'logarithmic compression' in the selective memory area of the left hemisphere in women. The latter may open the possibility of use of *f*TCD and *f*TCDS to determine early onset of memory deficits in patients with neurodegenerative disorders. Another practical clinical implication of the findings is that, in the structuring of tests of color vision, one eye has to be tested at a time, since binocular interaction may inhibit the responses from color processing neurons due to multiplexing responses in ocular dominance hypercolumns, rather than responses evoked from ocular dominance columns (blobs) [15].

In conclusion, gender differences in color processing implicated right hemisphere wavelength-differencing in men, but left hemisphere frequency-differencing in women. Future research using *f*TCDS technique should explore clinical applications of color processing in stroke rehabilitation, and monitoring of drug effects. Genetic and comparative animal experiments, as well as brain lesion studies are needed to further elucidate mechanisms of gender differences in color processing.

4.2. Gender-related asymmetry during facial processing

Facial perception occurred in the cortical region of the right hemisphere in men, but in the left in women. Similar observations have been made using transcranial Doppler [27], and electrophysiological techniques [28]. Similar gender-related hemisphere differences have been observed at the amygdale for emotionally related stimuli [29], and for performance-related processing [30-32]. Men showed a right lateralization during object processing, but women showed a right tendency or bilateral activation. The observed category-specific face effect was consistent with the concept of category-specific model, which posits a neural module for face category as distinct from non-face [59, 75, 76, 77]. However, others have advocated the existence of alternative models [33, 34].

The *f*TCD technique presumes that, the neuronal assemblies processing light information share analogous topological organization as their blood flow supply, then dark would elicit the least effect, followed by Paradigm 1, Paradigm 2, and Paradigm 3. This type of summation of responses related to stimulus complexity could be presumed as evidence for topological organization of these cortical areas in men. It has been posited that the latter extends from the area implicated in object perception to a much greater area involved in facial perception [26]. This agrees with the object form topology hypothesis proposed by Ishai and colleagues [33]. However, the relatedness of object and facial perception was process-based, and appears to be associated with their common holistic processing strategy in the right hemisphere. Moreover, when the same men were presented with facial Paradigm 3 requiring analytic processing, the left hemisphere was activated. This agrees in principle with the suggestion made by Gauthier that the extrastriate cortex contains areas that are best suited for different computations, and described as the process-map model [34]. Therefore, the proposed models are not mutually exclusive, and this underscores the fact that facial processing does not impose any new constraints on the brain other than those used for other stimuli. It may be suggested that each stimulus was mapped by category into face or non-face, and by process into holistic or analytic. Therefore, a unified category-specific process-mapping system was implemented for either right or left cognitive styles.

Furthermore, in women, the neuronal assemblies may not have the same orderly topological arrangement as in men; rather the neurons involved in processing cone and rod vision were segregated within the right hemisphere cortical region. Hence, in women the right hemisphere responded to luminance effect and object perception, but showed no category-specific face effect. The latter arrangement explains the observed right lateralization for non-face Paradigm 1, but left lateralization for facial Paradigms 2 and 3. In other words, similar to men, women showed a tendency for holistic mechanism for processing object stimulus in the right hemisphere, but in contrast to men, they preferred the analytic mechanism for facial perception in the left hemisphere. Therefore, one major observed gender-related difference was that, while men employed a category-specific process-mapping system for facial processing in the right hemisphere, women used a category-specific process-mapping system for facial processing in the left hemisphere. In conclusion, it could be said that men and women use different hemispheres with complimentary mechanisms to perceive the essence of facial expressions that we come across in our daily life.

Author details

Philip C. Njemanze

Address all correspondence to: info@chidicon.com

International Institutes of Advanced Research and Training, Chidicon Medical Center, Owerri, Imo State, Nigeria

References

[1] Albers J: Interaction of color. New Haven: Yale University Press; 1963, 20-21.

[2] Daw N: Goldfish retina: organization for simultaneous color contrast. Science 1968, 158:942-944.

[3] Land EH, McCann JJ: Lightness and retinex theory. J Opto Soc Am 1971, 61:1-11.

[4] Livingstone MS, Hubel DH: Anatomy and physiology of color system in the primate visual cortex. J Neurosci 1984, 4:309-356.

[5] Dufort PA, Lumsden CJ: Color categorization and color constancy in a neural network model of V4. Biol Cybern 1991, 65:293-303.

[6] Foster DH, Nascimento SMC: Relational color constancy from invariant cone-excitation ratios. Proc R Soc Lond B Biol Sci 1994, 257:115-121.

[7] Kraft JM, Brainard DH: Mechanisms of color constancy under nearly natural viewing. Proc Natl Acad Sci USA 1999, 96:307-312.

[8] Conway BR: Spatial structure of cone inputs to color cells in alert Macaque primary visual cortex (V-1). J Neurosci 2001, 21:2768-2783.

[9] Itten J: The art of color; the subjective experience and objective rationale of color. Edited by: van Haa E translator. New York: Reinhol; 1966.

[10] Zeki S: A vision of the brain, plate 16. Cambridge MA: Blackwell Scientific; 1993.

[11] Njemanze PC: Asymmetric neuroplasticity of color processing during head down rest: a functional transcranial Doppler spectroscopy study. J Grav Physiol 2008, 15:49-59.

[12] Njemanze PC: Gender-related asymmetric brain vasomotor response to color stimulation: a functional transcranial Doppler spectroscopy study. Exp Transl Stroke Med 2010, 2:21-27.

[13] Jacobs GH, Neitz J: Color vision in squirrel monkeys: sex-related differences suggest the mode of inheritance. Vision Res 1985, 25:141-143.

[14] McCann JJ, Houston KL: Color sensation, color perception and mathematical models of color vision. In Color Vision: Physiology and Psychophysics. Edited by: Mollon JD, Sharpe LT. London: Academic Press; 1983.

[15] Gouras P: Cortical mechanisms of color vision. In The Perception of Color: Vision and Dysfunction. Edited by: Gouras P. England: Macmillan; 1991:179-197.

[16] Kentridge RW, Heywood CA, Weiskrantz L: Color contrast processing in human striate cortex. Proc Natl Acad Sci USA 2007, 104:15129-15131.

[17] Njemanze PC. Gender-related differences in physiologic color space: a functional transcranial Doppler (fTCD) study. Exp Transl Stroke Med 2011, 3:1-8.

[18] Lueck CJ, Zeki S, Friston KJ, Deiber MP, Cope P, Cunningham VJ, Lammertsma AA, Kennard C, Frackowiak RS: The color centre in the cerebral cortex of man. Nature 1989, 340:386-389.

[19] Till JS: Opthalmologic aspects of cerebrovascular disease. In Cerebrovascular Disorders. Edited by: Toole JF. New York, NY: Raven Press; 1984:231-250.

[20] Njemanze PC, Gomez CR, Horenstein S: Cerebral lateralisation and color perception: A transcranial Doppler study. Cortex 1992, 28:69-75.

[21] Zeki S, Marini L: Three cortical stages of color processing in the human brain. Brain 1998, 121:1669-1685.

[22] Njemanze PC: Asymmetry of cerebral blood flow velocity response to color processing and hemodynamic changes during -6 degrees 24-hour head-down bed rest in men. J Grav Physiol 2005, 12:33-41.

[23] Gray H, Clemente CD: Gray's anatomy of the human body. Philadelphia: Lippincott Williams and Wilkins;, 30 1984.

[24] Bliss TVP, Lomo T: Long-lasting potentiation of synaptic transmission in the dentate area of the anesthetized rabbit following stimulation of the preforant path. J Physiol 1973, 232:331-356.

[25] Ito M: Long-term depression. Ann Rev Neurosci 1989, 11:85-102.

[26] Njemanze PC: Cerebral lateralisation for facial processing: Gender-related cognitive styles determined using Fourier analysis of mean cerebral blood flow velocity in the middle cerebral arteries. Laterality 2007, 12:31-49.

[27] Njemanze, P C: Asymmetry in cerebral blood flow velocity with processing of facial images during head-down rest. Aviat Space Environ Med, 2004, 75:800-805.

[28] Everhart DE, Shucard JL, Quatrin T, Shucard DW: Sex-related differences in event-related potentials, face recognition, and facial affect processing in prepubertal children. J Neuropsychol, 2001, 15:329-431.

[29] Cahill L, Uncapher M, Kilpatrick L, Alkire MT, Turner J: Sex-related hemispheric lateralisation of amygdala function emotionally influences memory: An fMRI investigation. Learn Memory, 2004, 11:261-266.

[30] Njemanze PC: Cerebral lateralisation and general intelligence: Gender differences in a transcranial Doppler study. Brain Lang, 2005, 92:234-239.

[31] Tranel D, Damasio H, Denburg NL, Bechara, A: Does gender play a role in functional asymmetry of ventromedial prefrontal cortex? Brain 2005, 128:2872-2881.

[32] Jung RE, Haier RJ, Yeo RA, Rowland LM, Petropoulos H, Levine AS, Sibbitt WS, Brooks WM: Sex differences in N-acetylaspartate correlates of general intelligence: An 1H-MRS study of normal human brain. Neuroimage, 2005, 26:965-972.

[33] Ishai A, Ungerleider LG, Martin A, Schouten JL, Haxby JV: Distributed representation of objects in the human ventral visual pathway. Proc Natl Acad Sci USA 1999, 96:9379-9384.

[34] Gauthier I: What constrains the organisation of the ventral temporal cortex? Trends Cogn Sci 2000, 4:1-2.

[35] Bartley SH: Central mechanisms of vision. In J. Field, H. W. Magoun, & V. E. Hall (Eds.), Handbook of physiology, Section 1: Neurophysiology 1959, (Ch. 30, pp. 738-739). Washington, DC: American Physiological Society.

[36] Marinoni M, Ginanneschi A, Inzitari D, Mugnai S, Amaducci L. Sex-related differences in human cerebral hemodynamics. Acta Neurol Scand, 1998, 97:324-327.

[37] Muller HR, Brunholzl C, Radu E. W, Buser M. Sex and side differences of cerebral arterial caliber. Neuroradiology, 1991:33:212-216.

[38] McDonald DA. Blood flow in arteries 1974, pp. 311-350. Baltimore: Williams & Wilkins Co

[39] Meinders JM, Kornet L, Brands PJ, Hoeks AP. Assessment of local pulse wave velocity in arteries using 2D distension waveforms. Ultrasonography Imaging, 2001, 23:199-215.

[40] Kang HS, Han MH, Kwon BJ, Kwon OK, Kim SH, Chang KH. Evaluation of the lenticulostriate arteries with rotational angiography and 3D reconstruction. AJNR, 2005, 26:306-312.

[41] Campbell KB, Lee LC, Frasch HF, Noordergraaf A. Pulse reflection sites and effective length of the arterial system. Am J Physiol, 1989, 256:H1684-H1689.

[42] Peters M: Description and validation of a flexible and broadly usable hand preference questionnaire. Laterality 1998, 3:77-96.

[43] Frisén L: Clinical Tests of Vision. New York: Raven Press; 1990.

[44] Stroobant N, Vingerhoets G: Transcranial Doppler ultrasonography monitoring of cerebral hemodynamics during performance of cognitive tasks. A review. Neuropsychol Rev 2000, 10:213-231.

[45] Toole JF: Cerebrovascular Disorders. New York, NY: Raven Press; 1984.

[46] Knecht S, Deppe M, Drager B, Bobe L, Lohmann H, Ringelstein E, et al. (2000). Language lateralisation in healthy right-handers. Brain 2000, 123:74-81.

[47] Njemanze PC. Cerebral lateralisation in linguistic and nonlinguistic perception: Analysis of cognitive styles in the auditory modality. Brain Lang 1991, 41:367-380.

[48] Njemanze PC. Cerebral lateralisation in random letter task in the visual modality: A transcranial Doppler study. Brain Lang 1996, 53:315-325.

[49] Bowling A. Measuring disease (2nd ed.), 2001. Buckingham, UK: Open University Press.

[50] Spielberger CD, Ritterband LE, Sydeman SJ, Reheiser EC, Unger KK. Assessment of emotional states and personality traits: Measuring psychological vital signs. In J. N. Butcher (Ed.), Clinical personality assessment: Practical approaches. New York: Oxford University Press, 1995.

[51] Bartley SH: Central mechanisms of vision. In Handbook of Physiology, Section I: Neurophysiology. Edited by: Field J, Mogoun HW, Hall VE. Washington, D.C.: American Physiological Society; 1959:738-739.

[52] Thompson RF: Brain: A Neuroscience Primer. New York: Worth Publishers; 3, 2000.

[53] LeVay S, Wiesel TN, Hubel DH: The development of ocular dominance columns in normal and visually deprived monkeys. J Comp Neurol 1980, 191:1-51.

[54] Dacey DM: Parallel pathways for spectral coding in primate retina. Ann Rev Neurosci 2000, 23:743-775.

[55] Bear MF, Connors BW, Paradiso MA: Neuroscience: exploring the brain. Baltimore: Lippincott Williams & Wilkins;, 2 2001, 314-348.

[56] Kodak E: Kodak Photographic Filters Handbook Publication No. B-3. Rochester, New York: Eastman Kodak Company; 1990.

[57] Kim JJ, Andreasen NC, O'Leary DS,Wiser AK, Boles-Ponto, LL, Watkins GL, et al. Direct comparison of the neural substrates of recognition memory for words and faces. Brain 1999, 122:1069-1083.

[58] Sinha P, Poggio TI. I think I know that face. Nature 1996, 348:404.

[59] Allison T, Ginter H, McCarthy G, Nobre A, Puce A, Luby M, et al. Face recognition in human extrastriate cortex. J Neurophysiol 1994, 71:821-825.

[60] Jonsson P, Sonnby-Borgstrom M. The effects of pictures of emotional faces on tonic and phasic autonomic cardiac control in women and men. Biological Psychology 2003, 62:157-173.

[61] Bloomfield P. Fourier analysis of time series. An introduction . New York: Wiley, 1976.

[62] Brigham EO. The fast Fourier transform. New York: Prentice-Hall, 1974.

[63] Simmons WK, Ramjee V, Beauchamp MS, McRae K, Martin A, Barsalou LW: A common neural substrate for perceiving and knowing about color. Neuropsychol 2007, 45:2802-2810.

[64] Slotnick SD: Memory for color reactivates color processing region. NeuroReport 2009, 20:1568-1571.

[65] Squire LR: Memory and the hippocampus: a synthesis from findings with rats, monkeys, and humans. Psychol Rev 1992, 99:195-231.

[66] Schacter DL, Norman KA, Koutstaal W: The cognitive neuroscience of constructive memory. Annu Rev Psychol 1998, 49:289-318.

[67] Slotnick SD: Visual memory and visual perception recruit common neural substrates. Behav Cogn Neurosci Rev 2004, 3:207-221.

[68] Tootell RB, Hamilton SL: Functional anatomy of the second visual area (V2) in the macaque. J Neurosci 1989, 9:2620-2644.

[69] Jakobson LS, Pearson PM, Robertson B: Hue-specific colour memory impairment in an individual with intact colour perception and colour naming. Neuropsychologia 2008, 46:22-36.

[70] Kamiya A, Iwase S, Michikami D, Fu Q, Mano T, Kitaichi K, Takagi K: Increased vasomotor sympathetic nerve activity and decreased plasma nitric oxide release after head-down bed rest in humans: disappearance of correlation between vasoconstrictor and vasodilator. Neurosci Lett 2000, 281:21-24.

[71] Okamura TK, Ayajiki H, Fujioka K, Shinozaki K, Toda N: Neurogenic cerebral vasodilation mediated by nitric oxide. Jap J Pharmacol 2002, 88:32-38.

[72] Haghikia A, Mergia E, Friebe A, Eysel UT, Koesling D, Mittmann T: Longterm potentiation in the visual cortex requires both nitric oxide receptor guanylyl cyclases. J Neurosci 2007, 27:818-823.

[73] Xie X, Barrionuevo G, Berger TW: Differential expression of short-term potentiation by AMPA and NMDA receptors in dentate gyrus. Learn Mem 1996, 3:115-123.

[74] Escobar ML, Derrick B: Long-Term Potentiation and Depression as Putative Mechanisms for Memory Formation. In Neural Plasticity and Memory: From Genes to Brain Imaging. Edited by: Bermudez-Rattoni F. Boca Raton (FL): CRC Press; 2007

[75] Clark VP, Keil K, Maisog JM, Courtney S, Ungerleider LG, Haxby JV. (1996). Functional magnetic resonance imaging of human visual cortex during face matching: A comparison with positron emission tomography. Neuroimage 1996, 4:1-15.

[76] Haxby JV, Ungerleider LL, Horwitz B, Maisog JM, Rapoport SI, Grady CL. Face encoding and recognition in the human brain. Proc Natl Acad Sci USAS, 1996, 93:922-927.

[77] Puce A, Allison T, Asgari M, Gore JC, McCarthy G. Differential sensitivity of human visual cortex to faces, letter strings, and textures: A functional magnetic resonance imaging study. J Neurosci 1996, 16:5205-5215.

Chapter 7

Follicle Detection and Ovarian Classification in Digital Ultrasound Images of Ovaries

P. S. Hiremath and Jyothi R. Tegnoor

Additional information is available at the end of the chapter

http://dx.doi.org/10.5772/56518

1. Introduction

Some of the successful applications of the image processing techniques are in the area of medical imaging. The development of sophisticated imaging devices coupled with the advances in algorithms specific to the medical image processing both for diagnostics and therapeutic planning is the key to the wide popularity of the image processing techniques in the field of medical imaging. Ultrasound imaging is one of the methods of obtaining images from inside the human body through the use of high frequency sound waves. The reflected sound wave echoes are recorded and displayed as a real time visual image. It is a useful way of examining many of the body's internal organs including heart, liver, gall bladder, kidneys and ovaries. The detection of follicles in ultrasound images of ovaries is concerned with the follicle monitoring during the diagnostic process of infertility treatment of patients.

For women undergoing assisted reproductive therapy, the ovarian ultrasound imaging has become an effective tool in infertility management. Among the many causes, ovulatory failure or dysfunction is the main cause for infertility. Thus, an ovary is the most frequently ultrasound scanned organ in an infertile woman. Determination of ovarian status and follicle monitoring constitute the first step in the evaluation of an infertile woman. Infertility can also be associated with the growth of a dominant follicle beyond a preovulatory diameter and subsequent formation of a large anovulatory follicle cyst. The ovary is imaged for its morphology (normal, polycystic or multicystic), for its abnormalities (cysta, dermoids, endometriomas, tumors etc), for its follicular growth in ovulation monitoring, for evidence of ovulation and corpus luteum formation and function. Ovulation scans allow the doctor to determine accurately when the egg matures and when it ovulates. Daily scans are done to visualize the growing follicle, which looks like a black bubble on the screen of the ultrasound imaging machine.

1.1. Ovarian types

The outcome of ovarian evaluation is the classification of the ovary into one of the three types of ovaries, namely, normal ovary, cystic ovary and polycystic ovary, which are described below :

i. Normal ovary with antral/dominant follicles

A normal ovary consists of 8-10 follicles from 2mm to 28mm in size [1]. The group of follicles with less than 18mm in size are called antral follicles, and the size in the range of 18-28mm are known as dominant follicles. In a normal menstrual cycle with ovulation, a mature follicle, which is also a cystic structure, develops [2]. The size of a mature follicle that is ready to ovulate is about 18-28mm in diameter. During the past 50 years, it has been accepted that folliculogenesis begins with recruitment of a group or cohort of follicles in the late luteal phase of the preceding menstrual cycle followed by visible follicle growth in the next follicular phase [3]. The group or cohort of follicles begins growth and by the mid-follicular phase, around day 7, a single dominant follicle appears to be selected from the group for accelerated growth [4]. The dominant follicle continues to grow at a rate of about 2mm per day. In women, a preovulatory follicle typically measures 18–28mm when a surge of luteinizing hormone (LH) is released from the pituitary to trigger ovulation; ovulation occurs approximately 36 hours after LH release [5]. The Figure 1 shows an ultrasound image of normal ovary with dominant follicles.

ii. Ovarian cyst

An ovarian cyst is simply a collection of fluid within the normal solid ovary. There are many different types of ovarian cysts, and they are an extremely common gynaecologic problem. Because of the fear of ovarian cancer, cysts are a common cause of concern among women. But, it is important to know that the vast majority of ovarian cysts are not cancer. However, some benign cysts will require treatment, in that they do not go away by themselves, and in quite rare cases, others may be cancerous [6]. The most common types of ovarian cysts are called functional cysts, which result from a collection of fluid forming around a developing egg. Every woman who is ovulating will form a small amount of fluid around the developing egg each month. The combination of the egg, the special fluid-producing cells, and the fluid is called a follicle and is normally about the size of a pea. For unknown reasons, the cells that surround the egg occasionally form too much fluid, and this straw colored fluid expands the ovary from within. If the collection of fluid gets to be larger than a normal follicle, about three-quarters of an inch in diameter, a follicular cyst is said to be present. If fluid continues to be formed, the ovary is stretched as if a balloon was being filled up with water. The covering of the ovary, which is normally white, becomes thin and smooth and appears as a bluish-grey. Rarely, though, follicular cysts may become as large as 3 or 4 inches [7]. The Figure 2 shows an ultrasound image of cystic ovary.

iii. Polycystic ovary

The typical polycystic appearance is defined by the presence of 12 or more follicles measuring less than 9mm in diameter arranged peripherally around a dense core of stroma [8]. Other ultrasound features include enlarged ovaries, increased number of follicles and density of

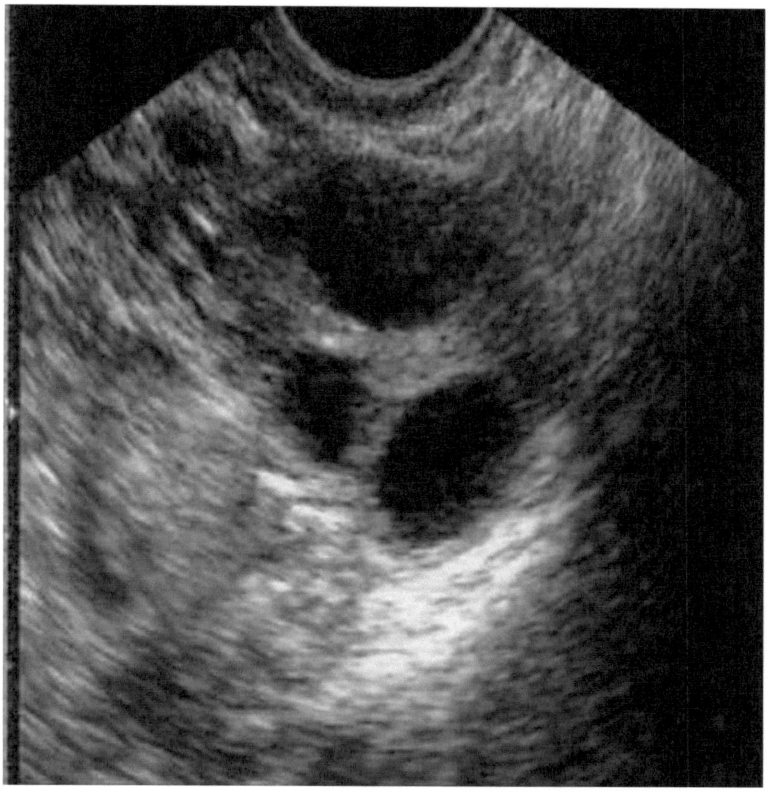

Figure 1. Ultrasound image of a normal ovary with dominant follicles

ovarian stroma. The current ultrasound guidelines supported by ESHRE/ASRM consensus characterize the polycystic ovary as containing 12 or more follicles measuring 2–9mm [9]. The basic difference between polycystic and normal ovaries is that, although the polycystic ovaries contain many small antral follicles with eggs in them, the follicles do not develop and mature properly, and hence, there is no ovulation [10]. The infertility incidence with polycystic ovaries is very high. These women usually will have difficulty in getting pregnant and, hence, invariably require treatment to improve chances for pregnancy. In a polycystic ovary, the numerous small cystic structures, also called antral follicles, give the ovaries a characteristic "polycystic" (many cysts) appearance in ultrasound image. It is referred to as polycystic ovarian syndrome (PCOS/PCOD) [11]. Since women with polycystic ovaries do not ovulate regularly, they do not get regular menstrual periods. The Figure 3 shows an ultrasound image of ovary with PCOD.

A computer assisted diagnostic procedure is desirable because of tedious and time consuming nature of the manual follicle segmentation and ovarian classification done by medical experts. In the present book chapter, the objective of study is to design algorithms for follicle detection and ovarian classification in ultrasound ovarian images in order to assist medical diagnosis in infertility treatment using digital image processing techniques.

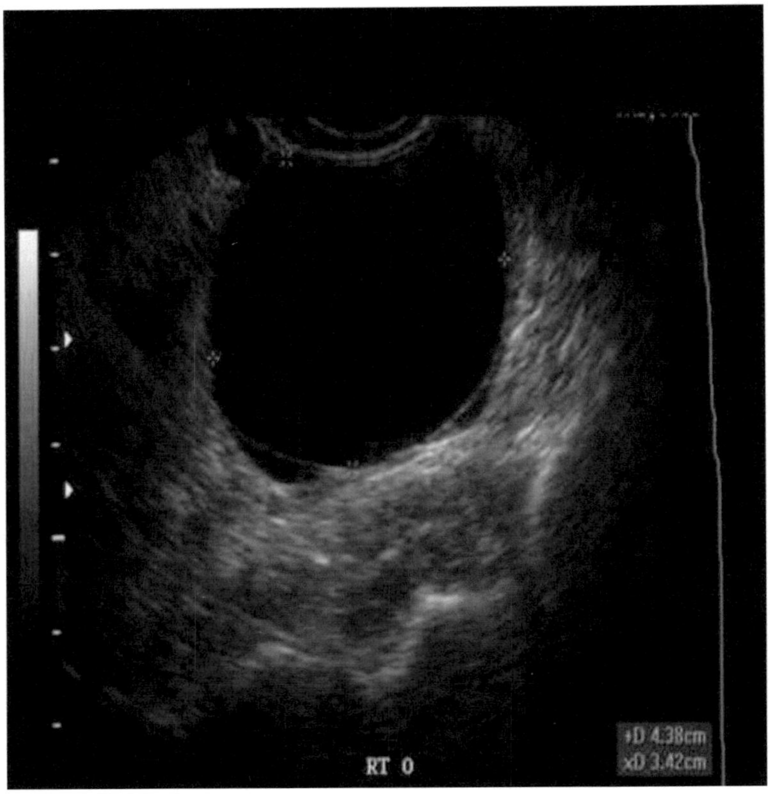

Figure 2. Ultrasound image of a cystic ovary

1.2. Background literature

In [12,13], follicular ultrasound images are segmented using an optimal thresholding method applied to coarsely estimated ovary. However, this fully automated method, using the edges for estimation of ovary boundaries and thresholding as a segmentation method, doesn't give optimal results. In [14], this method has been upgraded using active contours and, consequently, the segmentation quality of recognized follicles is considerably improved. Edges of recognized objects were much closer to the real follicle boundaries. However, the determination of suitable parameters for snakes automatically is problematic. In [15], region growing based segmentation method is used for the follicle detection. In [16], a semi automated method is proposed for the outer follicle wall segmentation, wherein a frequent manual tracing of the inner border of all follicles is done. In [17], cellular automata and cellular neural networks are employed for the follicle segmentation. The results are found to be very promising but an obvious drawback of these two methods is the difficulty in determination of the required parameters for follicle segmentation. In [18], the authors have determined the inner border of all follicles using watershed segmentation techniques. Watershed segmentation was applied on smoothed image data which merged some small adjacent follicles. Therefore binary mathematical morphology was employed to separate such areas adhoc in some steps. In [19],

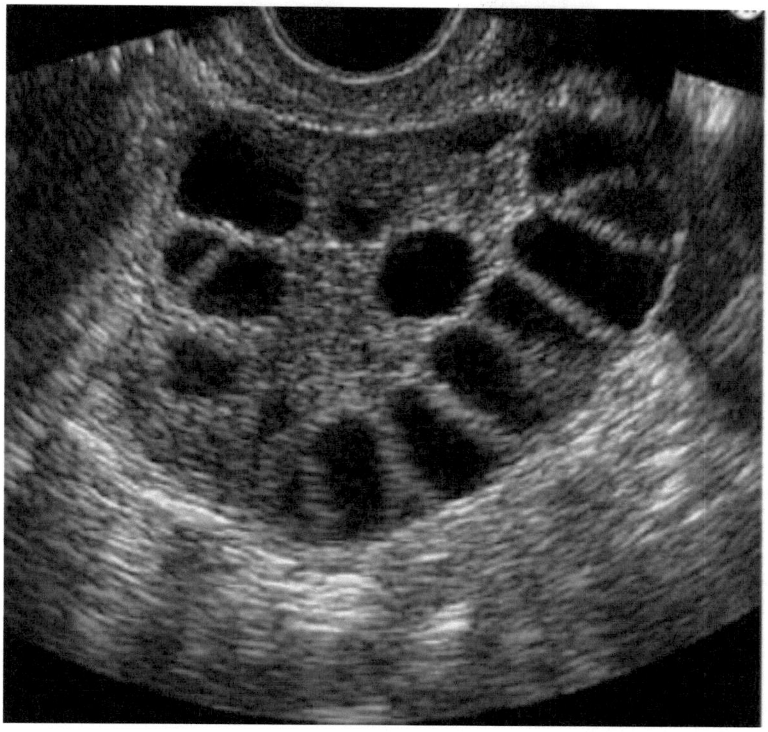

Figure 3. Ultrasound image of an ovary with PCOD

the authors have reported follicle segmentation based on modified region growing method for the follicle segmentation and linear discriminant classifier for the purpose of classification. In [20], the scanline thresholding method is used for the follicle detection and the segmentation performance is measured in terms of the mean square error (MSE).

The follicles are the regions of interest (ROIs) in an ovarian ultrasound image, which need to be detected by using image processing techniques. This is basically an object recognition problem. Thus, the basic image processing steps, namely, preprocessing, segmentation, feature extraction and classification, apply. In the literature, the authors have employed various techniques for ultrasound image processing, as shown below:

1. Preprocessing

   – Gaussian low pass filter

   – Homogeneous region growing mean filter (HRGMF)

   – Contourlet transform

2. Segmentation

   – Optimal thresholding

   – Edge based method

- Watershed transform
- Scanline thresholding
- Active contour method

3. Feature extraction
   - Geometric features
   - Texture features

4. Classification
   - 3σ interval based classifier.
   - K-NN classifier
   - Linear discriminant classifier
   - Fuzzy classifier
   - SVM classifier

1.3. Image data set

For the purpose of experimentation, the databases D1, D2 and D3, of ultrasound images of ovaries are prepared in consultation with the medical expert, namely, Radiologist and Gyneocologist, for the present study of the follicle detection and ovarian classification in ovarian images. Some of the images are captured by the Toshiba [Model SSA-320A/325A] diagnostic ultrasound system with the transvaginal transducer frequency 26 Hz. Some of the images are obtained from the publicly available websites [www.radiologyinfo.com; www.ovaryresearch.com]. The image dataset D1 consists of the 80 ultrasound ovarian images, with the size 256x256. The image dataset D2 consists of the 90 ultrasound ovarian images, with the size 512x512. The image dataset D3 consists of the 70 ultrasound ovarian images, with the size 512x512. It contains the images of 30 normal (healthy) ovaries, 20 polycystic ovaries and 20 cystic ovaries.

2. Follicle detection

The methods employed by [Hiremath and Tegnoor] for follicle detection based on different segmentation, feature extraction and classification techniques are described below:

a. Edge based method

The automatic method for the detection of follicles in ultrasound images of ovaries using edge based method uses, Gaussian lowpass filter for preprocessing, canny operator for edge detection for segmentation, 3σ-intervals around the mean for the purpose of classification [21]. The experimentation has been done using sample ultrasound images of ovaries and the results

http://dx.doi.org/10.5772/56518

are compared with the inferences drawn by medical expert. Initially, the image is processed with Gaussian low pass filter yielding denoised image. Then canny operator is applied to detect the edges from the denoised image. Morphological dilation is performed by using the disk shaped structuring element with radius 1 to fill the weak edges. which yields the segmented image. Possible holes inside the segmented regions are filled. Any spurious regions due to noise are eliminated by morphological erosion. The regions in segmented image having smaller area than the threshold T (empirical value) are removed. The segmented regions are labeled. Set all the nonzero pixels of the border of segmented image to zero, which yields the final segmented image. Thus the plausible follicle regions are the labeled segments.

The geometric features are extracted for the known follicle regions. The main aim of geometric feature extraction is to recognize geometric properties of ovarian follicles in ultrasound images. The ovarian follicles are oval shaped compact structures, which resemble the circular/ellipse and are, thus, characterized by the seven geometric features, namely, the area A, the ratio R of majoraxislength to minoraxislength, the compactness Cp, the circularity Cr, the tortousity Tr, the extent E and the centriod $Y = \frac{1}{B^2} \sum_{i,j=1}^{B} CS_{-i,-j}\left(F^{-1}(\Lambda(F(CS_{i,j}(X))))\right)$.

The classification stage comprises two steps, namely, the training phase and the testing phase.

Training phase: In the training phase, the geometrical features, are computed for regions known to be follicles in the training images in consultation with the medical expert. Then, the sample means and standard deviations of the geometric parameters R, Cp, Cr, Tr, E and, $C = (Cx, Cy)$ are computed which are used to set the rules for classification of labelled segments into follicles and non-follicles. The $\overline{R}$, $\overline{Cp}$, $\overline{Cr}$, $\overline{Tr}$, $\overline{E}$, $(\overline{Cx}, \overline{Cy})$ denote the mean values, and, the σ_R, σ_{Cp}, σ_{Cr}, σ_{Tr}, σ_E, $(\sigma_{Cx}, \sigma_{Cy})$ denote the standard deviation values, of the geometric parameters R, Cp, Cr, Tr, E and C=(Cx,Cy).

Now, the classification rules for follicle recognition are formulated as following: A region with area A, ratio R, compactness Cp, circularity Cr, Tortousity Tr, extent E, and centriod $C = (Cx, Cy)$, is classified as a follicle, if the following conditions are satisfied:

$$A > T_A \tag{1}$$

$$\overline{R} - \alpha\sigma_R < R < \overline{R} + \alpha\sigma_R \tag{2}$$

$$\overline{Cp} - \alpha\sigma_{Cp} < Cp < \overline{Cp} + \alpha\sigma_{Cp} \tag{3}$$

$$\overline{Cr} - \alpha\sigma_{Cr} < Cr < \overline{Cr} + \alpha\sigma_{Cr} \tag{4}$$

$$\overline{Tr} - \alpha\sigma_{Tr} < Tr < \overline{Tr} + \alpha\sigma_{Tr} \tag{5}$$

$$\overline{E} - \alpha\sigma_{E} < \mathrm{E} < \overline{E} + \alpha\sigma_{E} \tag{6}$$

$$\overline{Cx} - \alpha\sigma_{Cx} < Cx < \overline{Cx} + \alpha\sigma_{Cx} \tag{7}$$

$$\overline{Cy} - \alpha\sigma_{Cy} < Cy < \overline{Cy} + \alpha\sigma_{Cy} \tag{8}$$

The constants T_A and α are empirically determined. In our experiments, we have determined that the empirical values are T_A =30, α=3. The equations (1) to (8) constitute the 3σ-classifier, which is to be used in the testing phase.

Testing phase : During the testing phase, the area A, the ratio R, the compactness Cp, the circularity Cr, the tortousity Tr, the extent E and the centriod, $C=(Cx, Cy)$ are computed for a region of the segmented image and apply the above classification rules to determine whether it is a follicle or not. The comparison of the experimental results for the two sample images with the manual segmentation done by medical expert is presented in the Figure 4. There is good agreement between the segmented image and the manual segmentation done by the medical expert, which demonstrates the efficiency of the edge based method. The manual segmentation is done by the team of three medical experts (Radiologists (2) and Gynaecologist (1)).

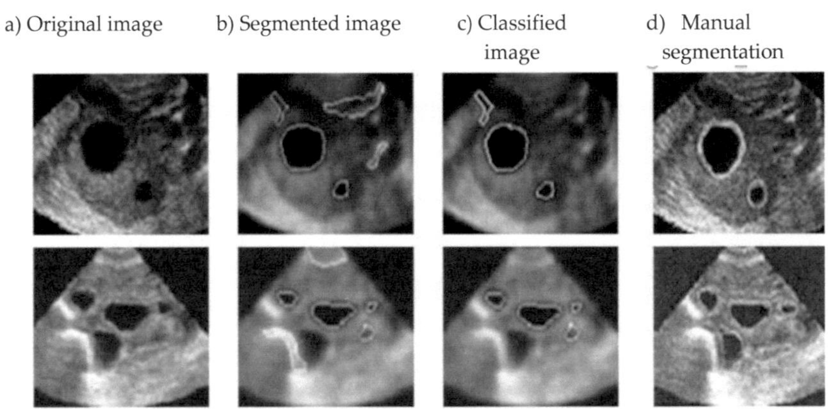

Figure 4. Some typical results: a) Original images, b) Segmentation by edge based method, c) Classified image, d) Manual segmentation by medical expert.

http://dx.doi.org/10.5772/56518

b. Watershed segmentation method

The follicle detection in ultrasound images of ovaries using watershed segmentation method uses the watershed transform for segmentation, geometric features for feature extraction and 3σ-intervals around the mean for the purpose of classification [22]. We follow three steps in the segmentation, first, the internal marker image is obtained, second, external marker image is obtained, and third, modifying gradient of the original image, by mask. In next phase, segmentation is carried out by applying marker controlled watershed transform to modified gradient image, region filling and clearing the border. Finally, preserve the regions which are most probably appear as follicles, while all other regions are removed. The feature extraction is based on seven geometric parameters of the follicles and the classification of regions for follicle detection is based on 3σ intervals around the mean. The experimental results are in good agreement with the manual follicle detection by medical experts.

c. Optimal thresholding method

In the automatic detection of follicle in ultrasound images of ovaries using optimal thresholding method, sobel operator and morphological opening and closing is used for preprocessing, optimal thresholding for segmentation and 3σ-intervals around the mean for classification are used [23]. Initially, the image is processed with finding the gradient by using sobel operators in horizontal direction. For the gradient image morphological opening and closing is applied by using appropriate structuring element. Then thresholding is applied to the filtered image by optimal thresholding method [24]. In the process, many undesired spurious regions are also obtained (e.g., regions inside the endometrium). These spurious regions must be removed as much as possible and all regions touching the borders are removed, which yields the segmented image. The feature extraction is based on seven geometric parameters of the follicles and the classification of regions for follicle detection is based on 3σ intervals around the mean. The experimental results are in good agreement with the manual follicle detection by medical experts.

2.1. HRGMF and thresholding

Ultrasound ovary images show planar sections through the follicles. These images are characterized by specular reflections and edge information, which is weak and discontinuous. Therefore, traditional edge detection techniques (e.g. Sobel, Prewitt) are susceptible to spurious responses when applied to ultrasound imagery. The main reason, that the follicle segmentation using solely edge information is rather unsuccessful, is a high level of added speckle noise [25]. The follicles being fluid-filled sacs appear as dark oval regions because they display similar fluid echotextures, which are more or less darker than their neighbourhood. The follicles could therefore be treated as homogeneous dark regions.

The main idea behind the HRGMF based method is as follows: [26]: In the first phase, the homogeneous region growing mean filter (HRGMF) is applied [27]. By using this filter, first homogeneous region can be identified and then this region is grown until it satisfies the similarity criteria. The value of filtering point is replaced by arithmetic mean of the grown region. In next phase, segmentation is carried out, by binarising the filtered image with three different thresholds, T1, set as standard deviation of the input image, T2, set as mean of the input image, T3, set as abs(T2-T1). The resultant images are combined after thresholding. The components are labelled, the holes inside the regions are filled, the borders if any are cleared. Finally, the regions which most probably appear as follicles are preserved, while all other regions are removed. The feature extraction is based on seven geometric parameters of the follicles and the classification of regions for follicle detection is based on 3σ intervals around the mean.

The experimentation has been done using two datasets D1 and D2. The D1 set consists of the 80 sample ultrasound ovarian images of size 256x256, out of which 40 images are used for training and 40 for testing. The D2 set consists of 90 sample ultrasound images of ovaries of size 512x512, out of which 45 images are used for training and 45 for testing. The ten-fold experiments are performed for the classification and the average follicle detection rate is computed.The Table 1 shows the classification results of the proposed method after ten-fold experiments for both the data sets D1 and D2. The average detection rates for the proposed method with D1 and D2 sets are 79.77% and 68.86%, false acceptance rates (FAR) are 25.99% and 28.41%, and false rejection rates (FRR) are 20.52% and 31.12%, respectively.

	Classification results for ten-fold experiments	
Data set	D1 set	D2 set
Classification rate	79.77%	68.86%
Type I error (FAR)	25.99%	28.41%
Type II error(FRR)	20.52%	31.12%

Table 1. Classification results of proposed method after ten-fold experiments.

The proposed HRGMF based method for follicle detection is more effective as compared to the edge based method, watershed based segmentation method and optimal thresholding methods. The experimental results are in good agreement with the manual follicle detection by medical experts, and thus demonstrate efficacy of the method. Thus, the proposed HRGMF based method for follicle segmentation is effective in computer assisted fertility diagnosis by the experts.

2.2. Contourlet transform and scanline thresholding

The follicle detection rate in the homogeneous region growing mean filter (HRGMF) based method is considerably improved. However, due to speckle noise, finding the object boundaries is difficult and thus leads to poor segmentation. To improve the segmentation accuracy, the contourlet transform is used for despeckling the ultrasound image followed by histogram equalization, and, thereafter, the horizontal and vertical scanline thresholding (HVST) method is employed for follicle detection using geometric parameters.

Contourlet transform : The first step of the algorithm is denoising the image, since ultrasound images are invariably noisy due to the mode of the image acquisition itself. (e.g. head of the ultrasound device is not moist enough). Especially, a disturbing type of noise is the speckle noise. Therefore the more efficient speckle reduction method based on the contourlet transform is used for denoising medical ultrasound images [28]. The contourlets can be loosely interpreted as a grouping of nearby wavelet coefficients since their locaters are locally correlated due to smoothness of the boundary curve [29, 30]. The contourlet transform is a multiscale and multidirectional framework of discrete image [31]. It is the simple directional extension for wavelet that fixes its subband mixing problem and improves its directionality. In this transform, the multiscale and multidirectional analyses are separated in a serial way. The laplacian pyramid (LP), is first used to capture the point discontinuities followed by a directional filter bank (DFB) to link point discontinuities into linear structure. Thus, we perform a wavelet like transform for edge detection, and then a local directional transform for contour segment detection. In other words, the contourlet transform comprises a double filter bank approach for obtaining sparse expansions for typical images with contours.

The contourlet transform exploits smoothness of contour effectively by considering variety of directions following contour. The contourlet transform can be designed to be a tight frame along with thresholding in order to achieve denoising of the image more effectively. The algorithm for contourlet transform method is as follows [32,33] : Firstly, apply the log transform to the input ultrasound image. Then, apply the contourlet transform on the log transformed image upto n levels of Laplacian pyramidal decomposition and m directional decompositions at each level, where n and m depend on the image size. Next, perform thresholding of contourlet transformed image. Lastly, the despeckled image is obtained by performing inverse contourlet transform on the thresholded image. Then, histogram equalization is applied to enhance the contrast of the despeckled image.

i. Horizontal and Vertical Scanline (HVST) based method

Firstly, all the pixels which are darker than their neighborhood row wise (horizontal scan) and then column wise (vertical scan) is collected. Then, the two resultant images are added to yield a segmented image. The regions with area less than a threshold value are removed. The holes inside the region are filled. The nonzero pixels touching the image border are set to zero [34,35].

Horizontal Scanline Thesholding (HST) : The follicle region will have more or less same grey level value for all the pixels within it. The horizontal scanline thresholding method is described as follows; Consider the input image f of the size MxN. The sample mean m_i and standard deviation σ_i of the ith row subimage of f are given by the equations 9 and 10 :

$$m_i = \frac{1}{N}\sum_{j=1}^{N} f(i,j) \tag{9}$$

$$\sigma_i = \sqrt{\left(\frac{1}{N}\sum_{j=1}^{N}(f(i,j) - m_i)^2\right)} \tag{10}$$

Now, set T4 = m_i and T5 = σ_i. Then multiply T4 and T5 by positive scale factors K1 and K2 (empirically fixed). Binarize ith row subimage using the thresholds K1T4 and K2T5 separately. This procedure is carried out for the rows i=1,...,M and obtain the horizontal mean (standard deviation) thresholded image fhm (fhsd).

Vertical Scanline Thresholding (VST): The VST method is described as follows; Consider the input image f of the size MxN. The sample mean m_j and standard deviation σ_j of the jth column subimage are given by the equations 11 and 12:

$$m_j = \frac{1}{M}\sum_{i=1}^{M} f(i,j) \tag{11}$$

$$\sigma_j = \sqrt{\frac{1}{M}\sum_{i=1}^{M}(f(i,j) - m_j)^2} \tag{12}$$

Now, set T6 = m_j and T7 = σ_j. Then multiply T6 and T7 by positive scale factors K3 and K4 (empirically fixed), respectively. Binarize jth column subimage using thresholds K3T6 and K4T7 separately. This procedure is carried out for the columns j=1,...,N and obtain the vertical mean (standard deviation) thresholded image fvm (fvsd).

Image Fusion: The resultant images fhm and fvm are combined, to yield the image fhvm. Any region touching the borders are removed. The resultant images fhsd and fvsd are combined, to yield the image fhvsd. Any region touching the borders are removed. Finally, the resultant images fhvm and fhvsd are combined, to yield the segmented image fseg, which contains segmented regions in it. The regions in fseg having smaller area than the threshold T8 are removed. The regions are labeled (identified) and possible holes inside them are filled.

The geometric features are extracted and then 3σ-intervals around the mean are used for classification. The Table 2 shows the classification results of the HVST based method after ten-fold experiments for both the data sets D1 and D2. The average detection rates for the proposed Method I with D1 and D2 sets are 90.10% and 92.76%, false acceptance rates (FAR) are 11.71% and 9.89%, and false rejection rates (FRR) are 21.55% and 7.23%, respectively.

	Classification results for ten-fold experiments	
Data set	D1 set	D2 set
Classification rate	90.10%	92.76%
Type I error (FAR)	11.71%	21.55%
Type II error(FRR)	9.89%	7.23%

Table 2. Classification results of proposed method after ten-fold experiments.

ii. *Edge based method:* The edge based segmentation method, which is described in the section 2 (a), is applied to the histogram equalized image obtained after despeckling the input image using contourlet transform [36]. The follicle detection rate is improved in the edge based segmentation after applying contourlet transform and histogram equalization, as compared to the method in the section 2(a) which employs Gaussian low pass filter and edge based segmentation.

The HVST based method for the follicle detection is more effective as compared to edge based segmentation after applying contourlet transform and histogram equalization.

3. Active contour method for follicle detection

The active contour method is used for segmentation of ultrasound image to increase the follicle detection accuracy. Either 3σ intervals based classifier or fuzzy classifier may be employed for follicle detection.

i. Active contour method with 3σ intervals based classification

The follicle detection in ultrasound images of ovaries using active contour method uses the contourlet transform based method for preprocessing, active contour method for segmentation and 3σ-intervals around the mean for classification [37]. Initially, the input image is despekled by using the contourlet transform method. Next, histogram equalization is applied to enhance the contrast of the despeckled image. Further, the negative transformation is applied on the histogram equalized image [38], as the proposed segmentation method works on high intensity valued objects. In the segmentation stage, the active contour without edges method is used [39]. The resulting image after applying active contour method contains segmented regions with it. The geometric features are extracted and then 3σ-intervals around the mean is used for classification.

The Figure 5 (a) depicts sample original ultrasound image of the ovary. The resultant images obtained at different steps of the proposed method are shown in the Figure 5 (b)-(e). Many undesired spurious regions are also obtained (e.g., regions inside the endometrium). These spurious regions must be removed as much as possible. Therefore, the regions having an area less than T (empirical value) are removed (Figure 5(f)). The Figure 5(g) depicts the segmented follicles (outlined in white) superimposed on the original image. The Figure 5(h) depicts the recognized follicles after applying the classification rules and the Figure 5(i) shows the follicles annotated manually by the medical expert.

The Figure 6 depicts comparison of the active contour method with the HVST based segmentation method. In the Figure 6, (a) and (e) are two original images, while (b) and (f) are their corresponding segmented images by HVST method. Similarly, (c) and (g) are segmented images of active contour method. It is observed that the follicles, which were not detected by HVST based segmentation method (Figure 6 (b) and (f)), are correctly identified by the active contour method (Figure 6 (c) and (g)). The Figure 6 (d) and (h) show the manual segmentation rendered by the medical expert. Hence, the classification accuracy is improved in the active

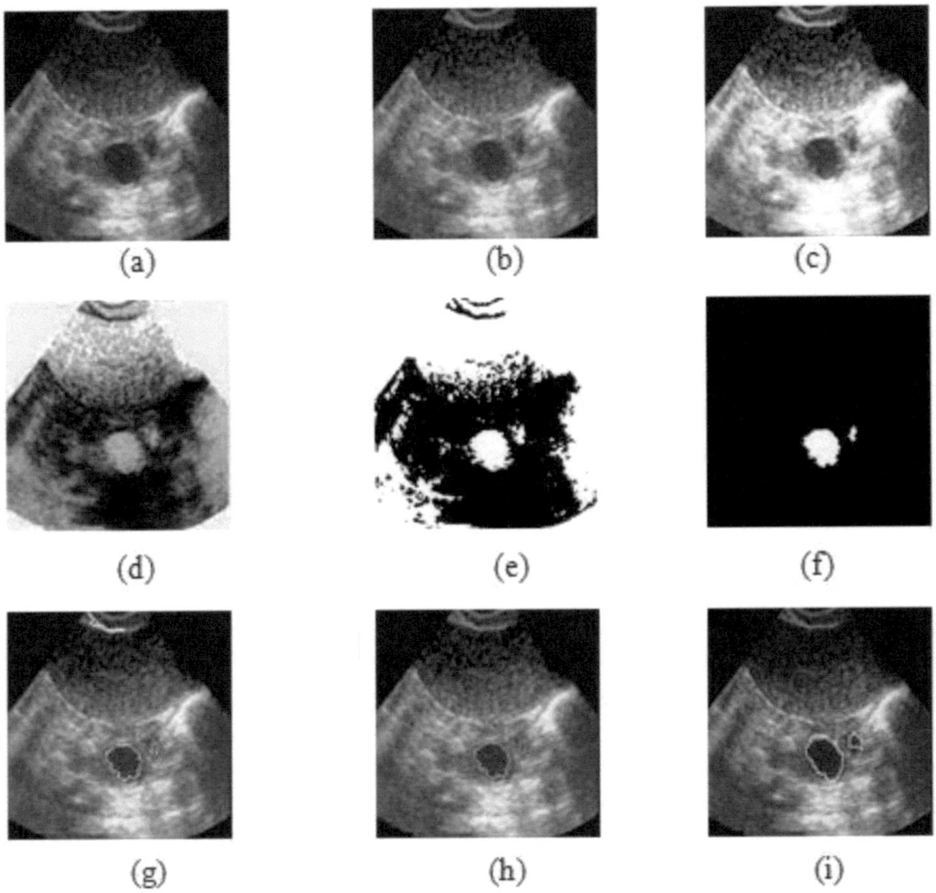

Figure 5. Original ultrasound image of the ovary and resultant images at different steps of proposed method. a) Original image, b) Contourlet transformed image (despeckling), c) Histogram equalized image, d) Image after applying negative transformation, e) Image after applying active contour without edges method, f) Segmented image after clearing the border, filling the holes and removing the small regions, g) Image showing recognized follicles(outlined in white) super imposed on the original image, h) Output image after classification, i) Manual segmentation of follicles by medical expert.

contour method as compared to HVST based segmentation method. The Table 3 presents the comparison of the experimental results of active contour method and HVST based method obtained for the original images in Figure 6. It is observed that the HVST based method leads to higher false acceptance rate (FAR) and false rejection rate (FRR). Further, the active contour method is found to yield more accurate results.

The Table 4 shows the comparison of classification results of the active contour method and the HVST based method after performing ten-fold experiments for both the data sets D1 and D2. The average detection rates for the active contour method using D1 and D2 sets are 92.3% and 96.66%, false acceptance rates (FAR) are 13.90% and 15.04%, and false rejection rates (FRR)

http://dx.doi.org/10.5772/56518

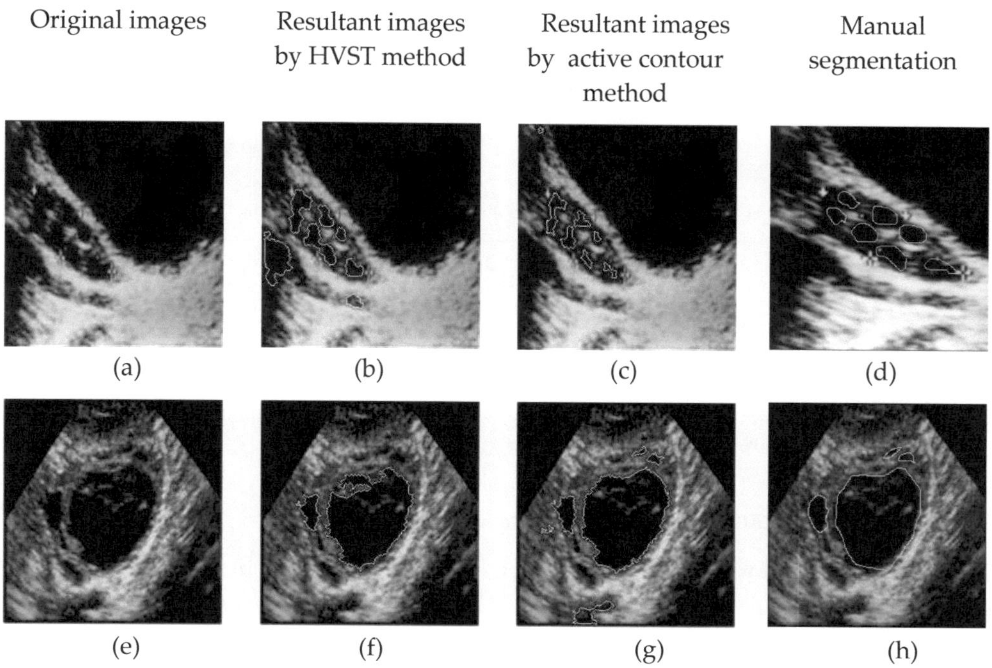

Figure 6. Comparison of resultant images of the active contour method with the HVST based method for two different original images. (a) and (e) original image, (b) and (f) resultant images of HVST method, (c) and (g) resultant images of the active contour method, (d) and (h) manual segmentation by medical expert.

Original Image	Number of follicles detected						
	Active contour method			HVST based method			Manual (by medical expert)
	Total	Correct	False	Total	Correct	False	
Figure 6 (a)	6	6	-	6	5	1	7
Figure 6 (e)	6	4	2	2	2	-	4

Table 3. Comparison of experimental results of active contour method and HVST based method for original images in Figure 6.

are 7.62% and 3.33%, respectively. The average detection rates for the HVST based method using D1 and D2 sets are 90.29% and 92.76%, false acceptance rates (FAR) are 14.10% and 21.55%, and false rejection rates (FRR) are 9.60% and 7.23%, respectively. Clearly, the method based on active contours outperforms the HVST based method.

Classification results				
Data set	**D1 set**		**D2 set**	
Method	Active contour method	HVST based method	Active contour method	HVST based method Based Method
Classification rate	92.3%	90.29%	96.66%	92.76%
Type I error (FAR)	13.90%	14.10%	15.04%	21.55%
Type II error (FRR)	7.62%	9.60%	3.33%	7.23%

Table 4. Comparison of average classification results of the active contour method with the HVST based method after performing ten-fold experiments.

ii. Active contour method with fuzzy classification

To improve the performance of follicle detection in ultrasound images of ovaries, a new algorithm using fuzzy logic is developed. The method employs contourlet transform for despeckling, histogram equalization and negative transformation in the preprocessing step, the active contours without edges method for segmentation and fuzzy logic for classification. The seven geometric features are used as inputs to the fuzzy logic block of the Fuzzy Inference System (FIS). The output of the fuzzy logic block is a follicle class or non follicle class. The fuzzy-knowledge-base consists of a set of physically interpretable if-then rules providing physical insight into the process. The experimentation has been done using sample ultrasound images of ovaries and the results are compared with the inferences drawn by 3σ interval based classifier and also those drawn by the medical expert. The experimental results demonstrate the efficacy of the fuzzy logic based method [40].

Fuzzy set theory has been successfully applied to many fields, such as pattern recognition, control systems, and medical applications [41,42]. It has also been effectively used to develop various techniques in image processing tasks including ultrasound images [43]. The existence of inherent "fuzziness" in the nature of these images in terms of uncertainties associated with definition of edges, boundaries, and contrast makes fuzzy set theory an interesting tool for handling the ultrasound imaging applications [44]. Fuzzy logic was initiated in 1965 by L. A. Zadeh [45-48].

Training phase: The fuzzy inference system (FIS) of sugeno type is employed using the fuzzy input variables the ratio R of majoraxislength to minoraxislength, the compactness Cp, the circularity Cr, the tortuousity Tr, the extent E and the centriod C= (Cx, Cy) and output variables: follicle and non follicle classes. The Gaussian membership function is used for each of the fuzzy input variables with mean and standard deviation of the corresponding variables. Let mfr, mfcp, mfcr, mftr, mfe, mfcx and mfcy be the Gaussian membership functions of the fuzzy input variables R, Cp, Cr, Tr, E and C=(Cx,Cy), respectively, belonging to the follicle class. Let mfr1, mfcp1, mfcr1, mftr1, mfe1, mfcx1 and mfcy1 be the Gaussian membership functions of these input variables belonging to the non-follicle class.

During the training phase, the geometrical features, namely, R, Cp, Cr, Tr, E and C=(Cx,Cy), are computed for regions known to be follicles in the training images in consultation with the medical expert. Then, the mean and standard deviation of each of the geometric parameters R, Cp, Cr,Tr, E and C=(Cx,Cy), are computed which are used to set the rules for classification of follicles. The mean and standard deviation of these parametric values are stored as knowledge base which is shown in the Table 5. These values are used as the pattern (parameters) in FIS membership function design.

	Mean value	**Standard deviation**
Ratio(R)	1.82	0.58
Compactness (C_p)	37.35	10.16
Circularity (C_r)	0.37	0.09
Tortousity (T_r)	0.27	0.03
Extent (E)	0.51	0.09
Centriod C=(Cx,Cy)	(251, 55)	(201,70)

Table 5. The knowledge base of mean and standard deviation of parametric values of geometric features or the follicle regions

The construction of the membership functions for the output variables is done in the similar manner. Since this is Sugeno-type inference (precisely, zero-order Sugeno), constant type of output variable fits the best to the given set of outputs (1 for follicle and 0 to non-follicle classes). Based on the descriptions of the inputs (the ratio R of majoraxislength to minoraxislength, the compactness Cp, the circularity Cr, the tortousity Tr, the extent E and the centriod C=(Cx,Cy)) and output variables (follicle and non follicle). The fuzzy rules for classification procedure in verbose format are as follows:

i. IF (R is input to mfr) AND (Cp is input to mfcp) AND (Cr is input to mfcr) AND (Tr is input to mftr) AND (E is input to mfe) AND (Cx is input to mfcx) AND (Cy is input to mfcy) THEN (class is follicle)

ii. IF (R is input to mfr1) AND (Cp is input to mfcp1) AND (Cr is input to mfcr1) AND (Tr is input to mftr1) AND (E is input to mfe1) AND (Cx is input to mfcx1) AND (Cy is input to mfcy1) THEN (class is non-follicle).

At this point, the fuzzy inference system has been completely defined, in that the variables, membership functions and the rules necessary to determine the output classes are in place.

Testing phase: During the testing phase, the geometric features R, Cp, Cr, Tr, E and C= (Cx, Cy) are computed for each segmented region of the input image and then the above fuzzy classification rules are applied to determine whether the region is a follicle or not a follicle.

Experimental results: The ten-fold experiments are performed for the classification and the average follicle detection rate is computed. The Figure 7 (a) depicts an original ultrasound image of the ovary and the resultant images at different steps of fuzzy based method are shown in Figure 7(b)-(e). Many undesired spurious regions are also obtained (e.g., regions inside the endometrium). These spurious regions must be removed as much as possible. Therefore, the regions having an area less than T are removed (Figure 7(f)). The Figure 7 (g) depicts the segmented follicles (outlined in white) superimposed on the original image. The Figure 7 (h) depicts the recognized follicles after applying classification rules and Figure 7 (i) shows the follicles annotated manually by the medical expert.

The Figure 8 depicts comparison of the fuzzy logic based classification with the 3σ intervals based classification [section 3(i)]. In the Figure 8 (a) and (d) are two original images, (b) and (e) are their corresponding resultant images by the 3σ intervals based method. and, (c) and (f) are resultant images of fuzzy based method. It is observed that the regions which are misclassified as follicles, by the method in [section 3(i)] (Figure 8 (b) and (e)), are correctly classified by the fuzzy logic based method (Figure 8 (c) and (f)). Hence, the classification accuracy of the fuzzy logic based method is improved as compared to the method in [section 3(i)]. The Table 6 presents number of follicles detected in the results of the fuzzy based method and the method in [section 3(i)] corresponding to the original images in the Figure 8.

	Number of follicles detected						
Method	**fuzzy based method**			**3σ intervals based method [section 3(i)]**			**Manual (by medical expert)**
Input original image	Total	Correct	False	Total	Correct	False	
Figure 8(a)	3	3	-	5	3	2	3
Figure 8(d)	1	1	-	3	1	2	1

Table 6. Comparison of experimental results of proposed fuzzy logic based classification and 3σ interval based classification based method for original images in the Figure 8.

The Table 7 shows the comparison of classification results of fuzzy based method and the method in [section 3(i)] after ten-fold experiments for both the data sets. The average detection rates for the fuzzy based method with D1 and D2 sets are 98.18% and 97.61%, false acceptance rates (FAR) are 4.52% and 9.05%, and false rejection rates (FRR) are 1.76% and 2.37%, respectively. The average detection rates for the method in the Section 3(i) with D1 and D2 sets are 92.3% and 96.66%, false acceptance rates (FAR) 13.6% and 15.04%, and false rejection rates (FRR) are 7.62% and 3.33%, respectively. It is observed that the false acceptance rate (FAR) is reduced and the classification accuracy is improved in case of the fuzzy logic based method as compared to that in the 3σ intervals based method [section 3(i)] for classification.

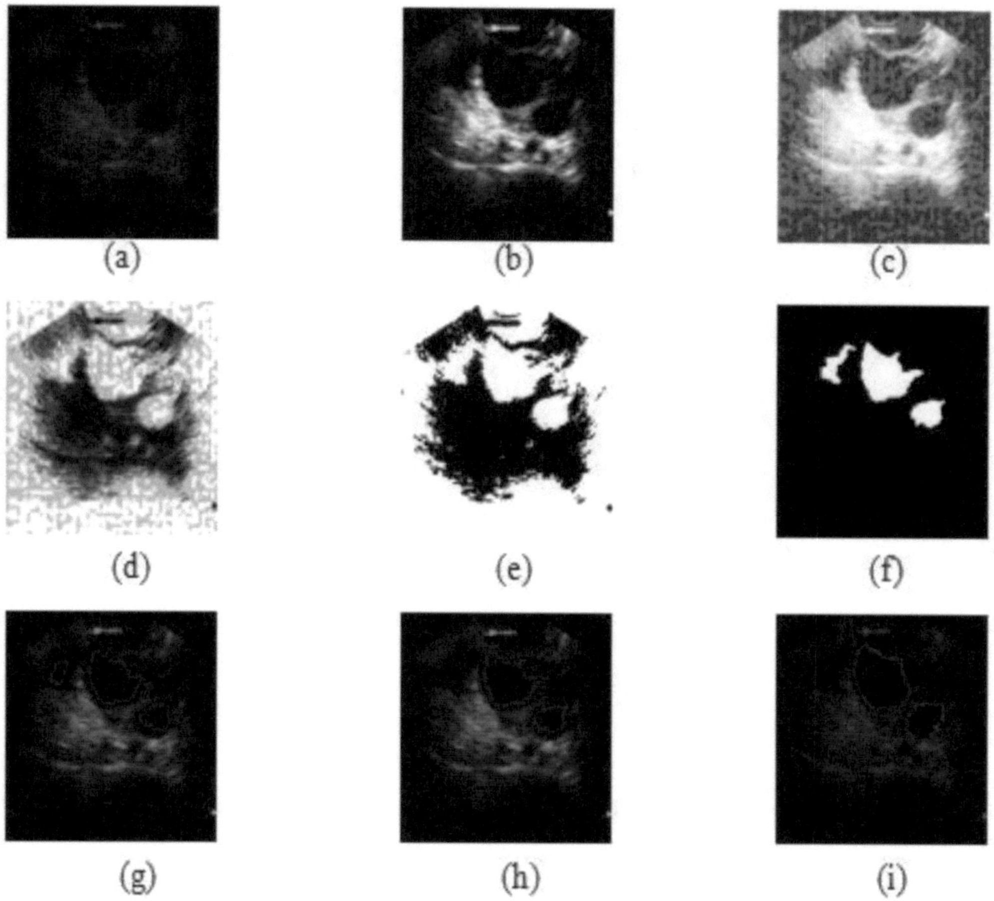

Figure 7. Original ultrasound image of the ovary and resultant images at different steps of fuzzy based method. a) Original image, b) Contourlet transformed image (despeckling), c) Histogram equalized image, d) Image after applying negative transformation, e) Image after applying active contour without edges method, f) Segmented image after clearing the border, filling the holes and removing the small regions, g) Image showing recognized follicles(outlined in white) super imposed on the original image, h) Output image after fuzzy classification, i) Manual segmentation of follicles by medical expert.

4. Ovarian classification

The ovaries are classified into three types based on the number and size of the follicles. Ovary is scanned, follicles are identified by using the method described the section 3, and the size of the follicles are measured and the number of follicles are counted.

There are three categories :

- The ovary containing 1-2 follicles with size measuring greater than 28mm in size, is a cystic ovary.

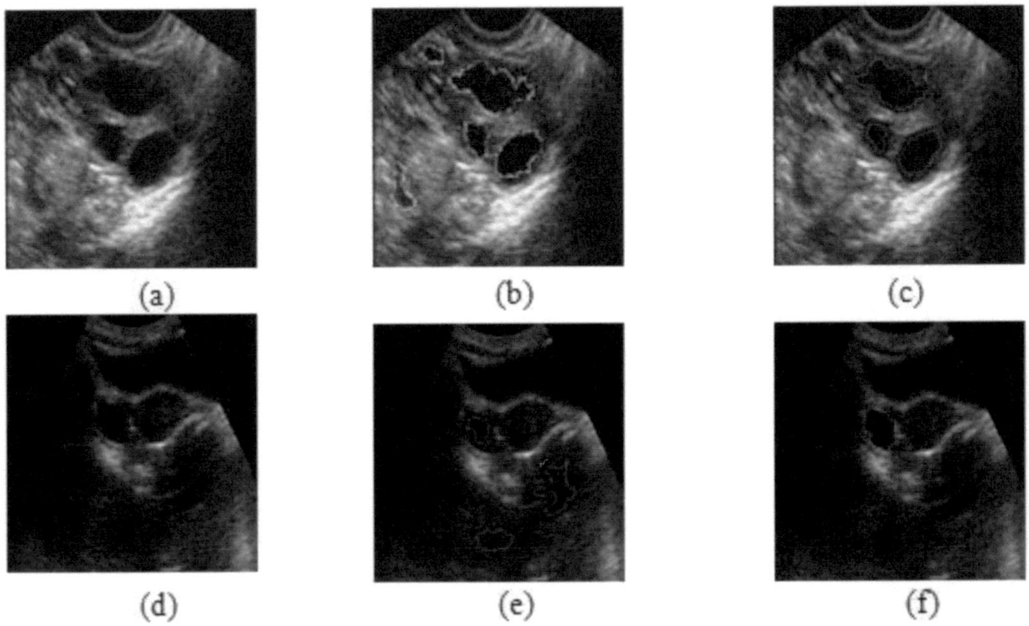

Figure 8. Comparison of resultant images of the fuzzy based method with the 3σ intervals based classification for two different original images. (a) and (d) original images, (b) and (e) resultant images of 3σ intervals based, (c) and (f) resultant images of fuzzy based method.

- The ovary containing 12 or more follicles with size measuring less than 10mm, is a polycystic ovary.
- The ovary containing 1-10 follicles with size measuring 2-10mm, are antral follicles and with the 10-28mm size, are dominant follicles, is a normal ovary with m number of antral follicles and n number of dominant follicles.

The two ovarian classification methods are discussed below [Hiremath and Tegnoor, 2012]:

i. Fuzzy ovarian classification

Training phase: The fuzzy inference system (FIS) of sugeno type is employed using the fuzzy input variables the number of follicles NN and the size of the follicle S and output variables: normal, cystic and polycystic ovarian classes. The Trapezoidal membership function is used for each of the fuzzy input variables with minimum and maximum value of the corresponding variables. Let mfn1 and mfs1, mfn2 and mfs2, and mfn3 and mfs3, be the trapezoidal membership functions of the fuzzy input variables NN and S respectively, belonging to the normal ovarian class, cystic ovarian class, polycystic ovarian class.

During the training phase, the parameters, namely, NN and S, are computed for the ovarian images known to be healthy, cystic and polycystic ovary in the training images in consultation with the medical expert, which are used to set the rules for classification of ovarian images.

We denote,

n1 - number of follicles of normal ovary

sz1 - size of the follicles in the normal ovary

n2 - number of follicles of cystic ovary

sz2- size of the follicles in the cystic ovary

n3 - number of follicles of polycystic ovary

sz3 - size of the follicles in the polycystic ovary

The number of follicles and size of follicles of these three classes are stored as knowledge base which is shown in the Table 8.

Classification results				
Data set	**D1 set**		**D2 set**	
Methods	Fuzzy logic method	3σ interval based method [section 3(i)]	Fuzzy logic method	3σ interval based method [section 3(i)] Based Method
Classification rate	98.18 %	92.3 %	97.61%	96.66%
Type I error (FAR)	4.52 %	13.6 %	9.05%	15.04%
Type II error (FRR)	1.76 %	7.62 %	2.37 %	3.33 %

Table 7. Comparison of classification results of fuzzy based classification method with 3σ intervals based method after ten-fold experiments.

The construction of the membership functions for the output variables is done in the similar manner. Since this is Sugeno-type inference (precisely, zero-order Sugeno), constant type of output variable fits the best to the given set of outputs (0 for normal ovary and 0.5 for cystic ovary and 1 for polycystic ovary). Based on the descriptions of the inputs (the number of the follicles NN and size of the follicles S) and output variables (normal ovary, cystic ovary, polycystic ovary). The fuzzy rules for classification procedure in verbose format are as follows:

i. IF (n1 is input to mfn1) AND (sz1 is input to mfs1) THEN (class is normal ovary)

ii. IF (n2 is input to mfn2) AND (sz2 is input to mfs2) THEN (class is cystic ovary)

iii. IF (n2 is input to mfn3) AND (sz3 is input to mfs3) THEN (class is polycystic ovary)

At this point, the fuzzy inference system has been completely defined, in that the variables, membership functions and the rules necessary to determine the output classes are in place.

Image type	Number of follicles	Size of the follicle
Normal ovary	1-10	15-10000
Cystic ovary	1-2	4300-75000
Polycystic ovary	12-20	15-9000

Table 8. The knowledge base of number of follicles and size of follicles of all the three classes

Testing phase: During the testing phase, we compute the number of follicles NN, and the size of each follicle S, for an ovary with the detected follicles and apply the above classification rules to determine whether an ovary is normal, cystic, and polycystic.

Experimental results: The experimentation is done using image data set D3. The D3 set consists of 70 sample ultrasound ovarian images of size 512x512, out of which 35 images are used for training and 35 for testing. In the first step, the ten-fold experiments for the follicle detection are done and then the average follicle detection rate is computed. Further, in the second step, for the ovary classification, 70 sample images of the detected follicles are used, of which 35 are used for training and 35 are used for testing. The ten-fold experiments for the ovarian classification are done and the average classification rate for the ovarian type is computed. The Figure 9 shows the sample results for the ovarian classification method. detection method after performing ten-fold experiments for the image data set. The Table 9 shows the average classification results of follicle detection method after performing ten-fold experiments for the image data set. The follicle detection method (Section 3(ii)) yields the average detection rate for the fuzzy based method 98.47%, false acceptance rate (FAR) 2.61% and false rejection rate (FRR) 1.47%.

Classification rate	Type I error (FAR)	Type II error (FRR)
98.47%	2.61%	1.47%

Table 9. Average classification results after ten-fold experiments

The Table 10 shows the ten-fold experimental results of the ovarian classification based on fuzzy inference rules. It is observed that the average normal ovary cyst ovary and polycystic ovary is 100%, with zero false acceptance rate is (FAR) and false rejection rate (FRR). Although, the proposed ovarian classification method yields 100% classification results, it is to be noted that these results are with reference to the limited data set used for experimentation. However, in case of different data sets, with varying image resolution, image sizes and numbers, the classification accuracy may be less than 100%.

http://dx.doi.org/10.5772/56518

Ovarian class	Number of images	Number of correctly classified images	Manual detection	Type I error	Type II error
Normal ovary	15	15	15	-	-
Cystic ovary	10	10	10	-	-
Polycystic ovary	10	10	10	-	-

Table 10. Experimental results for classification accuracy for all the three classes

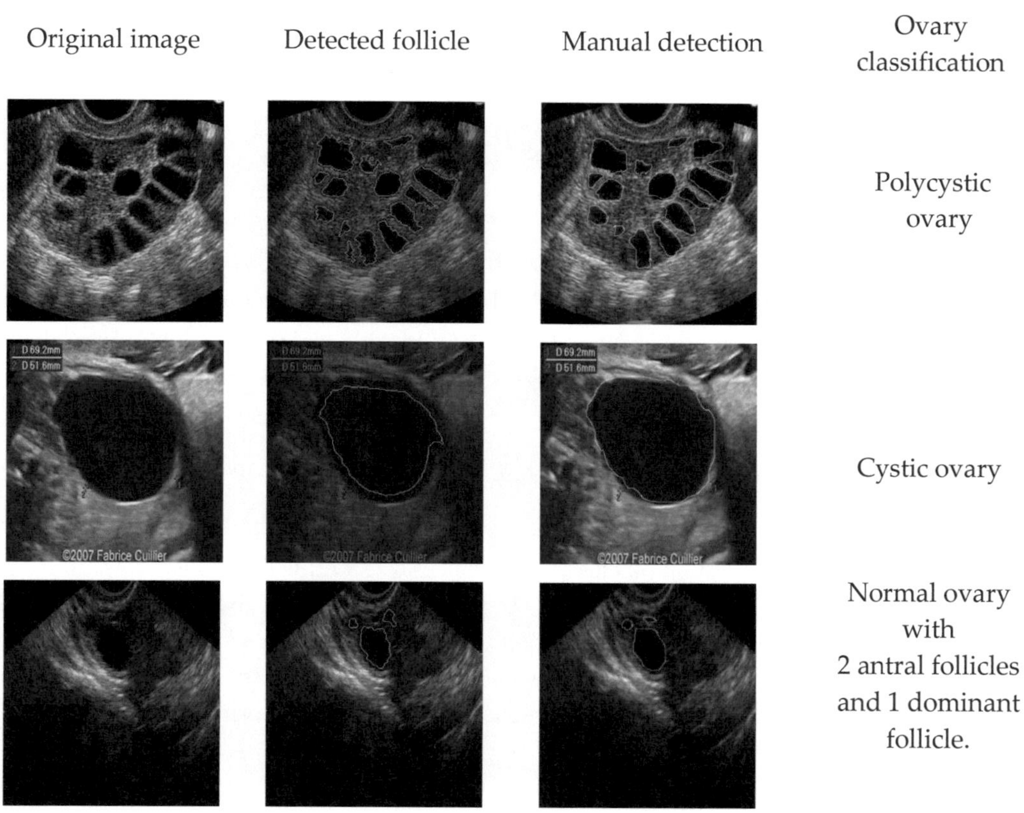

Figure 9. Sample results for proposed ovarian classification method

ii. Ovarian classification by using SVM

The aim of support vector machine (SVM) is to devise a computationally efficient way of learning separating hyper planes in a high dimensional feature space [49]. The SVMs have been shown to be an efficient method for many real-world problems because of its high generalization performance without the need to add a priori knowledge. Thus, SVMs have much attention as a successful tool for classification [50,51], image recognition [52,53] and bioinformatics [54]. The SVM model can map the input vectors into a high-dimensional feature space through some non-linear mapping, chosen a priori. In this space, an optimal separating hyperplane is constructed. SVM is the implementation of the structural risk minimization principle whose object is to minimize the upper bound on the generalization error. Given a set of training vectors (l in total) belonging to separate classes, (x1, y1), (x2, y2), (x3, y3),..., (xl, yl), where $x_i \in R^n$ denotes the ith input vector and $y_i \in \{+1, -1\}$ is the corresponding desired output. The maximal margin classifier aims to find a hyperplane w: wx + b = 0 to separate the training data. In the possible hyperplanes, only one maximizes the margin and the nearest data point of each class. The Figure 10 shows the optimal separating hyperplane with the largest margin. The support vectors denote the points lying on the margin border. The solution to the classification is given by the decision function in the equation 13.

$$f(x) = sign\left(\sum_{i=1}^{N_{SV}} \alpha_i y_i k(s_{i,} x) + b \right) \tag{13}$$

where α_i is the positive Lagrange multiplier, s_i is the support vector (N_{SV} in total) and $k(s_i, x)$ is the function for convolution of the kernel of the decision function. The radial kernels perform best in our experimental comparison, and, hence, are chosen in the proposed diagnosis system. The radial kernels are defined as (equation 14).

$$k(x, y) = \exp\left(-\gamma (x - y)^2 \right) \tag{14}$$

By using the SVM method, firstly, follicles are detected and secondly, the ovarian classification is performed [55]. During the training phase, the parameters, namely, the number of follicles NN and the size of the follicle S, are determined for the ovarian images known to be normal, cystic and polycystic ovary in the training images in consultation with the medical expert. The quadratic kernel is used for training the three-class SVM classifier; normal, cystic and polycystic ovary being the three classes.

During the testing phase, the parameters, namely, the number of follicles NN and the size of follicles S, are determined, and then, the SVM classifier is used to determine whether an ovary is normal, cystic, or polycystic.

Experimental results: The Table 11 shows the comparison of classification results of SVM based method and the fuzzy based method in [section 4(i)] after ten-fold experiments. The average follicle detection rate for the SVM method is 98.89%, false acceptance rate (FAR) is 1.61 % and false rejection rate (FRR) is 1.10%. The average detection rate for the method in [section 4(i)] is 98.47%, false acceptance rate (FAR) is 2.61% and false rejection rate (FRR) is 1.47%. It is observed that the classification accuracy is improved in the SVM based method as compared to the fuzzy based method [section 4(i)].

http://dx.doi.org/10.5772/56518

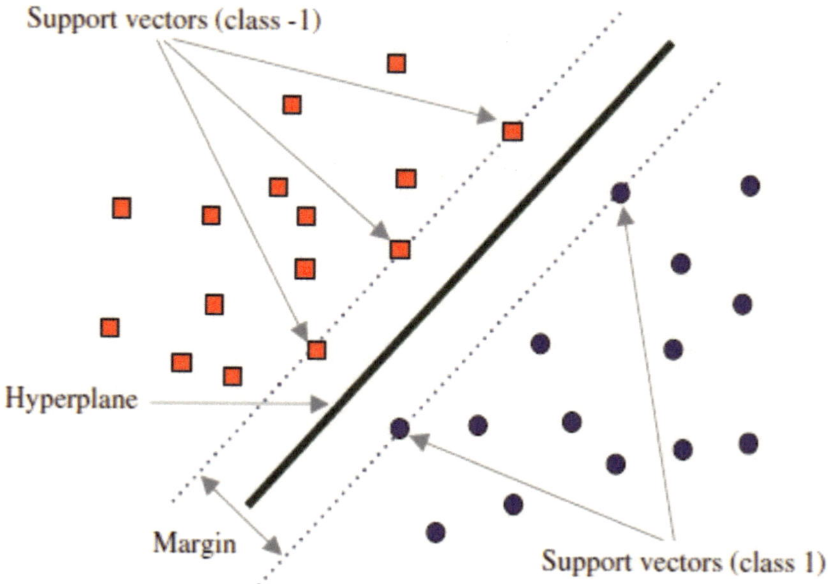

Figure 10. Optimal hyperplane for support vector machine

	Classification accuracy (%) of follicle detection	
Method	**SVM based method**	**Fuzzy based method [4(i)]**
Classification rate	98.89 %	98.47%
Type I error (FAR)	1.61 %	2.61%
Type II error (FRR)	1.10 %	1.47%

Table 11. Comparison of classification results of SVM based method and fuzzy based method [section 4(i)] for follicle detection after ten-fold experiments

The Table 12 shows the ten-fold experimental results of the ovarian classification based on SVM. It is observed that the average classification rates for normal ovary, cystic ovary and polycystic ovary are 100%, with zero false acceptance rate (FAR) and zero false rejection rate (FRR). It is observed that both the proposed SVM based method and the fuzzy based method [section 4(i)] yield 100% accuracy in ovarian classification, although the SVM outperforms the fuzzy method [section 4(i)] in follicle detection.

The Table 13 shows the comparison of all the follicle detection and ovarian classification methods developed in the present study and the other follicle detection methods available in the literature.

Ovary type	Number of images	Number of correctly classified images		Manual detection by expert	Type I error (FAR)		Type II error (FRR)	
		SVM	Fuzzy [4(i)]		SVM	Fuzzy [4(i)]	SVM	Fuzzy [4(i)]
Normal ovary	15	15	15	15	0	0	0	0
Cystic ovary	10	10	10	10	0	0	0	0
Polycystic ovary	10	10	10	10	0	0	0	0

* Type I Error: Regions are not follicles, but they are recognized as follicles.

**Type II Error: Regions are follicles, but they are not recognized as follicles.

Table 12. Experimental results for classification accuracy of the SVM based method for the three classes of ovaries in comparison with the fuzzy based method [section 4(i)]

Method	Data set used	Classification accuracy
Edge based method with Gaussian lowpass filter	D1	62.3%
	D2	45.2%
Watershed segmentation method	D1	49.55%
	D2	50.68%
Optimal thresholding method with Sobel operator	D1	50.77%
	D2	61.82%
HRGMF based thresholding method	D1	79.47%
	D2	68.86%
Edge based method with contourlet transform method	D1	75.2%
	D2	59.95%
HVST based method	D1	90.10%
	D2	92.76%
Active contour with 3σ interval based method	D1	92.37%
	D2	96.66%
Active contour with fuzzy classification	D1	98.18%

Method	Data set used	Classification accuracy
	D2	97.61%
Active contour with fuzzy classification of ovary	D3	98.47%
Active contour with SVM classification of ovary	D3	98.47%
Modified region growing and LD classifier [Maryruth et al., 2007]	(70)	83.25%
Region growing method [Potocnik and Zazula, 2000]	(50)	78%
Cellular neural network [Cigale and Zazula, 2000]	(50)	60%
Edge based method [Potocnick et al., 2002]	(50)	61%
Prediction based method [Potocnick and Zazula, 2002]	(50)	78%
Note : D1, D2 and D3 are image data sets.		

Table 13. Comparison of the proposed method with all the other methods proposed in the present study and also with the other methods in the literature.

5. Conclusion

The main significant research contributions that fulfill the objectives set in the present chapter are :

i. Automatic detection of follicles using better segmentation and classification methods.

ii. Automatic ovarian classification into three categories, namely: normal ovary, cystic ovary and polycystic ovary.

The performance comparison of the various methods proposed in the present study and other methods in the literature is summarized in the Table 13. It is observed that :

i. the proposed method using contourlet transform based despeckling, active contour without edges based segmentation, geometric feature extraction and fuzzy logic or SVM based classifier, has yielded better follicle detection results; and,

ii. the proposed method for ovarian classification using fuzzy or SVM has yielded better classification results.

These research contributions are expected to be useful for the design and development of the software tool to support the medical experts, namely, Gynecologists and Radiologists, in their effort for ovarian image analysis and to implement the same in automated diagnostic systems. Further, these research contributions serve as the basis for design of automatic systems for the detection of the follicles inside the ovary under the examination during the entire female cycle and to study the ovarian morphology and, thus, help the medical experts for monitoring follicles and identifying the ovarian type during the course of infertility treatment of patients. The burden of the experts is significantly reduced in their everyday routine, without sacrificing the accuracy of diagnosis and prognosis.

The future research in this direction would be to take up the analysis of ovarian images captured at regular intervals for various subjects undergoing drug susceptibility tests. Further, the image processing methods could be developed in the detection of ovarian cancer stages.

Acknowledgements

Authors are thankful to Mediscan Diagnostics Care, Gulbarga, for providing the ultrasound images of ovaries. We are indebted to Dr. Suchitra C. Durgi, Radiologist, Dr. Chetan Durgi, Radiologist and Dr. Suvarna M. Tegnoor, Gynaecologist, Gulbarga, for helpful discussions and for rendering manual detection of follicles and ovarian classification in ultrasound images of ovaries.

Author details

P. S. Hiremath* and Jyothi R. Tegnoor*

*Address all correspondence to: hiremathps53@yahoo.com

*Address all correspondence to: jyothi_rt1@yahoo.co.in

Dept of Computer Science, Gulbarga University, Gulbarga, India

References

[1] Gougeon A. and Lefevre B. Evolution of the Diameters of the Largest Healthy and Atretic Follicles During the Human Menstrual Cycle, Reproduction and Fertility 1983;69: 497-502.

http://dx.doi.org/10.5772/56518

[2] Gougeon A., Adashi E. and Leung P. Dynamics of Human Follicular Growth, a Morphologic Perspective: Comprehensive Endocrinology, The Ovary, Raven Press, New York, 1993: 21-39.

[3] Pellicer A., Gaitán P., Neuspiller F., Ardiles G., Albert C., Remohí J. and Simón C., Ovarian Follicular Dynamics: From Basic Science to Clinical Practice, Journal of Reproductive Immunology 1998; 39(1-2) 29-61.

[4] Hanna M. D., Chizen D. R. and Pierson R. Characteristics of Follicular Evacuation During Human Ovulation, J Ultrasound Obstet Gynaecol 1994; 4(6) 488-493.

[5] Pierson R. and Chizen D. Ultrasonography of Normal and Aberrant Ovulation. Imaging in Infertility and Reproductive Endocrinology, 1994;155-166.

[6] Bal A. and Mohan H. Malignant Transformation in Mature Cystic Teratoma of the Ovary: Report of Five Cases and Review of the Literature, Arch Gynecol Obstet, 2007; 275(3)179-182.

[7] Yamanaka Y. and Tateiwa Y. Preoperative Diagnosis of Malignant Transformation in Mature Cystic Teratoma of The Ovary, Eur J Gynaecol Oncol 2005; 26(4)391-392.

[8] Battaglia C., Artini P. G., Genazzani A. D., Gremigni R., Slavatori M. R. and Sgherzi M. R., Color Doppler Analysis in Oligo and Amenorrheic Women with Polycystic Ovary Syndrome. Gynecolog Endocrinto, 1997;11:105-110.

[9] Balen Adam H., Joop S. E. Laven, Seang-Lin Tan and Didier Dewailly, Ultrasound Assessment of the Polycystic Ovary: International Consensus Definitions, Human Reproduction, 2003;9(6)505-511.

[10] Pache T. D., Wladimiroff J. W., Hop W. C. and Fauser B. C. How to Discriminate Between Normal and Polycystic Ovaries: Transvaginal US Study. Radiology 1992;183(2) 421-423.

[11] Kelsey T.W. and Wallace W. H. B. Ovarian Volume Correlates Strongly with Number of Non Growing Follicles in the Human Ovary, Obstretics and Gynocology International, 2012; Article-id 305025.

[12] Potocnik B., Zazula D., Korze D. Automated Computer-Assisted Detection of Follicles in Ultrasound Images of Ovary. Journal of Medical Systems 1997; 21(6) 445-457.

[13] Potocnik B., Viher B. and Zazula D. Computer assisted detection of ovarian follicles based on ultrasound images, Proc. of a szamitastechnika orvosies biological alkalmazasai, Verzprem, Hungary, pp. 24-34; 1998.

[14] Potocnik B. and Zazula D. Aktivne krivulje-nadgradnja razpoznavalnih sistemov (Active contours-an extension of recognition systems). Proceedings of 7th Electrotechnical and Computer Science Conference ERK 98, Portoroz, Slovenia, Vol. B, 1998; 249-252.

[15] Potocnik B. and Zazula D. Automated Analysis Of Sequence of Ovarian Ultrasound Images, Part I: Segmentation of Single 2D Images. Image Vision and Computing 2002; 20(3) 217-225.

[16] Sarty G. E., Liang W., Sonka M. and Pierson R. A. Semiautomated Segmentation of Ovarian Follicular Ultrasound Images Using a Knowledge Based Algorithm. Ultrasound in Medicine and Biology, 1998; 24(1)27-42.

[17] Cigale B. and Zazula D. Segmentation of Ovarian Ultrasound Images Using Cellular Neural Networks, International Journal of Pattern Recognition and Artificial Intelligence, 2004; 18, 563-581.

[18] Krivanek and Sonka M. Ovarian Ultrasound Image Analysis Follicle Segmentation. IEEE Transactions on Medical Imaging, 1998; 17(6) 935-944.

[19] Maryruth, Lawrence J. and Eramian Mark G. Computer Assisted Detection of Polycystic Ovary Morphology, Ultrasound Images 2007; 23(2) 306-309.

[20] Mehrotra P., Chakraborthy C., Ghoshdastidar B. and Ghostidas S. Automated Ovarian Follicle Detection for Polycystic Ovarian Syndrome, Proc. of IEEE International Conference on Image Information Processing (ICIIP), 3-5 Nov 2011, Himachal Pradesh, India, 1-4; 2011.

[21] Hiremath P. S. and Tegnoor J. R. Automatic Detection of Follicles in Ultrasound Images of Ovaries, Proc. of Second International Conference on Cognition and Recognition (ICCR-08), 15-17 Apr. 2008, Mysore, India, pp 468-473; 2008.

[22] Hiremath P. S. and Tegnoor J. R. Automatic Detection of Follicles in Ultrasound Images of Ovaries, Proc. of Third International Conference on Systemic, Cybernetics and Informatics (ICSCI-09), 07-10 Jan. 2009, Hyderabad, India, pp. 327-330; 2009.

[23] Hiremath P. S. and Tegnoor J. R. Automatic Detection of Follicles in Ultrasound Images of Ovaries by Optimal Threshoding Method, International Journal of Computer Science and Information Technology 2010; 3(2) 217-220.

[24] Gonzalez R. C. and Woods R. E. Digital Image Processing, Second Edition, Pearson Edu; 2002.

[25] Jing Hanm B S., Shin D. V., Arthur G. L. and Chi-Ren Shyu, 2010, Multiresolution Tile Based Follicle Detection Using Colour and Textural Information of Follicular Lymphoma IHC Slides, Proc. of IEEE International Conference on Biomedicine Workshop., 18-21 Dec. 2010, Hong Kong, China, pp. 886-87; 2010.

[26] Hiremath P. S. and Tegnoor J. R. Automatic Detection of Follicles in Ultrasound Images of Ovaries using HRGMF Based Segmentation, International Journal of Multimedia, Computer Vision and Machine Learning (IJMCVML) 2010; 1(1) 83-87.

[27] Koo Ja. I. and Song B. Park. Speckle Reduction with Edge Preservation, Medical Ultrasonics 1991; 3(13) 211-237.

[28] Srinivasrao Ch., Srinivaskumar S. and Chattergi B. N. Content Based Image Retrieval Using Contourlet Transform, ICGST-GVIP Journal 2007;7(3) 9-15.

[29] Jainping Zhou, Arthur L. Cunha and Minh N. Do, Non subsampled Contourlet Transform: Construction and Application in Enhancement, Proc. of IEEE International Conference on Image Processing, 11-14 Sept. 2005, Genoa, Italy, pp. 469-72; 2005.

[30] Do Minh N. and Vetterli Martin, The Contourlet Transform: An Efficient Directional Multiresolution Image Representation, IEEE Transaction on Image Processing 2005; 14(12)2091-2106.

[31] Eslami Ramin and Hayder Radha, 2006, Translation invariant contourlet transform and its application image denoising, IEEE Transactions on Image Processing 2005;15(11) 3362-74.

[32] Hiremath P. S., Akkasaliger P. and Badiger S., 2009, Despeckling medical ultrasound images using the contourlet transform, Proc. of Indian International Conferance on Artificial Intelligence, 16-18 Dec. 2009, Tumkur, India, pp. 1814-1827.

[33] Hiremath P. S., Akkasaliger P. and Badiger S., Performance Comparision of Wavelet Transform and Contourlet Transform Based Method for Despekling Medical Ultrasound Images, International Journal of Computer Applications, 2011, 26(9)34-41.

[34] Hiremath P. S. and Tegnoor J. R. Automatic Detection of Follicles in Ultrasound Images of Ovaries using Horizontal and Vertical Scanline Thresholding Method, Proc. of Second International Conference on Signal and Image Processing (ICSIP-09), 12-14 Aug. 2009, Mysore, India, pp 468-473;2009.

[35] Hiremath P. S. and Tegnoor J. R. Recognition of Follicles in Ultrasound Images of Ovaries using Geometric Features, Proc. of Second IEEE International Conference on Biomedical and Pharmaceutical Engineering (ICBPE-09), 2-4 Dec. 2009, Singapore, ISBN 978-1-4244-4764-0/09; 2009.

[36] Hiremath P. S. and Tegnoor J. R. Automatic Detection of Follicles in Ultrasound Images of Ovaries using Edge based Method, International Journal of Computer Applications (IJCA), Special Issue on "Recent Trends in Image Processing and Pattern Recognition", RTIPPR, pp 120-125, ISSN 0975-8887; 2010.

[37] Hiremath P. S. and Tegnoor J. R. Automatic Detection of Follicles in Ultrasound Images of Ovaries using Active Contours Method, International Journal of Service Computing and Computational Intelligence (IJSCCI) 2011; 1(1) pp 26-30, ISSN 2162-514X.

[38] Jahne B., Digital Image Processing. Berlin, Germany Springer–Verlag; 1993.

[39] Chan Tony F. and Vese Luminita A., Active Contours Without Edges, IEEE Transactions on Image Processing 2001; 10(2) 266-277.

[40] Hiremath P. S. and Tegnoor J. R. Fuzzy Logic Based Detection of Follicles in Ultrasound Images of Ovaries, Proc. of Fifth Indian International Conference on Artificial

Intelligence (IICAI-2011), 14-16 Dec 2011, Tumkur, Karnataka, India, pp 178-189, ISBN: 978-0-9727412-8-6; 2011.

[41] Sourabh Dash, Raghunathan Rengaswamy and Venkat Subramanian. Fuzzy-Logic Based Trend Classification for Fault Diagnosis of Chemical Processes, International Journal of Computers and Chemical Engineering 2003; 27(3)347-362.

[42] Nedeljkovic I., Image Classification Based on Fuzzy Logic, The International Archives of the Photogrammetry, Remote Sensing and Spatial Information Sciences 2004, 34: 173-179,

[43] Kerre E. E. and Nachtegael M. Fuzzy Techniques in Image Processing. Springer, Heidelberg; 2000.

[44] Khademi A., Sahba F., Venetsanopoulos A. and Krishnan S., 2009, Region, Lesion and Border-Based Multiresolution Analysis of Mammogram Lesions, Proc. of the Sixth International Conference on Image Analysis and Recognition (ICIAR), 6-8 July 2009, Halifex, Canada, pp. 802-813.

[45] Zadeh L. A. Fuzzy Sets, Information and Control,1965; 8: 333-335.

[46] Zadeh L.A. Outline of a New Approach to the Analysis of Complex Systems and Decision Processes, IEEE Transactions on Systems, Man, and Cybernatics 1973; 3(1).

[47] Zadeh L.A. Fuzzy algorithms, Info and Ctl. 1968, 12: 94-102.

[48] Zadeh L.A. Making Computers Think Like People, IEEE. Spectrum 1984; pp. 26-32.

[49] Christianini N. and Shawe-Taylor J. An Introduction to Support Vector Machines and Other Kernel-Based Learning Methods. Cambridge University Press, UK 12; 2000.

[50] Kim K. I., Jung K., Park S. H. and Kim H. J. Support Vector Machines for Texture Classification, IEEE Trans Pattern Anal Mach Intell 2002; 24(11) 1542-1550.

[51] Song Q., Hu W. J. and Xie W. F., 2002, Robust Support Vector Machine With Bullet Hole Image Classification, IEEE Trans. Systems, Man and Cybenetics, Part C: Applications and Review 2002; 32(4) 440-448.

[52] El Naqa I., Yang Y. Y., Wernick M. N., Galatsanos N. P. and Nishikawa R. M. A Support Vector Machine Approach for Detection of Micro Calcifications. IEEE Trans Med Imaging 2002; 21(2)1552-1563.

[53] Yang M. H., Roth D. and Ahuja N. A tale of two classifiers: SNoW vs. SVM in visual recognition, Proc. of Seventh European Conference on Computer Vision, Copenhagen, Denmark, 27 May-2 June 2002, pp. 688-699; 2002.

[54] Sun Y. F., Fan X. D. and Li Y. D., Identifying Splicing Sites in Eukaryotic RNA: Support Vector Machine Approach, Comput. Biol. Med 2003, 33(1)17–29.

http://dx.doi.org/10.5772/56518

[55] Hiremath P. S. and Tegnoor J. R. Automated Ovarian Classification in Digital Ultrasound Images using SVM, International Journal of Engineering Research and Technology 2012; 1(6).

Chapter 8

Speckle Noise Reduction in Medical Ultrasound Images

P.S. Hiremath, Prema T. Akkasaligar and
Sharan Badiger

Additional information is available at the end of the chapter

http://dx.doi.org/10.5772/56519

1. Introduction

The use of ultrasound imaging in medical diagnosis is well established because of its non-invasive nature, low cost, capability of forming real time imaging and continuing improvement in image quality. However, it suffers from a number of shortcomings and these include: acquisition noise from the equipment, ambient noise from the environment, the presence of background tissue, other organs and anatomical influences such as body fat, and breathing motion. Therefore, noise reduction is very important, as various types of noise generated limits the effectiveness of medical image diagnosis.

Ultrasound is a sound wave with a frequency that exceeds 20 kHz. It transports energy and propagates through several means as a pulsating pressure wave [1]. It is described by a number of wave parameters such as pressure density, propagation direction, and particle displacement. If the particle displacement is parallel to the propagation direction, then the wave is called a longitudinal or compression wave. If the particle displacement is perpendicular to the propagation direction, it is a shear or transverse wave. The interaction of ultrasound waves with tissue is subject to the laws of geometrical optics. It includes reflection, refraction, scattering, diffraction, interference, and absorption. Except from interference, all other interactions reduce the intensity of the ultrasound beam.

Ultrasound technique is mainly based on measuring the echoes transmitted back from a medium when sending an ultrasound wave to it. In the echo impulse ultrasound technique, the ultrasound wave interacts with tissue and some of the transmitted energy returns to the transducer to be detected by the instrument [2]. Further, the reflected waves are picked up by the transducer probe and relayed to the machine. The machine calculates the distance from the transducer probe to the tissue or organ (boundaries) using the speed of sound in tissue (1,540 m/s) and the time of the each echo's return (millionths of a second). The machine displays the distances and intensities of the echoes on the screen, forming a two dimensional image. Superficial structures such as muscles, tendons, testes, breast and the neonatal brain are imaged at a higher frequency (7- 18 MHz), which provides better axial and lateral resolution. Deeper structures such as liver and kidney are imaged at a lower frequency 1-6 MHz with lower axial and lateral resolution but greater penetration.

The usefulness of ultrasound imaging is degraded by the presence of signal dependent noise known as speckle. Speckle noise is multiplicative in nature. This type of noise is an inherent property of medical ultrasound imaging and because of this noise the image resolution and contrast become reduced, which effects the diagnostic value of this imaging modality [3]. So, speckle noise reduction is an essential pre processing step, whenever ultrasound imaging is used for medical imaging. Therefore, image despeckling is a very important task, and should be filtered out [4-6], without affecting important features of the image.

In ultrasound images, the noise content is multiplicative and non Gaussian. Such noise is generally more difficult to remove than additive noise, because the intensity of the noise varies with the image intensity. A model of multiplicative noise is given by

$$y_{ij} = X_{ij} n_i \tag{1}$$

where the speckle image y_{ij} is the product of the original image $X_{ij,}$ and the non-Gaussian noise $n_{ij.}$ The indices i, j represent the spatial position over the image. In most applications involving multiplicative noise, the noise content is assumed to be stationary with unitary mean and unknown noise variance σ^2. To convert multiplicative noise into an additive noise, as given in the Eq.(2), a logarithmic transformation is applied to the speckle image y_{ij} [7]. The noise component n_{ij} is then approximated as an additive zero mean gaussian noise.

$$\ln y_{ij} = \ln X_{ij} + \ln n_{ij} \tag{2}$$

The Discrete Wavelet Transform (DWT) is then applied to $\ln y_{ij}$ and the wavelet transformed image is subjected to thresholding. After applying the inverse DWT, the processed image is subjected to an exponential transformation, which is the inverse logarithmic operation,that yields a denoised image.

1.1. Image quality assessment

Image quality is important when evaluating or segmenting ultrasound images, where speckle obscures subtle details in the image [8]. In a recent study [9] it is shown that speckle reduction improves the visual perception of the expert in the assessment of ultrasound imaging of the human organs. The statistical parameters like Signal to Noise Ratio (SNR), Correlation Coefficient (CC), variance, Mean Square Error (MSE) and Peak Signal to Noise Ratio (PSNR) for image quality assessment are described below. The following metrics are calculated using the original image X and the despeckled image Y.

Variance: It determines the average dispersion of the speckle in the image. A lower variance gives a cleaner image as more speckles are reduced. The formula for calculating the variance is

$$\sigma^2 = \frac{1}{N^2} \sum_{i,j=0}^{N-1} \left(X_{ij} - \bar{X} \right)^2 \tag{3}$$

where $\bar{X}$ is the mean intensity value of the image X of size N×N.

Mean Square Error: The MSE measures the quality change between the original image (X) and denoised image (Y) of size N×N. It is given by

$$MSE = \frac{1}{N^2} \sum_{i,j=0}^{N-1} \left(X_{ij} - Y_{ij} \right)^2 \tag{4}$$

The MSE has been widely used to quantify image quality and, when used alone, it does not correlate strongly enough with perceptual quality. It should be used, therefore, together with other quality metrics and visual perception.

Signal to Noise Ratio: The SNR compares the level of desired signal to the level of background noise. The higher the ratio, the less obtrusive the background noise is. It is expressed in decibels (dB) as

$$SNR = 10 \log_{10} \left(\frac{\sigma^2}{\sigma_e^2} \right) \tag{5}$$

where, σ^2 is the variance of the original image and σ_e^2 is the variance of error (Difference between the original and denoised image i.e. $|X - Y|$).

Peak Signal-to-Noise Ratio: The PSNR is computed as

$$PSNR = 10 \log_{10} \left(\frac{S^2}{MSE} \right) \tag{6}$$

where S is the maximum intensity in the original image. The PSNR is higher for a good quality image and lower for a poor quality image. It measures image fidelity, that is, how closely the transformed image resembles the original image.

Correlation Coefficient: It represents the strength and direction of a linear relationship between two variates. The best known is the Pearson product moment correlation coefficient, which is obtained by dividing the covariance of the two variables by the product of their standard deviations, and it is given by

$$CC = \frac{N^2 \Sigma X_{ij} Y_{ij} - \Sigma X_{ij} \Sigma Y_{ij}}{\sqrt{N^2 \Sigma X_{ij}^2 - \left(\Sigma X_{ij}\right)^2} \sqrt{N^2 \Sigma Y_{ij}^2 - \left(Y_{ij}\right)^2}} \quad (7)$$

where the summations are done over both the indices i and j from 0 to N-1. If the correlation coefficient is near to +1, then there exists stronger positive correlation between the original image and despeckled image.

Computational time: The computational time (T_c) of a filter is defined as the time taken by a digital computing platform to execute the filtering algorithm when no other software, except the operating system, runs on it. Normally, T_c depends on the computing system's clock time period. But, in addition to the clock period, it depends on the memory size, the input data size, and the memory access time, etc. The computational time taken by a filter should be low for online and real time image processing applications. Hence, a filter with lower T_c is better than a filter having higher T_c value while all other performance measures remain identical.

1.2. Image data set

For the purpose of experimentation, a medical ultrasound image database is prepared in consultation with a medical expert for the present study. The images are acquired using the instrument GE LOGIQ 3 Expert system with 5 MHz transducer frequency, in JPEG format. The data set consists of 70 ultrasound images of size 512x512, of kidney and liver.

In the present Chapter, the aim of the study is to address, novel issues related to despeckling medical ultrasound images. It is envisaged that the results of this investigation would be used as a pre processing step for effective image segmentation or image registration techniques in other applications also.

The remaining part of this Chapter is organised into five sections. The section 2 deals with common speckle filters. The section 3 examines wavelet transform methods, while the section 4 investigates contourlet transform methods. The section 5 describes the Gaussian model of speckle noise. Finally, the section 6 gives the conclusions.

2. Common speckle filters

Speckle reducing filters are originated from the synthetic aperture radar community [10]. Later these filters are applied to ultrasound imaging since the early 1980s [11]. There are two major classifications of speckle reduction filters, viz. single scale spatial filters and transform domain multiscale filters. The spatial filter acts on an image by smoothing it; that is, it reduces the intensity variation between adjacent pixels. The simple sliding window spatial filter replaces the center value in the window with the average of all the neighboring pixel values including itself. By doing this, it replaces pixels, that are unrepresentative of their surroundings. It is implemented with a convolution mask, which provides a result that is a weighted sum of the values of a pixel and its neighbors. It is also called a linear filter. The mask or kernel is a square.

Often a 3× 3 square kernel is used. If the coefficients of the mask sum up to one, then the average brightness of the image is not changed. If the coefficients sum to zero, the average brightness is lost, and it returns a dark image.

The common speckle filters such as Lee, Kuan and Wiener filters are considered for the study. The brief definition and mathematical description of the standard spatial filters are discussed below:

Lee filter:

The Lee filter [12] is based on the approach that the smoothing is performed on the area having low variance. However, smoothing will not be performed on area of high variance, which is near edges. The Lee filter assumes that the image can be approximated by a linear model represented by Eq.(8)

$$Y_{ij} = \bar{K} + W^{*}(C - \bar{K}) \tag{8}$$

where Y_{ij} is the gray scale value of the pixel at (i, j) after filtering. If there is no smoothing, the filter will output, only the mean intensity value $\bar{K}$ of the kernel K, otherwise, the difference between the centre pixel C and $\bar{K}$ is calculated and multiplied with a weighting function W given in Eq.(9) :

$$W = \frac{\sigma_k^2}{(\sigma_k^2 + \sigma^2)} \tag{9}$$

and then summed with $\bar{K}$, where σ_k^2 is the variance of the pixel values within the kernel given by the Eq. (10):

$$\sigma_k^2 = \frac{1}{M^2} \sum_{u,v=0}^{M-1} (K_{uv} - \bar{K})^2 \tag{10}$$

where MxM is the size of the kernel and K_{uv} is the pixel value within the kernel at indices u and v, $\bar{K}$ is the mean intensity value of kernel. The parameter σ^2 is the variance of the image X, which is given by the Eq.(3). The main disadvantage of Lee filter is that it tends to ignore speckle noise in the areas closest to edges and lines.

Kuan filter:

The Kuan filter [13] is a generalization of the Lee filter. The Kuan filter converts the multiplicative model of speckle into an additive linear form. However, it is based on the equivalent number of looks (ENL), which is computed from an ultrasound image to determine a different weighting function W given by the Eq.(11):

$$W = \frac{(1 - C_u / C_i)}{(1 + C_u)}. \tag{11}$$

The weighting function is computed from estimated noise variation coefficient of the image, C_u given by the Eq.(12):

$$C_u = (ENL)^{-\frac{1}{2}} \tag{12}$$

and the variation coefficient C_i of the image given by the Eq. (13):

$$C_i = \sigma_k / \bar{K} \tag{13}$$

where ENL is given by the Eq.(14) :

$$ENL = \left(\frac{\bar{K}}{\sigma_k}\right)^2 \tag{14}$$

In the Eq.(14), the σ_k is the standard deviation of the kernel and $\bar{K}$ is the mean intensity value of the kernel. The only disadvantage of the Kuan filter is that the ENL parameter needs to be computed.

Wiener filter:

The Wiener filter [14] is a linear spatial domain filter. There are two alternatives : (i) Fourier transform method (frequency domain) (ii) mean squared method (spatial domain), for implementing the Wiener filter. The first alternative is used for denoising and deblurring, whereas the second alternative is used for denoising only. The frequency domain alternative of Wiener filtering requires a prior knowledge of noise power spectra and the original image. But, in the spatial domain alternative, no such prior knowledge is required. It is based on statistical least squared principle and minimizes the mean squared error between actual signal sequence and desired signal sequence.

In an image, the statistical properties differ too much from one region to another region. Thus, both global statistics (mean, variance, and higher order moments of entire image) and local statistics (mean, variance, and higher order moments of kernel) are important. Wiener filtering is based on both, global and local statistics and is given by

$$Y_{ij} = \bar{K} + \frac{\sigma_k^2}{\sigma_k^2 + \sigma^2}(K_{uv} - \bar{K}) \tag{15}$$

where Y_{ij} denotes the despeckled image, $\bar{K}$ is the local mean, σ_k^2 is the local variance, K_{uv} is $(u, v)^{th}$ pixel in the kernel K and σ^2 is the global variance. Let us consider kernel of size MxM, then local variance σ_k^2 is defined by Eq.(10). From the Eq.(15), it is observed that the filter output is equal to local mean if the centre pixel value equals local mean, or else it outputs the modified value different from local mean. Thus, filter output varies from the local mean

http://dx.doi.org/10.5772/56519

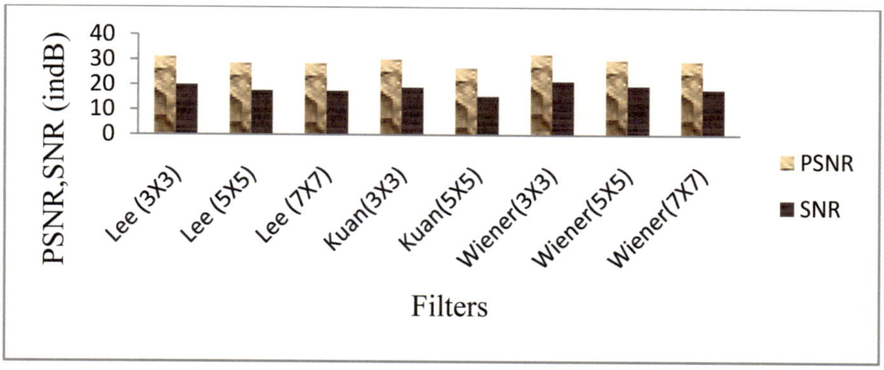

Figure 1. Performance of various despeckling filters, in terms of PSNR, SNR.

depending upon the local variance and thus tries to hold the true original value as far as possible.

The Lee filter and Wiener filter are implemented using kernel size 3x3, 5x5, 7x7 and Kuan filter using kernel size 3x3 and 5x5.The classical Wiener filter, is not adequate for removing speckle, since it is designed mainly for additive noise suppression. To address the multiplicative nature of speckle noise, a homomorphic approach is developed in [15], which converts the multiplicative noise into additive noise, by taking the logarithm of image and then applies the Wiener filter. The PSNR, SNR, CC, variance and MSE are considered as filter performance measures. The Figures 1.-4. show the average results obtained for 70 ultrasound images, which are despeckled using Kuan, Lee and Wiener filter. The optimality is determined by the criteria, namely (i) higher SNR and PSNR values, (ii) lower variance, MSE values and (iii) Correlation Coefficient is nearly equal to one. From the Figures 1.-4., it is observed that Wiener filter with kernel size 3x3 gives better results than other despeckling filters. The computational time of different filters are given in the Table 1. The filter having less computational time is usually required for online and real time applications. The least value of computation is highlighted. From the Table 1, it is observed that Wiener filter with kernel size 3x3 is better among all the filters compared here, for despeckling medical ultrasound images.

For proper judgement of performance of filters, the subjective evaluation should be taken into consideration. For subjective evaluation, the despeckled images of various filters are shown in the Figure 5. From the Figure 5, it is observed from visual inspection that all the three methods achieved good speckle suppression performance. However, Lee and Kuan filters lost many of the signal details and the resulting images are blurred. Further, Wiener filter with kernel size 3x3 yielded better visual enhancement of medical ultrasound images. However, the Lee filter smoothes away noise in flat regions, but leaves the fine details such as lines and texture unchanged.

Thus the main disadvantage of Lee filter is that, it tends to ignore speckle noise in the area closest to edges and lines. The Kuan filter is considered to be more superior to the Lee filter. It does not make an approximation on the noise variance within the filter window. The only

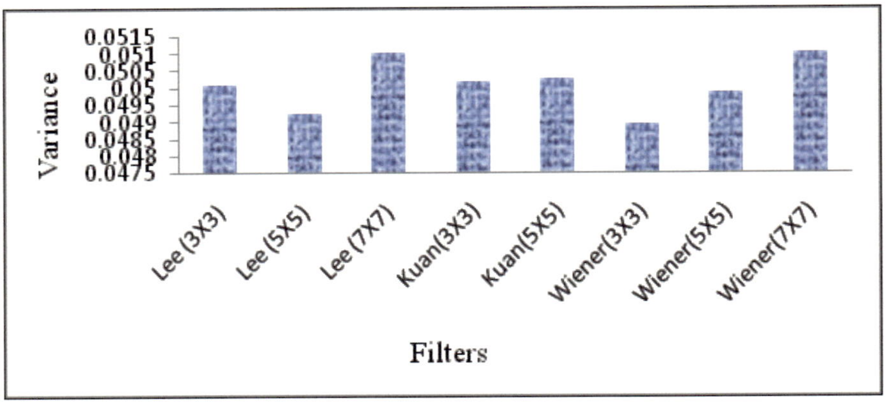

Figure 2. Performance of various despeckling filters, in terms of variance

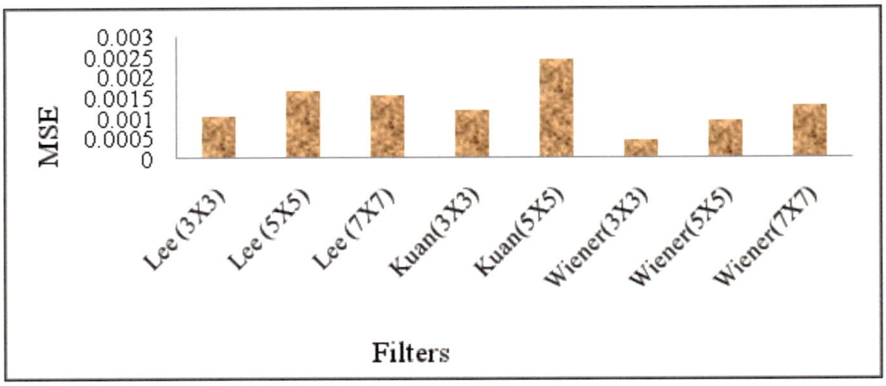

Figure 3. Performance of various despeckling filters, in terms of MSE.

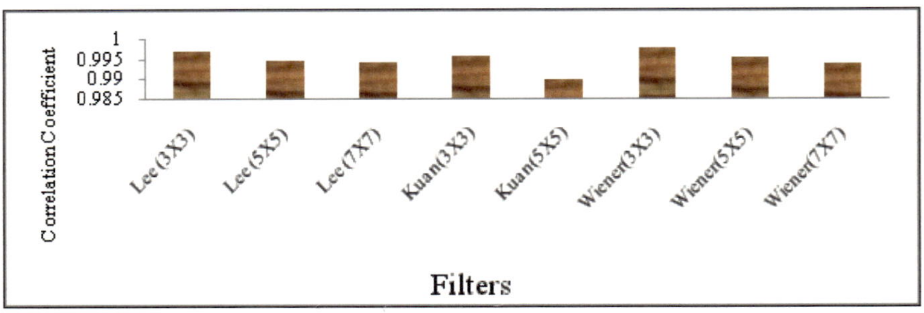

Figure 4. Performance of various despeckling filters, in terms of Correlation Coefficient

limitation of Kuan filter is the high computational time due to estimation of ENL parameter. The Wiener filter with kernel size 3×3 is effective in preserving the edges and other detailed information upto some extent. Further, when the various spatial domain filters are compared by visual inspection, it is observed that Wiener filter with kernel size 3×3 yielded better visual

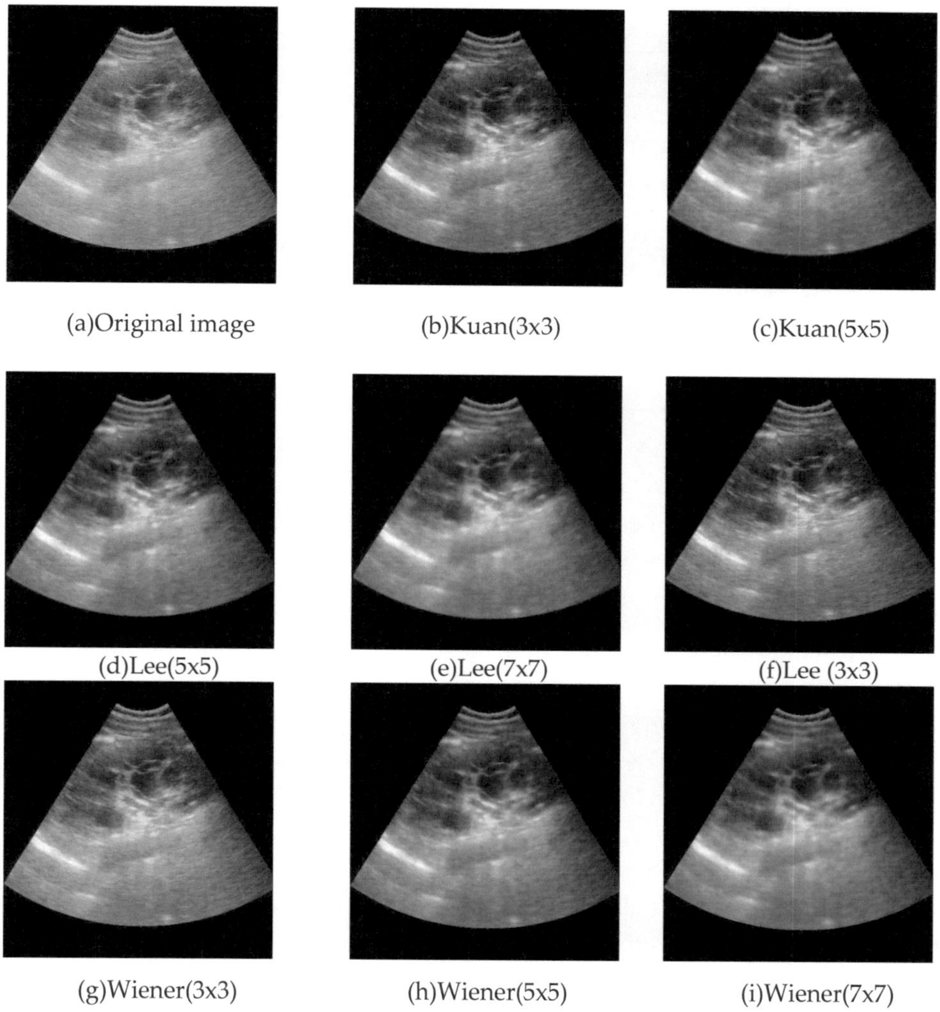

Figure 5. Performance comparison of various despeckling filters by visual inspection of an ultrasound image of kidney.

enhancement of medical ultrasound images. Further, for the complete removal of speckle without losing any data is not possible at the moment. This is because all of these filters rely on local statistical data related to the filtered pixel. An alternative approach is to use wavelet transform.

3. Wavelet transform method

The primary goal of speckle reduction is to remove the speckle without losing much detail contained in an image. To achieve this goal, we make use of the wavelet transform and apply multiresolution analysis to localize an image into different frequency components or useful

Despeckling filters	Computational Time (in Secs.)
Lee (3x3)	25.60
Lee (5x5)	25.63
Lee (7x7)	25.64
Kuan(3x3)	40.89
Kuan(5x5)	41.57
Wiener(3x3)	**4.14**
Wiener(5x5)	5.14
Wiener(7x7)	6.15

Table 1. Performance comparison of various despeckling filters based on computational time.

subbands and then effectively reduce the speckle in the subbands according to the local statistics within the bands. The main advantage of the wavelet transform is that the image fidelity after reconstruction is visually lossless.

A wavelet is a mathematical function used to decompose a given function or continuous-time signal into different frequency components and study each component with a resolution that matches its scale. A wavelet transform is the representation of a function by wavelets. The wavelets are scaled and translated copies (known as daughter wavelets) of a finite length or fast decaying oscillating waveform (known as mother wavelet). Wavelet transforms are classified into continuous wavelet transform (CWT) and discrete wavelet transform. The CWT analyzes the signal through the continuous shifts of a scalable function over a time plane. Because of computers discrete nature, computer programs use the discrete wavelet transform. The discrete transform is very efficient from computational point of view.

Image denoising using wavelet techniques is effective because of its ability to capture most of the energy of a signal in a few significant transform coefficients. Another reason of using wavelet transform is due to development of efficient algorithms for signal decomposition and reconstruction [16] for image processing applications such as denoising and compression. A survey of despeckling techniques is discussed in [17, 18] and many wavelet domain techniques are already available in the literature. In [19], the authors have presented a novel speckle suppression method for medical ultrasound images, in which it is shown that the subband decompositions of ultrasound images have significantly non Gaussian statistics that are best described by families of heavy tailed distributions such as the alpha stable. Then, a Bayesian estimator is designed to exploit these statistics. Alpha stable model is used to develop a blind noise removal processor that performs a nonlinear operation on the data. In [20], the authors have proposed a novel technique for despeckling the medical ultrasound images using lossy compression. In [21], authors have proposed a new wavelet based image denoising technique, in which the different threshold functions, namely universal threshold, Visu shrink, sure shrink, Bayes shrink and normal shrink are considered for the study. The threshold value is calculated using circular kernel, mean max threshold, nearest neighbour and new threshold function.

Any decomposition of an image into wavelets involves a pair of waveforms, one to represent the high frequencies corresponding to the detailed parts of an image (wavelet function ψ) and one for high frequencies are transformed with short functions (low scale). The result of WT is a set of wavelet the low frequencies or smooth parts of an image (scaling function ϕ) coefficients, which measure the contribution of the wavelets at different locations and scales. The WT performs multiresolution image analysis [22]. The scaling function for multiresolution approximation can be obtained as the solution to a two scale dilatational Eq.(16):

$$\phi(x) = \sum_{k} a_L(k)\phi(2x\text{-}k) \tag{16}$$

for some suitable sequence of coefficients $a_L(k)$. Once ϕ has been found, an associated mother wavelet is given by a similar looking Eq.(17):

$$\psi(x) = \sum_{k} a_H(k)\phi(2x\text{-}k). \tag{17}$$

Wavelet analysis leads to perfect reconstruction filter banks using the coefficient sequences $a_L(k)$ and $a_H(k)$. The input sequence X is convolved with high pass (HPF) and low pass (LPF) filters $a_H(k)$, $a_L(k)$ respectively. Further, each result is down sampled by two, yielding the transform signals x_H and x_L. The signal is reconstructed through upsampling and convolution with high and low synthesis filters s_H (k) and s_L (k). By cascading the analysis filter bank with itself a number of times, digital signal decomposition with dyadic frequency scaling known as DWT can be formed. The DWT for an image as a 2D signal can be derived from 1D DWT. The easiest way for obtaining scaling and wavelet functions for two dimensions is by multiplying two 1D functions. The scaling function for 2D DWT can be obtained by multiplying two 1D scaling functions: $\phi(x,y)=\phi(x)\phi(y)$representing the approximation subband image (LL). The analysis filter bank for a single level 2D DWT structure produces three detail subband images (HL, LH, HH) corresponding to three different directional orientations (Horizontal, Vertical and Diagonal) and a lower resolution subband image LL. The filter bank structure can be iterated in a similar manner on the LL channel to provide multilevel decomposition. The separable wavelets are also viewed as tensor products of one dimensional wavelets and scaling functions. If $\psi(x)$ is the one dimensional wavelet associated with one dimensional scaling function $\phi(x)$, then three 2D wavelets associated with three subband images, called as vertical, horizontal and diagonal details, are given by

$$\psi^{V}(x,y) = \varphi(x)\psi(y) \tag{18}$$

$$\psi^{H}(x,y) = \psi(x)\varphi(y) \tag{19}$$

$$\psi^D(x,y) = \psi(x)\psi(y) \tag{20}$$

which correspond to the three subbands LH, HL and HH, respectively [23]. The wavelet equation produces different types of wavelet families like Daubenchies, Haar, Symlets, Coiflets and Biorthogonal wavelets [24].

3.1. Thresholding techniques

There are two approaches to perform the thresholding after computation of the wavelet coefficients, namely, subband thresholding and global thresholding [25]. In subband thresholding, we compute the noise variance of the horizontal, vertical and diagonal sub bands of each decomposition level, starting from the outer spectral bands and moving towards inner spectral bands (decomposition from higher levels towards lower levels) and calculate threshold value using Bayes shrinkage or Visu shrinkage rule. In global thresholding, we determine the threshold value from only the diagonal band but we apply this threshold to the horizontal, vertical and diagonal sub bands. This approach assumes that the diagonal band contains most of the high frequencies components; hence the noise content in diagonal band should be higher than the other bands. Thresholding at the coarsest level is not done, because it contains the approximation coefficients that represent the translated and scaled down version of the original image. Thresholding at this level will cause the reconstruction image to be distorted.

Shrinkage scheme:

The thresholding approach is to shrink the detail coefficients (high frequency components) whose amplitudes are smaller than a certain statistical threshold value to zero while retaining the smoother detail coefficients to reconstruct the ideal image without much loss in its details. This process is sometimes called wavelet shrinkage, since the detail coefficients are shrunk towards zero. There are three schemes to shrink the wavelet coefficients, namely, the keep-or-kill hard thresholding, shrink-or-kill soft thresholding introduced by [26] and the recent semi soft or firm thresholding. Shrinking of the wavelet coefficient is most efficient if the coefficients are sparse, that is, the majority of the coefficients are zero and a minority of coefficients with greater magnitude that can represent the image [27]. The criterion of each scheme is described as follows. Given that λ denotes the threshold limit, X_w denotes the input wavelet coefficients and Y_t denotes the output wavelet coefficients after thresholding, we define the following thresholding functions:

Hard thresholding:

$$Y_t = T_{hard}(X_w) = \begin{cases} X_w & , \text{for } |X_w| \ge \lambda \\ 0 & , \text{for } |X_w| < \lambda \end{cases} \tag{21}$$

Soft thresholding:

http://dx.doi.org/10.5772/56519

$$Y_t = T_{soft}(X_w) = \begin{cases} \text{sign}\{X_w\}(|X_w| - \lambda) & , \text{for } |X_w| \geq \lambda \\ 0 & , \text{for } |X_w| < \lambda \end{cases} \tag{22}$$

Semi soft thresholding:

$$Y_t = T_{semisoft}(X_w) = \begin{cases} 0 & , \text{for } |X_w| \leq \lambda \\ \text{sign}\{X_w\}\dfrac{\lambda_1(|X_w| - \lambda)}{\lambda_1 - \lambda} & , \text{for } \lambda < |X_w| \leq \lambda_1 \\ X_w & , \text{for } |X_w| > \lambda_1 \end{cases} \tag{23}$$

where $\lambda_1 = 2\lambda$.

The hard thresholding procedure removes the noise by thresholding only the wavelet coefficients of the detail sub bands, while keeping the low resolution coefficients unaltered. The soft thresholding scheme shown in Eq. (22) is an extension of the hard thresholding. It avoids discontinuities and is, therefore, more stable than hard thresholding. In practice, soft thresholding is more popular than hard thresholding, because it reduces the abrupt sharp changes that occurs in hard thresholding and provides more visually pleasant recovered images. The aim of semi soft threshold is to offer a compromise between hard and soft thresholding by changing the gradient of the slope. This scheme requires two thresholds, a lower threshold λ and an upper threshold λ_1 where λ_1 is estimated to be twice the value of lower threshold λ.

3.2. Shrinkage rule

A very large threshold λ will shrink almost all the coefficients to zero and may result in over smoothing the image, while a small value of λ will lead to the sharp edges with details being retained but may fail to suppress the speckle. We use the shrinkage rules, namely, the Visu shrinkage rule and Bayes shrinkage rule for thresholding which are explained in the following:

3.2.1. Visu shrinkage rule

Visu shrinkage rule [28] is thresholding by applying universal threshold. The idea is to find

each threshold λ_i to be proportional to the square root of the local noise variance σ^2 in each subband of the ultrasound image after decomposition. If N_k is the size of the subband in the wavelet domain, then λ_i

$$\lambda_i = \sigma\sqrt{2\log(N_k)} \tag{24}$$

The estimated local noise variance, σ^2, in each subband is obtained by averaging the squares of the empirical wavelet coefficients at the highest resolution scale as

$$\sigma^2 = \frac{1}{N_k^2} \sum_{i,j=0}^{N_k-1} W_{ij}^2 \tag{25}$$

The threshold of Eq.(24) is based on the fact that, for a zero mean independent identically distributed (i.i.d.) Gaussian process with variance σ^2, there is a high probability that a sample value of this process will not exceed λ. Thus, the Visu shrink is suitable for applications with white Gaussian noise and in which most of the coefficients are zero. In such cases, there is a high probability that the combination of (zero) coefficients plus noise will not exceed the threshold level λ.

3.2.2. Bayes shrinkage rule

In Bayes shrink [29], an adaptive data driven threshold is used for image denoising. The threshold on a given subband W_k of the image X, is given by

$$\lambda_K = \frac{\sigma_n^2}{\sigma_x} \tag{26}$$

where σ_n, the estimated noise variance found as the median of the absolute deviation of the diagonal detail coefficients on the finest level (sub band HH_1), is given by

$$\sigma_n = \frac{\mathrm{median}\left(\left\{W_{ij} \in HH_1\right\}\right)}{0.67452} \tag{27}$$

This estimator is used when there is no a priori knowledge about the noise variance. The σ_x, which is the estimated signal variance in the wavelet domain, is given by

$$\sigma_x = \sqrt{\max\left(\sigma_y^2 - \sigma_n^2, 0\right)} \tag{28}$$

and σ_y^2, an estimate of the variance of the W_k, Since W_k is modeled as zero mean, σ_y^2 can be found empirically by,

$$\sigma_y^2 = \frac{1}{N_k^2} \sum_{i,j=0}^{N_k-1} W_{ij}^2 \tag{29}$$

in which N_k is the number of the wavelet coefficients W_k on the subband considered. In the Eq. (27), the value 0.67452 is the median absolute deviation of normal distribution with zero mean and unit variance. In the Eq.(26), if (σ_n /σ_x) << 1, the signal is much stronger than the noise. The normalized threshold is chosen to be small in order to preserve most of the signal and remove the noise. If (σ_n /σ_x)>> 1, the noise dominates the signal. The normalized threshold is chosen to be large to remove the noise more aggressively. In the Eq.(28), if $\sigma_n^2 \geq \sigma_y^2$, σ_x will become zero i.e. λ becomes infinity. Hence, for this case, λ =max ({| W_{ij} |}).

The experimentation is carried out for each filter order, for each family and the decompositions are performed upto 4 levels. The statistical features: variance, PSNR, MSE, SNR and correlation coefficient, computed for different wavelets: DW (db1, db5), CW (coif1, coif2, and coif5), SW (sym1, sym3, sym5) and BW (bior2.2, bior6.8). The BW family, where filters are of order 6 in decomposition and order 8 in reconstruction (BW6.8), gives the better results among all the filter types. The PSNR is calculated for bior 6.8 filter up to 4 decompositions. The PSNR value increases up to 3 decompositions and thereafter reduces. Hence, the optimal level of decomposition is 3. The results obtained for the different thresholding schemes are given in the Table 2 [27]. From Table 2, it is found that, there is significant improvement of the subband threshold approach in terms of image quality assessment parameters over the global threshold approach. This is because subband thresholding approach employs an adaptive thresholding approach to respond to the changes in the noise content of the different subbands. In contrast, the global thresholding relies on a Visu threshold to threshold all subbands. The label (written in the parenthesis) in the Table 2. indicates the global(I) and subband thresholding (II), Bayes' (1) or Visu (2) shrinkage rule and the hard (i), soft (ii) or semi soft (iii) thresholding function employed to generate that image. The optimal thresholding scheme with shrinkage rule and shrinkage function are determined by the criteria, namely, higher SNR and PSNR values, lower Variance, MSE values and Correlation Coefficient is nearly equal to one. From Table 2, it is observed that subband decomposition (II) with soft thresholding (ii) using Bayes shrinkage rule (1) gives better results than other techniques. Bayes shrinkage is better than the universal threshold because the universal threshold tends to be high, killing many signal coefficients along with the noise. The Figure 6. shows the visual quality of proposed method based on wavelet filter with Wiener filter. It is observed that the wavelet filter (bior6.8 with level 3(L3)) yields better visualization effect and denoised image than the Wiener filter. The Table 3. shows the performance comparison of proposed method based on wavelet filter with despeckle filter, namely Wiener filter. From Table 3, it is observed that the wavelet filter (bior6.8 with level 3) yields better visualization effect and denoised image than the wiener filter in terms of variance and computational time. But the method based on despeckling using wavelet transforms needs to be improved interms of image quality assessment parameters.

3.3. Laplacian pyramid transform

Several speckle reduction techniques based on multi scale methods (e.g. Wavelet transform, Laplacian pyramid (LP) transform) have been proposed [30-33]. The LP has the distinguishing feature that each pyramid level generates only one bandpass image (even for multidimensional cases), which does not have "scrambled" frequencies. This frequency scrambling happens in the wavelet filter bank when a high pass channel, after down sampling, is folded back into the low frequency band, and thus its spectrum is reflected. In the LP, this effect is avoided by down sampling the low pass channel only.

Bayes' Shrinkage rule(1)	Global thresholding (I)					Subband thresholding (II)				
	Variance	MSE	SNR	CC	PSNR	Variance	MSE	SNR	CC	PSNR
Hard (i)	0.0396	0.0023	16.89	0.991	26.38	0.0482	0.0015	18.94	0.994	28.48
Soft (ii)	0.0396	0.0025	14.83	0.992	26.02	0.0368	0.0012	19.06	0.995	29.94
Semi soft (iii)	0.0370	0.0024	16.04	0.992	26.17	0.0456	0.0016	17.94	0.993	28.56
Visu shrinkage rule (2)	**Global thresholding (I)**					**Subband thresholding (II)**				
Hard (i)	0.0431	0.0028	15.94	0.993	25.52	0.0392	0.0029	16.15	0.992	27.33
Soft (ii)	0.0461	0.0032	14.12	0.992	24.92	0.0372	0.0023	17.79	0.994	28.78
Semi soft (iii)	0.0481	0.0031	14.15	0.992	25.00	0.0385	0.0032	16.17	0.993	27.51

Table 2. Performance evaluation of different thresholding methods interms of variance, MSE,PSNR,SNR and CC values.

Denoising methods	PSNR	SNR	MSE	Variance	CC	Computational time (in Secs.)
WT-L3-ST (bior 6.8)	29.94	19.06	0.00121	0.0368	0.9954	2.80
Wiener (3x3)	32.34	21.53	0.00058	0.0489	0.9977	4.14

Table 3. Performance comparison of wavelet based despeckling method and Wiener filter.

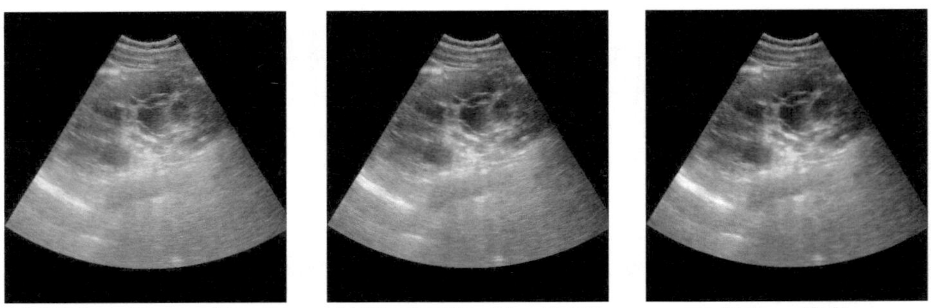

(a) Original ultrasound image (b) Wavelet filter(Bior 6.8,L3) (c) Wiener(3x3)

Figure 6. Despeckled images using Wiener filter and Wavelet filter

A speckle reduction method based on non linear diffusion filtering of band pass ultrasound images in the Laplacian pyramid domain has been proposed in [34], which effectively suppresses the speckle while preserving edges and detailed features. In [31], the authors have implemented a nonlinear multiscale pyramidal transform, based on non overlapping block

http://dx.doi.org/10.5772/56519

decompositions using the median operation and a polynomial approximation. It is shown that this structure can be useful for denoising of one and two dimensional (1-D and 2-D) signals. It can be used for the selection of thresholds for denoising applications.

In [33] the comparison of two multiresolution methods: Wavelet transform and Laplacian pyramid transform, for simultaneous speckle reduction and contrast enhancement for ultrasound images is given. As a lot of variability exists in ultrasound images, the wavelet method proves to be a much better method than the Laplacian one for an overall improvement. However, the Laplacian pyramid scheme need to be explored for achieving better despeckling results.

3.3.1. Laplacian pyramid scheme

One way of achieving a multiscale decomposition is to use a Laplacian pyramid (LP) transform [35]. In the first stage of the decomposition, the original image is transformed into a coarse signal and a difference signal. The coarse signal has fewer samples than the original image but the difference signal has the same number of samples as the original image. The coarse signal is a filtered and down sampled version of the original image. It is then up sampled and filtered to predict the original image. The prediction residual constitutes the detail signal. The coarse signal can be decomposed further and this process can be repeated a few times iteratively. Assuming the filters in LP are orthogonal filters, an image X is decomposed into J detail images d_j, j=1, 2,...,J and a coarse approximation image c_J. Then, we have

$$\|X\|^2 = \sum_{j=1}^{J} \|d_j\|^2 + \|c_J\|^2 \tag{30}$$

The Laplacian is then computed as the difference between the original image and the low pass filtered image. This process is continued to obtain a set of detail filtered images (since each one is the difference between two levels of the Gaussian pyramid). Thus the Laplacian pyramid is a set of detail filters. By repeating these steps several times, a sequence of images are obtained. If these images are stacked one above another, the result is a tapering pyramid data structure and, hence the name the Laplacian pyramid.

A speckle reduction method based on Laplacian pyramid transform for medical ultrasound image is illustrated using the block diagram shown in the Figure 7. In the Figure 7, a homomorphic approach such as the log transformation of the speckle corrupted image, converts the multiplicative noise of the original image into additive noise. Homomorphic operation simultaneously normalizes the brightness across an image and increases contrast. For every difference signal of N-level of Laplacian pyramidal decomposition a threshold value is calculated using Bayes' shrinkage rule. Further, thresholding is performed to reduce speckle. The exponential operation is performed on the filtered output to obtain the despeckled image.

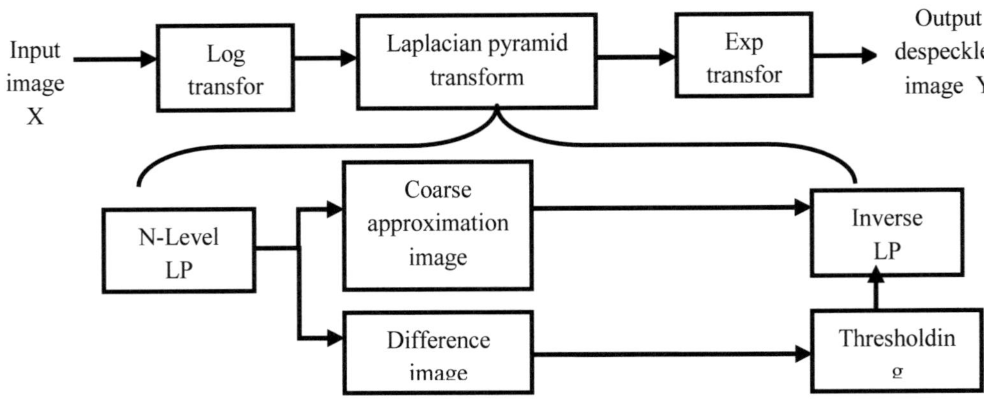

Figure 7. Block diagram of speckle noise suppression using Laplacian pyramid transform

The Laplacian pyramid transform is performed on the log transformed image. The Laplacian pyramidal decompositions up to six levels are obtained using biorthogonal filters with sufficient accuracy numbers such as the "9/7" and "5/3". Further, thresholding schemes such as hard thresholding, soft thresholding and semi soft thresholding is performed to reduce speckle. The threshold value is calculated using Bayes' shrinkage rule. The experimentation is carried out on 70 ultrasound images of liver and kidney. The performance evaluation of the proposed method is done in terms of variance, MSE, SNR, PSNR, CC values that are computed from despeckled image. The Laplacian pyramid transform with 1 level decomposition and hard thresholding is observed to be better than other thresholding methods.

The Table 4. shows the performance comparison of the proposed LP transform based despeckling method with the wavelet transform based despeckling method [36]. It is noticed that, in comparison with the despeckling medical ultrasound images based on WT, the despeckling based on LP method yields poor results. Because multiplicative noise is a particular type of signal dependent noise, in which the amplitude of the noise term is proportional to the value of the noise free signal having nonzero mean. Therefore, a band pass representation like LP is not suitable for multiplicative noise model, So the method needs to be improved.

In order to capture smooth contours in the images, the contourlet transforms, which allow directional decompositions, are employed for despeckling medical ultrasound images in the next section.

4. Contourlet transform method

The contourlet transform (CT) is a multiscale and multidirectional framework of discrete image. It is the simple directional extension for wavelet that fixes its subband mixing problem and improves its directionality. Among the "beyond wavelet" techniques, contourlet allows for different and flexible number of directions at each scale, while achieving nearly critical sampling. The desirable properties of CT for image representation includes multiresolution,

Despeckling methods	PSNR	SNR	MSE	Variance	CC	Computational time (in Secs.)
LP transform based despeckling method (LP-HT-L1)	28.44	18.23	0.00141	0.0416	0.9972	2.24
Wavelet transform based despeckling method (WT-L3-ST)	29.94	19.06	0.00121	0.0368	0.9954	2.80

Table 4. Performance comparison of the LP transform method and the wavelet transform based despeckling method

allowing images to be approximated in a coarse to fine fashion; localization of the basis vectors in both space and frequency; low redundancy, so as not to increase the amount of data to be stored; directionality, allowing representation with basis elements oriented in a variety of directions; and anisotropy, the ability to capture smooth contours in images, using basis elements that are a variety of elongated shapes with different aspect ratios [37].

The contourlet transform has been developed to overcome the limitations of the wavelets, and hence, the new algorithms based on the contourlet transform are more efficient than wavelet methods. In [38], the authors have presented a contourlet based speckle reduction method for denoising ultrasound images of breast. The double iterated filter bank structure and a small redundancy at most 4/3 using two thresholding methods shows a great promise for speckle reduction. In [39], the despeckling medical ultrasound images using contourlet transform using Bayes' shrinkage rule is investigated. The algorithm is also tested on ovarian ultrasound images to demonstrate improvements in the segmentation that yields good classification for follicle detection in an ovarian image [40].

In [41], speckle reduction based on contourlet transform using scale adaptive threshold for medical ultrasound image has been examined, where in the subband contourlet coefficients of the ultrasound images after logarithmic transform are modelled as generalized Gaussian distribution. The scale adaptive threshold in Bayesian framework is applied. The method is tested on both synthetic and clinical ultrasound images interms of S/MSE and edge preservation parameter. The proposed method exhibits better performance on speckle suppression than the wavelet based method, while it does well preserve the feature details of the image.

The contourlet transform can be divided into two main steps: Laplacian pyramid decomposition and directional filter banks. Contourlet transform is a multi scale and directional image representation that uses first a wavelet like structure for edge detection, and then a local directional transform for contour segment detection. A double filter bank structure of the contourlet obtains sparse expansions for typical images having smooth contours. In the double filter bank structure, the Laplacian pyramid is used to decompose an image into a number of radial subbands, and the directional filter banks decompose each LP detail subband into a number of directional subbands. The band pass images ($d_j\,[n]$) from the LP are fed into a DFB so that directional information can be captured. The scheme can be iterated on the coarse image

(c_j [n]). The combined result is a double iterated filter bank structure, named pyramidal directional filter bank (PDFB), which decomposes images into directional subbands at multiple scales. The general model for despeckling an image using contourlet transform is shown in the Figure 8.

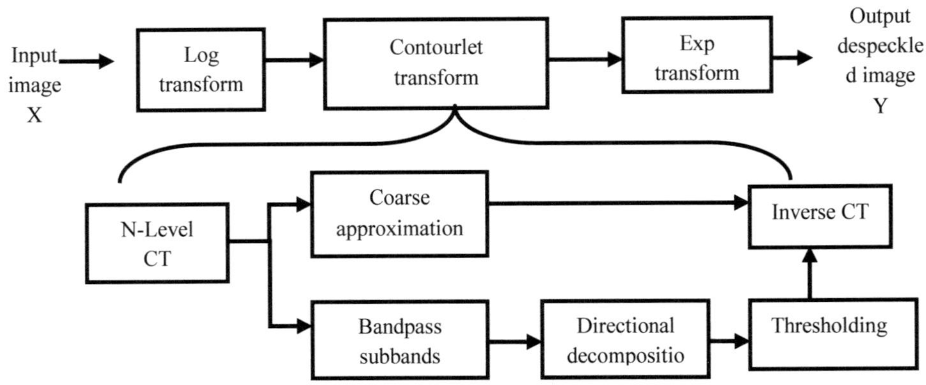

Figure 8. The general model for speckle reduction using contourlet transform.

In the Figure 8, the CT based despeckling method consists of the log transformed original ultrasound image being subjected to contourlet transform, to obtain contourlet coefficients. The transformed image is denoised by applying thresholding techniques on individual band pass sub bands using a Bayes shrinkage rule, derived from the local statistics of the signal in the transform domain. Bayes' shrink was proposed by [29]. The goal of Bayes' shrinkage method is to minimize the Bayesian risk, and hence its name, Bayes' shrink. Further, thresholding schemes such as hard thresholding, soft thresholding or semi soft thresholding is performed to reduce speckle. The exponential operation is performed on the filtered output to obtain the despeckled image.

The experimentation is carried out on 70 ultrasound images of liver and kidney. The six levels of Laplacian pyramidal decompositions are performed using biorthogonal filters with sufficient accuracy numbers such as the "9/7". The directional decompositions up to eight are performed in all the pyramidal levels, using two dimensional ladder filters. The contourlet transform uses the "9/7" filters in LP stage because, in the multiscale decomposition stage, it significantly reduces all inter scale, inter location and inter direction mutual information of contourlet coefficients. Similarly, in directional decomposition stage, the ladder structure PKVA filters [42] are more effective in localizing edge direction as these filters reduce the inter direction mutual information. Further, thresholding schemes such as hard thresholding, soft thresholding or semi soft thresholding is performed to reduce speckle. The threshold value is calculated using Bayes' shrinkage rule. The PSNR is calculated up to 6 LP decompositions. The PSNR value increases up to 2 decompositions using HT, ST and SST, and thereafter reduces. Hence, the optimal level of LP decomposition is 2. Further, it is observed from Table 5, that the 2-level Laplacian pyramidal decomposition and 4 directional bandpass subbands (2 at level 1, 2 at level 2) using hard thresholding yield better results than soft thresholding and semi soft thresholding techniques.

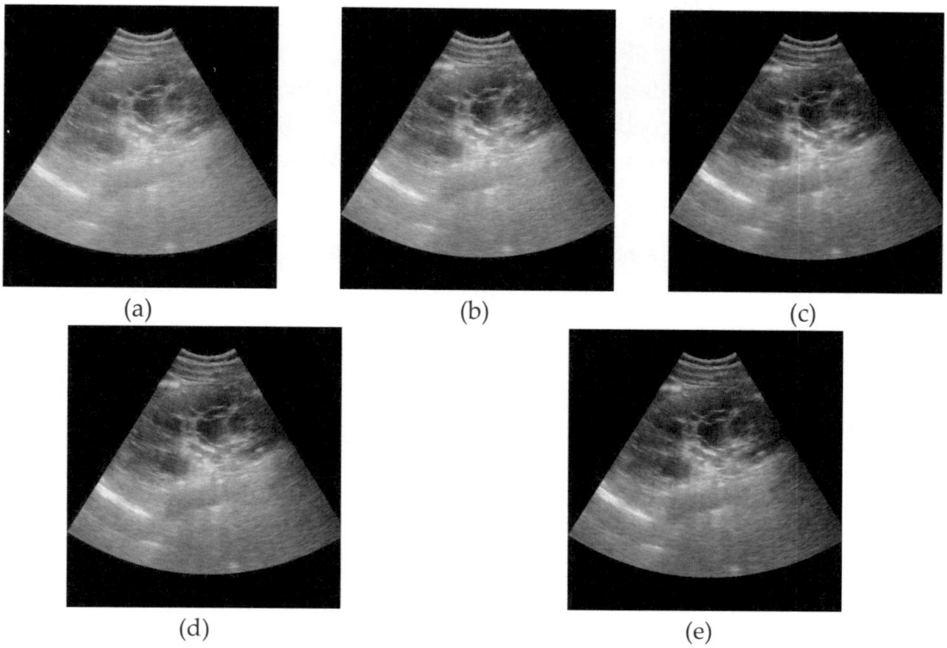

Figure 9. a) Original ultrasound image. (b) Despeckled image using wavelet transform using subband Bayes soft thresholding (level 3). (c) Despeckled image using contourlet transform using soft thresholding. (d) Despeckled image using contourlet transform using hard thresholcing. (e) Despeckled image using contourlet transform using semi soft thresholding.

Thresholding methods	Levels	PSNR	Variance	MSE	CC	SNR	Computational time(in Secs.)
Hard thresholding	L2-11	34.21	0.0203	0.00037	0.9990	27.74	1.64
Soft thresholding	L2-31	32.49	0.0382	0.00056	0.9983	24.14	1.68
Semi-soft thresholding	L2-11	33.31	0.0292	0.00046	0.9987	25.91	1.74

Table 5. The results obtained for the optimal optimal decomposition of LP levels and directional decompositions in terms of image quality assessment parameters using contourlet method based on different thresholding techniques with Bayes' shrinkage rule.

The frequency bands obtained by using optimal level L2-11 of contourlet decomposition are as follows: the 2nd level has 1 approximation band of size 128 x128 and 4 detail components (2 of 128 x 256, 2 of 256 x 512). The reconstructed image is the despeckled image. The hard thresholding is better than other thresholding methods, because small coefficients are removed while others are left untouched in HT, while in ST or SST coefficients above the threshold are shrunk by absolute value of threshold. Further, it is found that the despeckling based on contourlet transform gives better results than the speckle reduction method based on wavelet transform in particular. The wavelet based Bayes' shrink thresholding method is based on separable 2D wavelet transform that has limited directions (Horizontal, Vertical and Directional). Speckle noise in medical ultrasound images will generate significant coefficients in wavelet domain just like true detail features, such as edges. However, the speckle noise is less likely to generate significant coefficients in the contourlet method, and thus, it directly leads to better performance in suppressing noise than the wavelet based Bayes' shrink thresholding scheme.

Another way to analyze the effects of despeckling techniques is to study the despeckled images. In the Figure 9., the resultant images of a sample medical ultrasound image are presented to compare the results of different despeckling techniques by visual inspection. In the Figure 9(b) and (c), the speckle is reduced considerably, but the structures are blurred and some visible artifacts are introduced. However, in Figure 9(e), the speckle is reduced well and structures are enhanced. But some details are lost and some are over enhanced. It is encouraging to note that in the Figure 9(d), the speckle is effectively reduced and also structures are enhanced with almost no loss or noticeable artifact.

4.1. Cycle spinning based contourlet transform

The CT is not translation invariant. This means that the errors after denoising will be sensitive to the positions of discontinuities in the data. In order to avoid such effects, it is necessary to build translation invariant version of the transform. Translation invariance is achieved through several ways. For example, in [43], the time invariant schemes of wavelet based decompositions have been proposed and have been often referred to as cycle spinning. Unfortunately, due to the downsamplers and upsamplers present in the directional filter banks of CT, the CT is not shift invariant, which is important in image denoising by thresholding and normally causes pseudo-Gibbs phenomenon. In [44], the cycle spinning algorithm is utilized in developing a translation invariant contourlet based denoising technique. The experimental results clearly demonstrate the capability of the proposed scheme in image denoising, especially for detailed texture images. It is shown that most of the visual artifacts resulting from the contourlet transform denoising process are eliminated. In [45], a cycle spinning method is used to compensate for the lack of translation invariance property of sharp frequency localized contourlet. Experimental results demonstrate that cycle spinning is a simple and efficient way to average out the pseudo-Gibbs phenomena, which are around singularities and produced by the down sampling and up sampling of directional filter banks, and improve the denoising performance interms of visual quality and PSNR.

To compensate for the lack of translation invariance property of the contourlet transform, we apply the principle of cycle spinning to contourlets. Suppose X and Y are original and despeckled images, F and F^{-1} are forward and inverse contourlet transform, $S_{i,j}$ is the 2D circular shift in i^{th} row and j^{th} column directions, λ is the threshold operator in contourlet transform domain. The cycle spinning based contourlet transform for image denoising could be described as

$$Y = \frac{1}{B^2} \sum_{i,j=1}^{B} CS_{-i,-j}\left(F^{-1}\left(\lambda\left(F\left(CS_{i,j}(X)\right)\right)\right)\right) \tag{31}$$

http://dx.doi.org/10.5772/56519

where B is the series of bit shifts in the ith row and j^{th} column directions. If one decomposes an image of size (N, N) using the contourlet transform, the maximum number of decomposition levels in the LP stage will be B, and therefore, the maximum number of shifts are (B, B) in the row and column directions. After a B number of bit shifts, which depends on the level of decomposition, the transform output degrades. Hence, the cycle spinning has to be stopped after a certain number of bit shifts. The Figure 10. shows the block diagram for speckle reduction method based on contourlet transform with cycle spinning. The cycle spinning is applied to the log transformed image. It performs two dimensional circular shift in i^{th} row and j^{th} column directions. The circular shifting is performed up to B number of bit shifts, where B depends on the level of decomposition. The transform output degrades as B increases. Hence, the cycle spinning has to be stopped after a certain number of bit shifts. Then contourlet transform is performed using double filter bank structure. The six levels of Laplacian pyramidal decompositions are performed using biorthogonal filters with sufficient accuracy numbers such as the "9-7".The directional decompositions up to six is performed in the lowest pyramidal level, using two dimensional ladder filters designed in [42]. Further, a thresholding scheme either hard thresholding, soft thresholding or semi soft thresholding, is performed to reduce speckle. The threshold value is calculated using Bayes' shrinkage rule. The results obtained for the optimal bit shifts of cycle spinning using contourlet method based on hard thresholding, soft thresholding and semi soft thresholding using Bayes' rule are presented. The results obtained for different reconstruction methods are shown in Figures 11-15, which exhibit graphs of statistical features PSNR, SNR, variance, MSE and CC, respectively, for different levels of Laplacian pyramid decompositions and directional decompositions corresponding to optimal results of contourlet transform with cycle spinning based despeckling method [46]. The optimal reconstruction method is determined by the criteria, namely, lower variance and MSE, higher SNR and PSNR values, Correlation Coefficient is nearly equal to one. The contourlet transform with 2 level of pyramidal decomposition and two directional decompositions in the finest scale and hard thresholding technique with Bayes' shrinkage rule has yielded better results in comparison contourlet transform based methods [47]. In the Figures 11-15, the horizontal axis label CYC-HT-Bn indicates cycle spin (CYC), thresholding (HT,ST,SST), n number of bit shifts in cycle spinning. From Figures 11-15, it is observed that, 4 bit cycle spinning, having the 2-level of Laplacian pyramidal decomposition with 4 directional bandpass sub bands (2 at level 1, 2 at level 2) subject to soft thresholding, yields optimal results for speckle reduction. The computational time (in Secs.) of the cycle spinning based CT method is shown in Figure 15. The CT based despeckling method takes less computational time as compared to cycle spinning based CT method.

The Figure 16. illustrates the resultant despeckled images of an ultrasound image obtained by the cycle spinning based CT method using hard, soft and semi soft thresholding with Bayes' shrinkage rule, and also that obtained by the CT method [47], for comparison by visual inspection The despeckling method based on cycle spinning using contourlet coefficient shrinkage (Figure16.(b)) performs better and appears to be an improvement over direct contourlet transform based despeckling method.

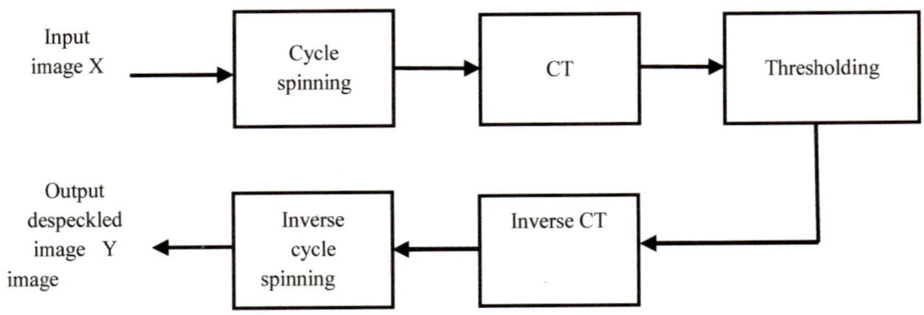

Figure 10. The block diagram of despeckling method based on contourlet transform with cycle spinning.

Among the transform domain filters developed in the previous sections, the contourlet transform with cycle spinning yields better visual quality enhancement of the despeckled images. However, there is still a need to remove Gaussian noise inherent in the medical ultrasound images, which is addressed in the next section.

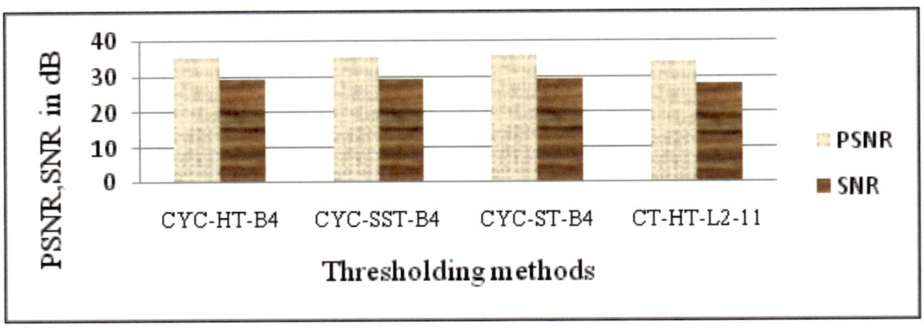

Figure 11. The values of PSNR and SNR for various thresholding methods obtained by cycle spinning based CT method and that by direct CT based method.

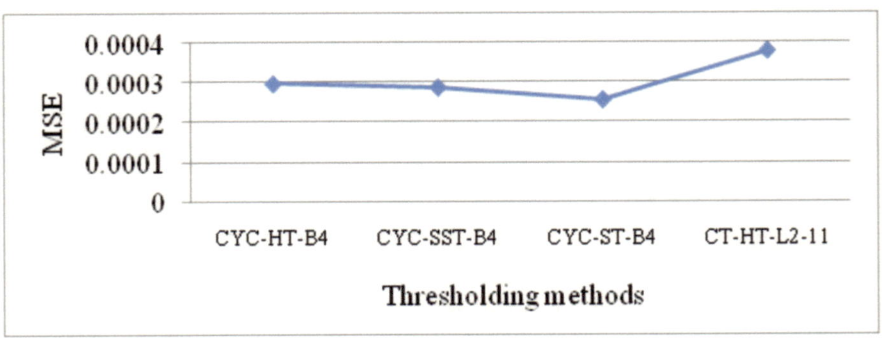

Figure 12. The values of MSE for various thresholding methods obtained by cycle spinning based CT method and that by direct CT based method.

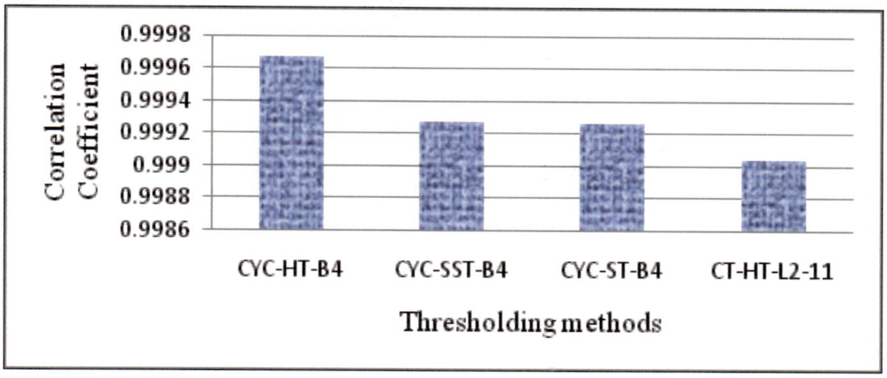

Figure 13. The values of Correlation Coefficient for various thresholding methods obtained by cycle spinning based CT method and that by direct CT based method.

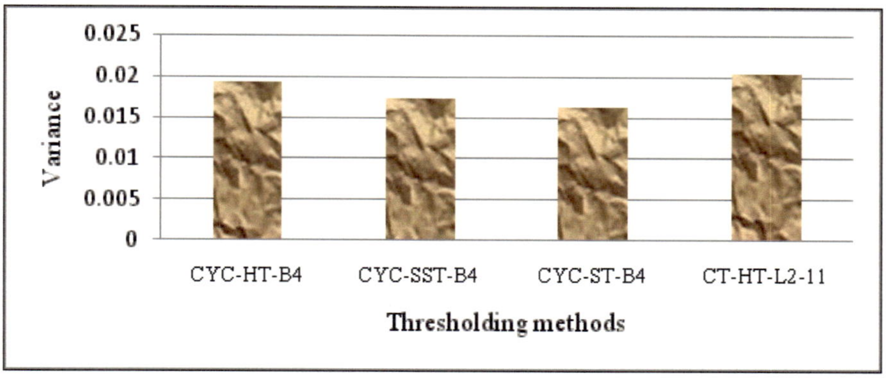

Figure 14. The values of variance for various thresholding methods obtained by cycle spinning based CT method and that by CT based method.

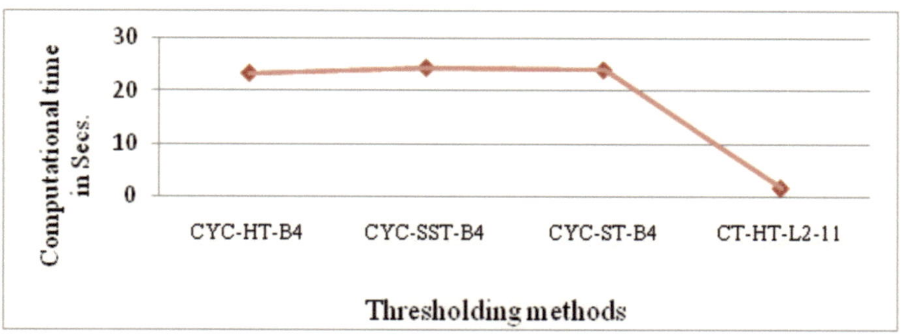

Figure 15. The values of computational time for various thresholding methods obtained by cycle spinning based CT method and that by CT based method.

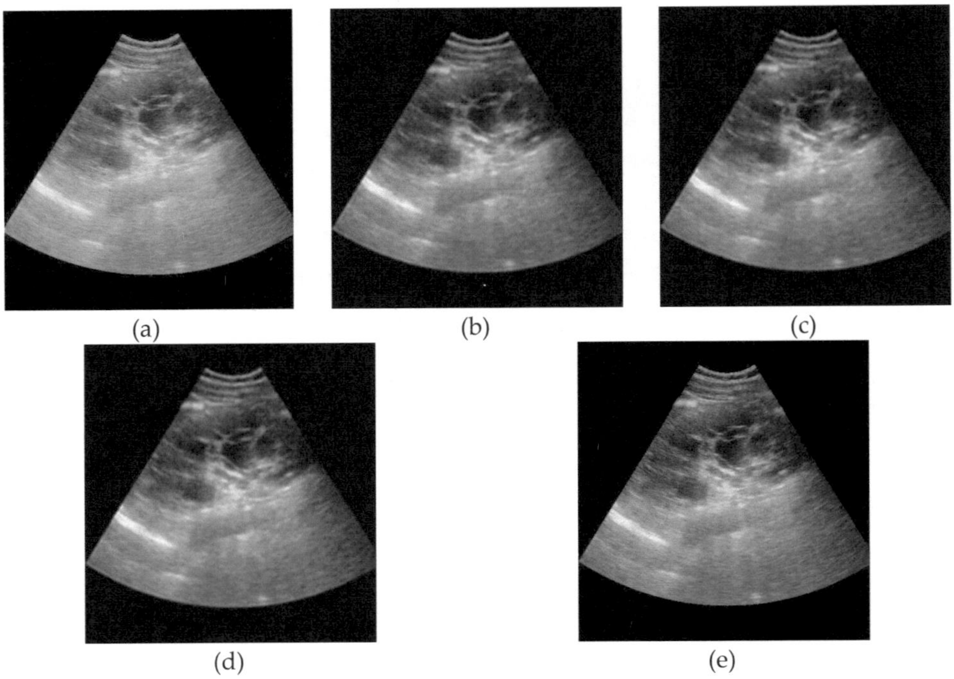

Figure 16. a) Original ultrasound image (b) Despeckled image using cycle spinning based CT using ST method. (c)Despeckled image using cycle spinning based CT using HT method. (d)Despeckled image using cycle spinning based CT using SST method. (e) Despeckled image using direct CT method.

5. Gaussian model for speckle noise

Gaussian probability density is often used in image filtering. The Gaussian has the unique ability not to create new edges as its scale (standard deviation) is increased. This property enables the extraction of edges that represent different levels of detail in an image. As the scale is increased, the number of extracted weak and false edges reduces. However, at the same time edges shift from their true positions. The amount of shift an edge makes not only depends upon the scale of the Gaussian filter, but also on the intensity distributions of the underlying image [48]. Mathematically, a Gaussian filter modifies the input signal by convolution with a Gaussian function. Smoothing is commonly undertaken using linear filters such as the Gaussian function (the kernel is based on the normal distribution curve), which tends to produce good results in reducing the influence of noise with respect to the image. The 2D Gaussian distributions, with standard deviation σ for image X, is given by Eq. (32) [49].

$$G(X, m, \sigma) = \frac{1}{\sigma\sqrt{2\pi}} e^{-\frac{1}{2}\left(\frac{X-m}{\sigma}\right)^2} \tag{32}$$

5.1. Pre- or post –processing

Usually, medical ultrasound images are affected by the mixed noise, which is the combination of speckle noise and Gaussian noise. There are two factors that influence the usefulness of a smoothing filter. The first reduces the range of resolutions over which variations in the output appear by the filter variation Δw, in the frequency domain be small and second factor is increase in spatial localization by a small spatial variance Δx. These localization requirements in the spatial and frequency domain are conflicting and related by the uncertainty principle given in Eq. (33)

$$\Delta w \ \Delta x \geq \frac{1}{4\pi} \tag{33}$$

It has been shown that Gaussian functions are the only ones that provide the optimal trade off between these conflicting requirements constrained by the Eq. (34) [50]..

$$\Delta w \Delta x = \frac{1}{4\pi} \tag{34}$$

So Gaussian filters are widely used in image filtering. In [51], the removal of mixed noise using order statistic filter and wavelet domain Wiener filter is proposed. Authors have evaluated two methods. The first method comprises, order statistic prefilter and empirical Wiener filter, which is used to reduce the Gaussian noise. The disadvantage of this method is the higher time consumption. The second method is, order statistic filter for each decomposition level, where decomposition is carried out by the wavelet transform, followed by thresholding. The drawback of this method is that its efficiency is less than that of the first method (about 1dB) in removing the mixed noise. In [52], denoising of mixed noise in ultrasound images is presented. Combined Bayesian maximum a posterior (MAP) estimator and ST-PCNN (Soft threshold pulse coupled neural networks) method has been used for mixed noise reduction. The method removes the speckle noise considerably than the Gaussian noise that degrades the ultrasound images. The drawback of the method is either Gaussian noise or speckle noise is removed. Hence we present a method to remove residual Gaussian noise from despeckled image.

Two alternative algorithms are developed for reducing mixed noise in medical ultrasound images [53]. In the first alternative, the denoising method reduces the Gaussian noise by applying Gaussian filter in pre processing stage, then despeckling is performed using either wavelet transform, Laplacian pyramid transform or contourlet transform. The noise model for the first alternative (i.e. Gaussian noise removal in pre processing followed by despeckling) is given by the Eq.(35).

$$X_{ij} = f_{ij} n_{ij} + g_{ij} \tag{35}$$

where X_{ij} represents the noisy pixel in the image X, f_{ij} represents the noise free pixel, n_{ij} and g_{ij} represent the multiplicative speckle noise and additive Gaussian noise, respectively. The indices i, j represent the spatial position over the image. We use transform domain filtering techniques [36,54,47] for despeckling along with Gaussian filter in pre processing stage for removal of Gaussian noise.

In the second alternative, the despeckling of medical ultrasound images is performed either using wavelet transform, Laplacian pyramid transform or contourlet transform and, then, it is followed by postprocessing stage in which Gaussian filter removes Gaussian noise from the despeckled image. However, the second alternative assumes the noise model given by the Eq.(36)

$$X_{ij}=(f_{ij}+g_{ij})\,n_{ij} \tag{36}$$

The second alternative is investigated for image quality enhancement, due to noise removal, in an ultrasound image.

The experimentation is carried out using various kernel sizes and different values of σ. Larger values of σ produce a wider peak influencing the greater blurring. Kernel size is increased with increasing σ to maintain the Gaussian nature of the filter. Gaussian kernel coefficients depend on the value of σ. The Figure 17. shows different convolution kernels that approximate a Gaussian with σ. Gaussians are locally sensitive and can be made more spatially localized by decreasing parameter σ. It is observed that the kernel size 3×3 with $\sigma = 0.5$ yields better results than other kernels. It is found that larger kernels of size 5×5 or 7×7 produce better denoising effect but make the image more blurred. Thus, the empirically determined kernel size 3×3 and σ=0.5 are used in two alternative methods (Gaussian filter in Pre or Post processing).The two alternative methods are evaluated in terms of filter assessment parameters, namely, PSNR, SNR, MSE, variance and CC. The comparisons of the performance of the both alternatives with the despeckling methods discussed in [36,54, 47] are given in the Table 6. From the Table 6, it is observed that the Gaussian filter in pre processing stage is found to be more effective than that in despeckling based on Laplacian pyramid transform and contourlet transform. However, the Gaussian filter in postprocessing stage is found to be more effective in despeckling based on wavelet transform. Thus, the Gaussian filter improves the performance of despeckling methods, because Gaussian noise is characterized by adding to each image pixel a value from a zero mean Gaussian distribution. The zero mean property of the distribution allows such noise to be removed by locally averaging pixel values [55]. Further, it is observed that, the Gaussian filter in pre processing stage followed by contourlet transform based despeckling method yields better visual enhancement than the other denoising methods, which is illustrated in the Figure 18. The denoising and visual enhancement techniques developed in this study lead to improvement in the accuracy and reliability of automatic methods for medical ultrasound imaging systems.

5.2. Linear regression model

We present a linear regression based approach for clinical ultrasound image despeckling in the spatial domain. We propose a linear regression model for Gaussian noise representation of speckle noise for medical ultrasound images. This approach introduces an adaptive filter,

0.0128	0.0876	0.0128
0.0876	0.5986	0.0876
0.0128	0.0876	0.0128

(a)

0.075	0.124	0.075
0.124	0.204	0.124
0.075	0.124	0.075

(b)

Figure 17. The 3x3 kernel with (a) σ = 0.5, (b) σ = 1.

Denoising methods	SNR	PSNR	CC	MSE	Variance	Computational time (in Secs.)
First alternative with wavelet transform	25.22	30.23	0.9992	0.00050	0.0128	0.91
First alternative with LP transform	20.07	31.66	0.9965	0.00106	0.0426	0.38
First alternative with CT transform	29.99	35.15	0.9998	0.00031	0.0071	1.62
Second alternative with WT transform	26.32	32.54	0.9995	0.00050	0.0120	0.89
Second alternative with LP transform	19.76	30.12	0.9959	0.00133	0.0440	0.76
Second alternative with CT transform	28.89	34.35	0.9996	0.00036	0.0088	2.25
Despeckling method (WT transform) [36]	19.06	29.94	0.9954	0.00121	0.0368	2.80
Despeckling method (LP transform) [54]	18.23	28.44	0.9972	0.00141	0.0416	2.24
Despeckling method (CT transform) [47]	27.74	34.21	0.9990	0.00037	0.0203	1.64

Table 6. Comparison of performance of denoising methods based on Gaussian filtering with despeckling methods.

well preserving edges and structures in the image. The parameters in the model are estimated through an efficient iterative scheme.

In [56], the authors have developed the adaptive weights smoothing algorithm, which is an iterative procedure in which the size of a neighbourhood is adaptive to the surface smoothness. In [57], the estimation of jump surfaces by local piecewise linear kernel smoothing is examined.

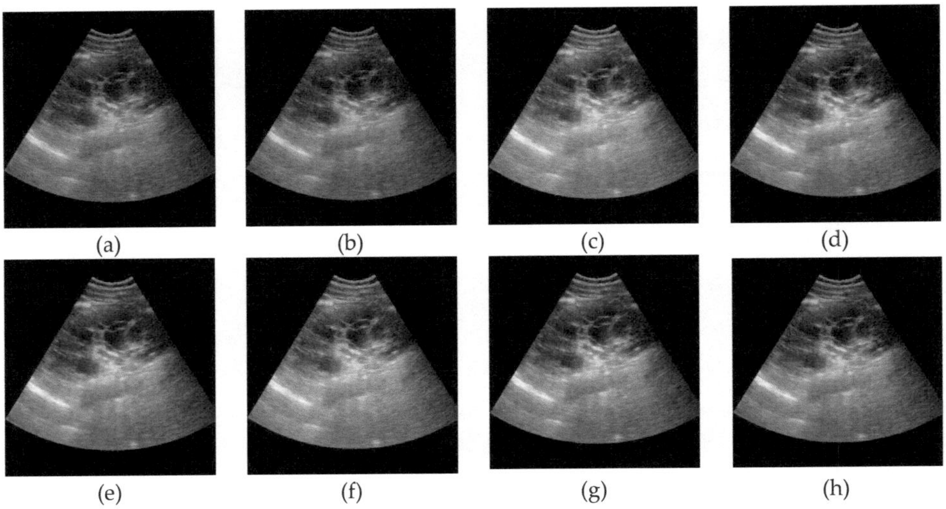

Figure 18. a) Original ultrasound image,(b) Denoised image using Gaussian filter, (c) Denoised image using 1st alternative with WT method (d) Denoised image using 1st alternative with LP method. (e) Denoised image using 1st alternative with CT method. (f) Denoised image using 2nd alternative with WT method. (g) Denoised image using 2nd alternative with LP method. (h) Denoised image using 2nd alternative with CT method.

In [58, 59], an anisotropic diffusion algorithm has been proposed for Gaussian noise removal. In [60], a bilateral filter to remove Gaussian noise is developed. In [61], a window based linear regression filter for echo cardiographic image denoising is proposed. The main draw backs of the above algorithms are that they need more computational time and complex circuit to implement them.

We consider a medical ultrasound image X and the corresponding despeckled image Y obtained by using the contourlet transform with cycle spinning [46]. The subtracted image Z=X-Y is the error image containing speckle noise. We find the mean m and standard deviation σ of Z and then simulate Gaussian noise G with these values of m and σ. The removal of this Gaussian noise G from despeckled image Y yields the new despeckled image $\hat{Y}$, i.e. $\hat{Y}$ =Y-G, which is further subtracted from the original image X to obtain the new error image Z containing the residual speckle noise. This procedure is repeated until the percentage of black pixels in error image Z reaches 99.9. We determine the maximum value of PSNR and the corresponding values of mean m and standard deviation σ using the iterated despeckled images $\hat{Y}$. This procedure is applied for all the medical ultrasound images X_i, i=1,..., 63, in the dataset, yielding the two sets of data points ($PSNR_i$,m_i) and ($PSNR_i$,σ_i), i=1,...,n_1 exhibits linear correlation. Using the method of least square errors, we obtain the lines of best fit for these data, namely:

$$m = a * PSNR + b \tag{37}$$

$$\sigma = c * PSNR + d \tag{38}$$

where a, b, c and d are the constants, which are the linear regression model parameters for Gaussian representation G(m, σ) of speckle noise in the medical ultrasound images. The Eqs. (37) and (38) represent the linear regression model for Gaussian representation G(m, σ) of speckle noise in a medical ultrasound image with its PSNR value determined already [62]. The steps involved in this procedure are given in the Algorithm 1.

Algorithm 1. Linear regression model for Gaussian representation G (m, σ) of speckle noise.

Input : Medical ultrasound image.

Output: Linear regression model parameters for Gaussian representation G (m, σ) of speckle noise.

Start

Step 1: Input medical ultrasound image X.

Step 2: Input despeckled ultrasound image Y obtained by using contourlet transform with cycle spinning.

Step 3: Find the error image Z as difference between X and Y (i.e. Z = X – Y).

Step 4: Find the percentage of black pixels in Z.

Step 5: Find the mean (m) and standard deviation (σ) of Z.

Step 6: Simulate the Gaussian noise G with mean m and standard deviation σ obtained in the Step 5.

Step 7: Subtract the simulated Gaussian noise G from despeckled image Y to obtain the resultant image ($\hat{Y}$), i. e. $\hat{Y}$ =Y-G.

Step 8: Find the PSNR, mean and standard deviation of the resultant image ($\hat{Y}$) obtained in the Step 7. Set Y = $\hat{Y}$.

Step 9: Repeat the Steps 3-8 until the percentage of black pixels in Z reach 99.9%.

Step 10: Find the maximum of the PSNR values obtained for the iterated despeckled images ($\hat{Y}$) and the corresponding values of m and σ. Store the values of maximum PSNR and corresponding values of m and σ.

Step 11: The Gaussian noise with mean m and standard deviation σ determined in the Step 10 is the modelled Gaussian noise for the image X.

Step 12: Repeat the Steps 1-11 for all the ultrasound images X and their corresponding despeckled images Y in the data set.

Step 13: Obtain the lines of best fit for the both PSNR vs. m and PSNR vs. σ obtained for all the ultrasound images (n_1) in the Step 12 using the method of least square errors. i. e. determine the constants a, b, c and d of the Eqs.(37) and (38), which are the lines of best fit that form the linear regression model for representing the speckle noise in ultrasound image as Gaussian noise. The lines of best fit are found using goodness of fit static.

Step 14: Output linear regression model parameters a, b, c and d of Eqs.(37) and (38).

Stop

The data points ($PSNR_i$,m_i) and ($PSNR_i$,σ_i), i=1,...,63 obtained for 63 typical ultrasound images of the image data set are stored and then used for regression of PSNR on m and also PSNR on σ. In the ultrasound image data set used for building regression model for Gaussian representation of speckle noise, we select a reference image X_{ref} for which the PSNR value is minimum. Given an arbitrary input medical ultrasound image X, we compute the PSNR of X with respect to the reference image X_{ref}. Using linear regression model (Eqs. (37) and (38)), we estimate the values of mean m and standard deviation σ of the Gaussian noise, which is removed from the input original image. The resultant image is the despeckled image (Y). The 'goodness of fit' statistic for the lines of regression is given by two quantities, namely, the sum of squares due to error of the fit (SSE) and root mean squared error (RMSE).The SSE is given by Eq. (39) :

$$SSE=\sum_{i=1}^{n}\left(Y_i-\hat{Y}_i\right)^2 \tag{39}$$

where Y_i=actual mean value of Gaussian noise, $\hat{Y}_i$= estimated mean value of Gaussian noise, and

n_1= total number of ultrasound images in the dataset.

The RMSE is given by Eq. (40) :

$$RMSE=\sqrt{\frac{SSE}{n_1}} \tag{40}$$

If the SSE and RMSE values are closer to zero, they indicate better fit. The general model for Gaussian noise estimation and removal in despeckling ultrasound image is shown in the Figure 19.

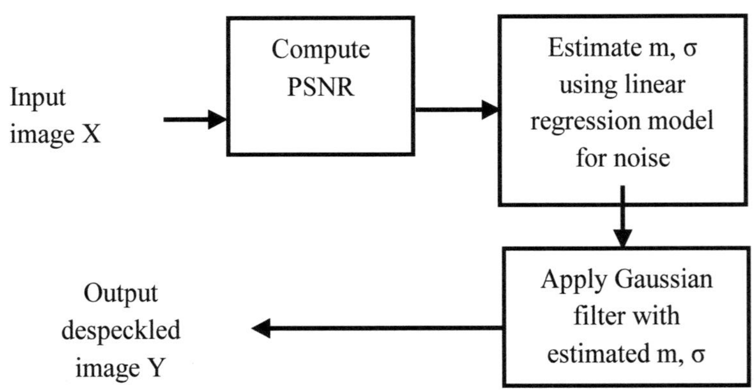

Figure 19. The general model for Gaussian representation of speckle noise.

The steps involved in the denoising process, shown in Figure 19 are given in the Algorithm 2.

Algorithm 2. Despeckling based on linear regression model for Gaussian noise estimation.

Input: Medical ultrasound image.

Output: Despeckled image.

Start

Step 1: Input medical ultrasound image X.

Step 2: Compute PSNR of image X with respect to the reference image X_{ref} prescribed by the regression model.

Step 3: Obtain Gaussian noise estimation G(m, σ) corresponding to the PSNR computed in the Step 2 using the regression model (Eqs.(37) and (38))

Step 4: Apply Gaussian filter with estimated mean (m) and standard deviation (σ), obtained n the Step 3, to the input image X, which yields the despeckled image Y.

Step 4: Apply Gaussian filter with estimated mean (m) and standard deviation (σ), obtained in the Step 3, to the input image X, which yields the despeckled image Y.

Step 5: Output the despeckled image Y.

Stop.

The linear regression model parameters a, b, c and d for Gaussian representation of speckle noise are computed for the dataset of 63 ultrasound images and the linear regression model equations are (Eqs.(37) and (38)),where a=-6.129e-007, b=2.742e-005, c=-0.0002192, d=0.01004, with the measures of 'best fit' are SSE=4.682e-009, RMSE=8.833e-006 for mean vs. PSNR and SSE=0.0006471, RMSE=0.003284 for standard deviation vs. PSNR. The Figures(20 and 21) show the lines of best fit for mean vs. PSNR and standard deviation vs. PSNR, respectively, which are used for Gaussian noise estimation and removal.

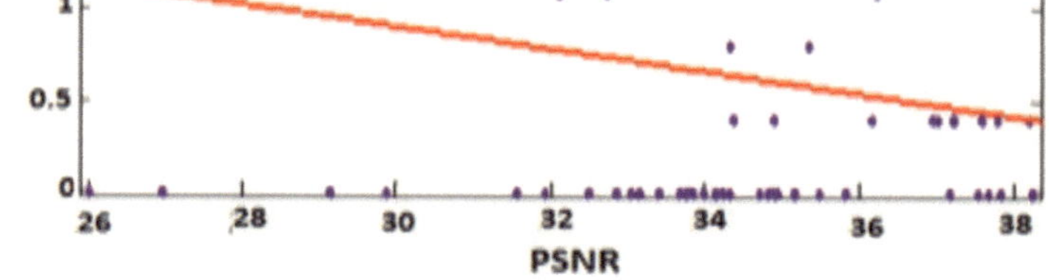

Figure 20. Linear regression of mean on PSNR

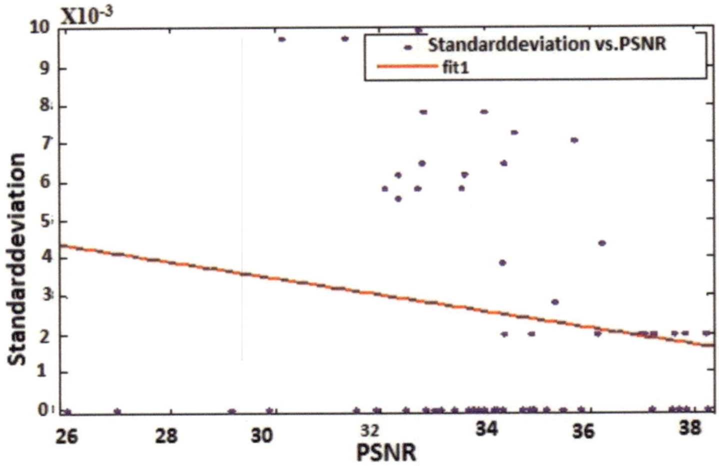

Figure 21. Linear regression of standard deviation on PSNR

The comparison of the results of the proposed method with the contourlet transform method (with cycle spinning) is given in the Table 7. It is observed that the image quality enhancement obtained by the despeckling method based on linear regression model is better than that obtained by the contourlet transform method in terms of PSNR and computational time required for denoising.

Denoising methods	PSNR (in dB)	Computational Time (in Secs.)
Contourlet transform using cycle spinning	35.91	24.09
Proposed method based on linear regression model	36.98	0.34

Table 7. Comparison of performance of despeckling based on contourlet transform and proposed method based on linear regression model.

The Figure 22. shows a sample medical ultrasound image, its despeckled image using contourlet transform with cycle spinning and the denoised image using the linear regression model respectively. The visual quality of image enhancement can also be observed from the sample image and its denoised image. The anatomical structures are more clearly visible in the Figure 22.(c) than that in Figure 22.(b). The box indicates the region of image in (b) and (c) showing prominent visual enhancement due despeckling methods.

The Figure 23 shows the visual enhancement due to various despeckling methods for comparison. (a) shows the sub image of original image, The Figure 23 (b)-(f) indicates the sub image showing visual enhancement due to different despeckling methods namely, Wiener filter with (3X3),wavelet transform method, contourlet transform method, cycle spinning based contour-

http://dx.doi.org/10.5772/56519

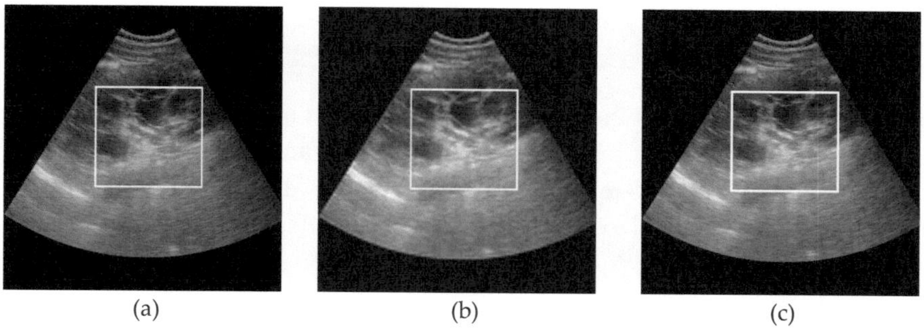

Figure 22. a) Original ultrasound image (b) Despeckled image using the contourlet transform with cycle spinning (c) Denoised image using the proposed linear regression model. The box Indicates the region of image in (b) and (c) showing prominent visual enhancement due to the despeckling.

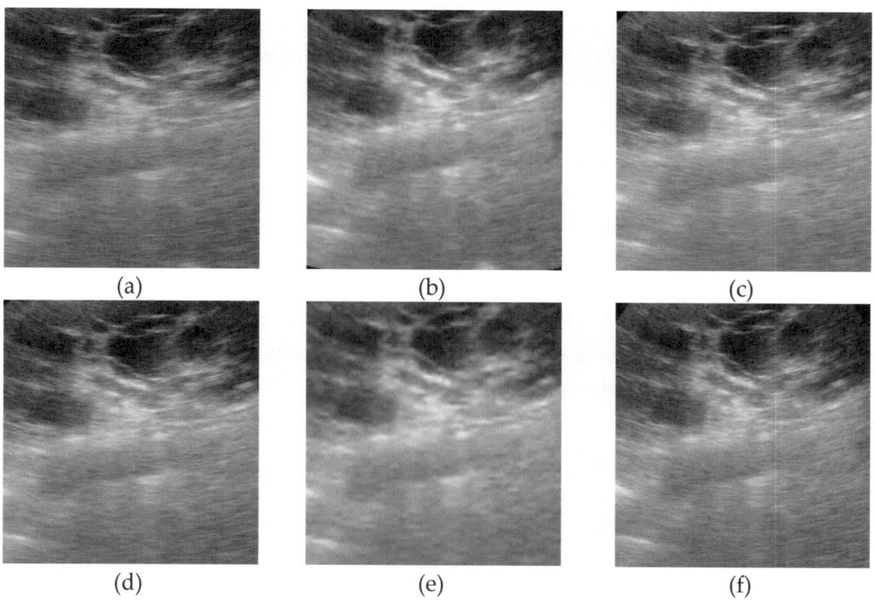

Figure 23. a) A sub image of original ultrasound image (b) sub image of despeckling using Wiener filter (c) sub image of despeckling using WT method (d) sub image of despeckling using CT method (e) sub image of despeckling using cycle spinning based CT method (f) sub image of despeckling using proposed linear regression model.

let transform method and proposed linear regression model. The prominent visual enhancement is observed using the proposed linear regression model.

The proposed method estimates the Gaussian noise content in the input medical ultrasound image for denoising the image efficiently. Hence, it is easily amenable for building embedded system software for ultrasound imaging equipments in order to display the high quality images, which helps the medical expert in the diagnosis with greater accuracy.

6. Conclusion

In this chapter, a despeckling method, based on a 2D directional non separable transform known as contourlet transform is presented. Conventional 2D wavelet transform is separable and thus cannot sparsely represent non separable structures of the image, such as directional curves. It is found that pyramidal directional filter bank feature of contourlet transform makes it a good choice for representation of curves and edges in the image. But, the contourlet transform, one of the recent geometrical image transforms, lacks the feature of translation invariance due to sub sampling in its filter bank structure. In cycle spinning, CT is improved by averaging the estimation of all translations of the degraded image. The Gibbs effect is considerably reduced by the contourlet transform with cycle spinning, because the average of different estimations of the image reduces the oscillations. In the literature, the authors [33,41,45,54,55,61] have considered ultrasound images (natural/synthetic) with artificially added speckle noise content and have proposed methods for despeckling such images. However, in the present study, we considered ultrasound images captured by the ultrasound equipment which contain inherent speckle noise and have proposed methods for removing the speckle noise more effectively.

When the noise characteristics of the images are unknown, it is proposed to denoise by a linear regression model, which is cost effective compared to the other methods. We have proposed a novel linear regression model for Gaussian noise estimation and removal in despeckling medical ultrasound images. The experimental results demonstrate its efficacy both in terms of speckle reduction and computational time required for denoising. Further, the proposed regression model is simple, generic and computationally inexpensive. Hence, it is easily amenable for building embedded system software for ultrasound imaging equipments in order to display the high quality images, which help the medical experts for speedy accurate image analysis and diagnosis. Further, the proposed regression model is simple, generic and computationally inexpensive.

Acknowledgements

Authors are grateful to the reviewers for their helpful comments which improved the quality of the paper. Further, authors are thankful to Dr. Ramesh Mankare, Radiologist, Sangamesh-

http://dx.doi.org/10.5772/56519

war Scanning Centre, Bijapur, Karnataka, India, for providing the ultrasound images of kidney, liver and also for helpful discussions.

Author details

P.S. Hiremath[1*], Prema T. Akkasaligar[2] and Sharan Badiger[3]

*Address all correspondence to: hiremathps53@yahoo.com

1 Dept. of P.G. Studies and Research in Computer Science, Gulbarga University, Gulbarga, Karnataka, India

2 Dept. of Computer Science and Engineering, B.L.D.E.A's Dr. P.G.H. College of Engineering, Bijapur, Karnataka, India

3 Dept. of Medicine, Sri.B.M.Patil Medical College, BLDE University, Bijapur, Karnataka, India

References

[1] Suetens Paul, Fundamentals of Medical Imaging, (1st Edition), Cambridge university, U.K.; 2002.p145-182.

[2] Hedrick W.R. and Hykes D.L., Image and signal processing in diagnostic ultrasound imaging, Journal of Diagnostic Medical Sonography 1989; 5(5): 231–239.

[3] Godman J.W., Some Fundamental Properties of Speckle, Jl. Opt. Soc. Am. 1976; 66 (11):1145-1149.

[4] Burckhardt C.B., Speckle in Ultrasound B Mode Scans, IEEE Trans. Sonics Ultrasonics 1978;25:1-6.

[5] Yongjian Y. and Acton S.T. Speckle reducing anisotropic diffusion, IEEE Trans. Image Processing. Nov. 2002; 11(11):1260–1270.

[6] Prager R.W., Gee A.H., Treece G.M., and Berman L., Speckle detection in ultrasound images using first order statistics, GUED/ F-INFENG/TR 415, University of Cambridge, Dept. of Engineering, July, 2002: 1–17.

[7] Zong X., Laine A. F., and Geiser E. A. Speckle reduction and contrast enhancement of echocardiograms via multiscale nonlinear processing, IEEE Trans.on Medical. Imaging., 1998;17:532-540.

[8] Netravati A.N. and Haskell B.G., Digital Pictures: Representation, Compression and standards, (2nd ed.) 2000, New York Plenum.

[9] Loizou C.P., Pattichis,Pantziaris M.,Tyllis T.,and Nicolaides A. Quality evaluation of Ultasound Imaging in the carotid Artery Based on Normalization and Speckle Reduction Filtering, International Federation for Medical and Biological Engineering, 2006; 414-426.

[10] Lee J.S. Speckle Analysis and Smoothing of Synthetic Aperture Radar Images, Comp. Graphics Image Processing 1981; 17: 24-32.

[11] Insana M., Hall T.J,Glendon., G.C., and Posental S.J., Progress in quantitative ultrasonic imaging, SPIE Vol. 1090 Medical Imaging III, Image Formation,1989; 2-9.

[12] Lee J.S. Refined filtering of image noise using local statistics Computer Graphic and Image Processing,1981;15: 380-389.

[13] Kuan D.T. Sawchuk A. A., Strand T. C., and Chavel P., Adaptive restoration of images with speckle IEEE Trans. ASSP, 1987; 35(3): 373-383.

[14] Wiener Norbert Extrapolation, Interpolation and Smoothing of Stationary Time Series, New York: Wiely, 1949.

[15] Jain A. K. 1989, Fundamental of Digital Image Processing. NJ: Prentice-Hall,

[16] Singh Y.K., Parui S.K., ISITRA: A generalized way of signal decomposition and reconstruction Digital Signal Processing, Elsevier, 2006, 16(1):3-23.

[17] Kalaivani Narayanan S. and Wahidabanu R.S.D., A View of Despeckling in Ultrasound Imaging., Int'l. Jl. of Signal Processing, Image processing and Pattern Recognition, 2009; 2(3): 85-98.

[18] Kaur Jappreet, Kaur Jasdeep, Kaur Manpreet, Survey of Despeckling Techniques for Medical Ultrasound Images, Int'l. Jl. Comp.Tech. Appl. 2011 July-august ;2(4): 1003-1007.

[19] Achim A., and Bezerianos A, Novel Bayesian Multiscale Method for Speckle Removal in Medical Ultrasound Images, IEEE Trans. on Medical Imaging, 2001; 20(8): 772-783.

[20] Nikhil gupta and Swamy M.N., Despeckling of Medical Ultrasound Images Using Data and Rate Adaptive Lossy Compression. IEEE Trans. Medical Imaging, 2005;24(6):682-695.

[21] Ruikar S.D. and Doye D.D., Wavelet Based Image Denoising Technique. Int'l. Jl. of Advanced Computer Science and Applications, March 2011; 2(3):49-53.

[22] Mallat S., A theory of multiresolution signal decomposition: The wavelet representation IEEE Trans. Pattern Anal. Machine Intell., July 1989; 11: 674-693.

[23] Gonzalez Rafael C., Woods Richard E., Digital Image Processing, 2nd Edition, Prentice Hall, Upper Saddle River, NJ, 2002; 350-402

[24] Cohen A., Daubechies I., and Feauveau J. C. Biorthogonal bases of compactly supported wavelets. Comm. Pure Appl. Math., 1992; 45:485-500.

[25] Mallat S. Wavelet tour of signal processing 3rd Edition, Academic press, 2009; 535-606.

[26] Donoho D.L., Johnstone I.M. De-noising by soft-thresholding. IEEE Trans. on Information Theory, 1995; 41(3):613-27.

[27] Hiremath P.S. Akkasaligar Prema T. and Badiger Sharan, Performance Evaluation of Wavelet Based Thresholding for Despeckling Medical Ultrasound Images,Proceedings of the Int'l Conf. on Cognition and Recognition(ICCR-08), 10th-12th April 2008, Mysore, Karnataka, India:574-579.

[28] Donoho, D.L., Johnstone I.M. Ideal Spatial Adaptation By Wavelet Shrinkage, Biometrika, 1994, 81:425-455.

[29] Chang S. G. Bin Yu and Martin Vetterli, Adaptive Wavelet Thresholding for Image Denoising and Compression, IEEE Trans. Image Processing, 2000, 9 (9): 1532-1546.

[30] Minh N. Do, Framing Pyramids, IEEE Trans. on Signal Processing, 2003 Sept, 51(9): 2329-2342.

[31] Vladimir P.M. Ilya Shmulevich, Karen Egiazarian, Jaakko Astola, Block Median Pyramidal Transform:Analysis and Denoising Applications IEEE Trans.on Signal Processing, 2001 Feb.; 49(2):364-372.

[32] Bruno Aiazzi, Luciano alparone and Stefano Baronti, Multiresolution Local - Statistics speckle filtering based on a ratio Laplacian pyramid, IEEE Trans. on Geosciences and Remote Sensing, 1998 Sept.; 36(5):1466-1476.

[33] Saad Ali, Visual enhancement of digital ultrasound images: Wavelet Versus Gauss-Laplace contrast Pyramid, Int'l. Jl. of Computer Assisted radiology and Surgery, 2007 Aug. ; 2(2),63-70:117-125.

[34] Zhang F.,Koh L.M., Yoo Y.M. and Kim Y.,2007, Nonlinear diffusion in Laplacian pyramid domain for ultrasonic speckle reduction, IEEE Trans. on Medical Imaging,26(2): 200-211.

[35] Burt P. J. and Adelson E. H., The Laplacian pyramid as a compact image code, IEEE Trans. on Commun,1983; 31(4):532-540.

[36] Hiremath P.S., Akkasaligar Prema T., Badiger Sharan, Visual Enhancement of Digital Ultrasound Images using Multiscale Wavelet Domain, Int'l. Jl. of Pattern Recognition and Image Analysis, 2010; 20(3): 303-315

[37] Do Minh N., Vetterli Martin, Framming pyramids, IEEE Trans. on Signal Processing,: 2003; 2329-2342

[38] Huang Mao yu, Huang yueh Min and Wang Ming-Shi, Dec. 15-17, 2004, Taipei, Taiwan. Speckle reduction of ultrasound image based on contourlet transform, Int'l. Computer Symposium :178-182.

[39] Hiremath P.S., Akkasaligar Prema T., Badiger Sharan, Despeckling Medical Ultrasound Images Using the Contourlet Transform,In: Proceedings of the 4th AMS Indian Int'l Conf. on Artificial Intelligence(IICAI-09),16-18 Dec. 2009,Tumkur, Karnataka,India,:1814-27.

[40] Hiremath P.S., Tegnoor Jyothi R., Automatic Detection of Follicles in Ultrasound Images of ovaries using Edge Based Method, IJCA Special Issue on Recent Trends in Image Processing and Pattern Recognition, 2010; 120-125.

[41] Song Xiao-yang, Chen Ya-zhu, Zhang Su, and Yang Wei, Speckle Reduction Based on Contourlet Transform Using Scale Adaptive Threshold for Medical Ultrasound Image, Jl. Shanghai Jiaotong Univ. (Sci), 2008; 13(5):553-558.

[42] Phoong S. M., Kim C. W., Vaidyanathan P. P., and Ansari R., A new class of two-channel biorthogonal filter banks and wavelet bases, IEEE trans. Signal Processing, 1995 Mar.; 43(3):649-665.

[43] Coifman R.R. and Donoho D.L., Translation invariant denoising, in Wavelets and statistics, Springer Lecture notes in Statistics, 103, Newyork, springer-Verlang,1994; 125-150.

[44] Eslami Ramin and Radha Hayder, The contourlet transform for image denoising using cycle spinning, Proceedings of Asilomar Conference on Signals, Systems and Computers, 2003;p1982-1986.

[45] Xiaobo Qu, Jingwen Yan, The cycle spinning based sharp frequency localized contourlet transform for image denoising, Proceedings of 2008 3rd Int'l. Conference on Intelligent System and Knowledge Engineering. 2008;p1247-1251.

[46] Hiremath P.S.,Akkasaligar Prema T.and Badiger Sharan, The Cycle Spinning Based Contourlet Transform for Despeckling Medical Ultrasound Image, Proc. Int,l Conf. on Trends in Information Technology and Applications, U.A.E., 11th-13th Dec. 2010, 72-76.

[47] Hiremath P.S., Akkasaligar Prema T. and Badiger Sharan, Speckle Reducing Contourlet Transform for Medical Ultrasound Images World Academy of Science, Engineering and Technology-Special Journal Issue, 2011; 80:1217 - 1224.

[48] Goshtasby Ardershir, On edge focusing Int'l. Jl. of Image and Vision Computing, 1994; 12(4):247-256.

[49] Fisher R., Perkins S., Walker A., Wolfart E.,2003, Gaussian Smoothing, Hypermedia image Processing Reference (HIPR2), Available from: URL: http:/ homepages. inf. ed.ac.uk / rbf/ HIPR2/gsmooth.html.

[50] Bracewell R., The Fourier transform and its applications, McGraw Hill: 1965; 160-163.

[51] Badulescu P. and Zaciu R. Removal of mixed-noise using order statistic filter and wavelet domain wiener filter. Semiconductor conference,Circuits And Systems'99 procedings, 1999;1:301-304.

[52] Saraswati J. S. and Mary brinda, Denoising of mixed noise in ultrasound images Int'l. Jl. of Computer Science Issues, July 2011; 8(4):517-523.

[53] Hiremath P.S., Akkasaligar Prema T. and Badiger Sharan, Removal of Gaussian Noise in Despeckling Ultrasound Images, The Int'l. Jl. of Computer Science and Applications (2278-1080), July 2012; 1(5): 25-35.

[54] Hiremath P.S., Akkasaligar Prema T. and Badiger Sharan, Performance Comparison of Wavelet Transform and Contourlet Transform based methods for Despeckling Medical Ultrasound Images Int'l. Jl. of Computer Applications (0975 - 8887), 2011; 26(9):34-41.

[55] Bamber J.C. and Daft C. Adaptive Filtering for Reduction of Speckle in Ultrasound Pulse Echoim ages. Ultrasonics, 1986: 41-44.

[56] Polzehl J. and Spokoiny V.G., Adaptative weights smoothing with applications to image restoration Journal of the Royal Statistical Society B-62: 2000; 335-354.

[57] Qiu P., The local piecewisely linear kernel smoothing procedure for fitting jump regression surfaces Technometrics 2004; 46:87-98.

[58] Perona P. and Malik J., Scale -space and edge detection using anisotropic diffusion, IEEE Trans. Pattern Anal. Machine Intell., 1990; 12:629-639.

[59] Black M.J., Sapiro Guillermo, Marimont David,and Heeger David, Robust Anisotropic Diffusion, IEEE Trans. on Image Processing, 1998; 7(3):421- 432.

[60] Black M.J., Fleet D., and Yacoob Y., Robustly Estimating changes in Image Appearance, Computer Vision and Image Understand, 2000; 78:8-31.

[61] Rajalaxmi S., Arun Kumar V., and Baskar P., Window Based Linear Regression Filter for Echocardiographic Image Denoising, Int'.l Jl. of Systems algorithms and Applications, May 2(ICRAET12), 2012, 180-183.

[62] Hiremath P.S., Akkasaligar Prema T., Badiger Sharan, Linear Regression Model for Gaussian Noise Estimation and Removal for Medical Ultrasound Images, Int'l. Jl. of Computer Applications (0975 - 8887), July 2012, 50(3),11-15.

Chapter 9

Strategies for Hardware Reduction on the Design of Portable Ultrasound Imaging Systems

D. Romero-Laorden, J. Villazón-Terrazas,
O. Martínez-Graullera and A. Ibáñez

Additional information is available at the end of the chapter

http://dx.doi.org/10.5772/55910

1. Introduction

In the last decade, ultrasonic imaging systems have been an essential tool for diagnosis in medical and industrial applications, especially in the Non Destructive Testing area (NDT). Conventional ultrasonic imaging devices produce high quality images with good resolution and contrast. However, these machines are usually associated to a high cost in hardware resources, as well as in the time required for the data acquisition and processing stages. This fact hinders the development of good quality, compact and low-power systems that can operate in a wide range of real-time applications.

In this sense, the Synthetic Aperture techniques (SAFT) have demonstrated to be an effective method to achieve these goals, minimizing the size of the systems and accelerating the image acquisition processes. Consequently, both power consumption and overall cost of the systems can be reduced making possible their miniaturization and portability. Conventional SAFT techniques are based on the sequential activation in emission and reception of every transducer element. Once all acoustic signals have been stored in memory, a beamforming process is applied in a post-processing stage in order to focus the image dynamically in emission and reception, obtaining the maximum quality at each image pixel. Despite of this, conventional SAFT techniques present some inconveniences which are summarized in the following points:

1. **Artifacts**. Conventional SAFT techniques produce grating lobes in the images due to the acquisition processes.
2. **Low contrast**. As a consequence of firing only one element at time the received signals have low signal-to-noise ratio, which results in low contrast images that are not feasible for regular imaging visualization (e.g. echography imaging needs very good images in order to reduce the fails in the diagnostic).

3. **Medium penetration**. And for the same reason, the penetration deep of ultrasound in the region of interest is smaller than the achieved using conventional imaging techniques (e.g. needed by cardiac imaging or industrial inspections).

In order to reduce some of these drawbacks, more sophisticated SAFT techniques have been proposed. Total Focusing Method (TFM) [1] is one of them, where each array element is sequentially used as a single emitter and all array elements are used as receivers. Thus, it is possible to obtain a set of $N \times N$ signals (Full Matrix Array capture, FMA) that is used to form the image. According to the description of professors Drinkwater and Wilcox [1–3], its name refers to the possibility of implementing dynamic focusing in emission and reception, which enables to obtain images perfectly focused at all points in the region of interest. However, the complexity of the acquisition process and the computational requirements of the beamforming make this method not appropriate for real-time purposes [1]. Other solutions that use an emission and reception sub-aperture have been also proposed [4–6], although they maintain a certain degree of hardware complexity (focussing is needed in emission and reception) and also require intensive computational capabilities to produce a real-time ultrasonic image.

To overcome the last inconveniences we propose a SAFT methodology based on a new paradigm, known as coarray [5, 6], which allows to use only one element in emission and a limited number of parallel channels in reception at each time. With the proposed solution, a strategy for a hardware reduction in ultrasonic imaging systems is possible, and it involves the following aspects:

- Optimization of the acquisition strategies to achieve the completeness of the coarray with a minimum number of hardware elements. In this sense, our objective is to establish a trade-off between the number of electronic channels, image quality and acquisition velocity [6].
- The use of pulse compression techniques to overcome the reduced capability of penetration when emission is limited to one element [5].
- The development of GPGPU[1] parallel beamforming techniques to achieve real time imaging [7].

This chapter is divided into two main sections. The first one is dedicated to analyse the use of the coarray paradigm as a tool for the design of ultrasonic imaging systems and to present several minimum redundancy coarray techniques. Moreover, Golay codes are presented and their integration within the presented SAFT methods is described. The second section presents the general ultrasonic imaging system's overview, its architecture and the parallel beamforming as a solution for ultrafast beamforming. Finally, we expose our conclusions and future research developments.

---

[1] General-purpose computing on Graphics Processing Units is the utilization of a graphics processing unit (GPU), which typically handles computation only for computer graphics, to perform computation in applications traditionally handled by the central processing unit (CPU). http://gpgpu.org

http://dx.doi.org/10.5772/55910

2. Coarray: New paradigm for the design of imaging systems

This section is focused on the development of ultrasonic imaging systems based on the pulse/echo aperture model which is known as coarray. In order to clarify this point, we are going to briefly review this mathematical concept and its principal implications.

The coarray is a mathematical tool that is often used by several authors as a way to quickly study the radiation properties of an imaging system [5, 6, 8, 9]. This concept is frequently referred to as *effective aperture* in ultrasound literature, and it basically is the virtual aperture which produces in one way the same beam pattern as the real aperture working in emission and reception as Figure 12 suggests.

Suppose a linear array with N elements. In far-field and assuming very narrow band signals, the radiation pattern could be written as:

$$f(u) = \sum_{n=0}^{N-1} a_n e^{jkx_n u} = \sum_{n=0}^{N-1} a_n e^{jkndu} = \sum_{n=0}^{N-1} a_n (e^{jkdu})^n \tag{1}$$

where a_n are the complex weights of the transducers and $u = sin(\theta)$ being θ the angle measured from the perpendicular to the array. Substituting e^{jkdu} by the complex variable z, the radiation pattern can be expressed as a polynomial, which corresponds with the Z-Transform of the sequence a_n. Thus, considering a pulse-echo system, the complex radiation pattern will be the product of two polynomials with degree $N-1$:

$$f_{total}(z) = Z\{c_n\} = \sum_{n=0}^{2N-2} c_n z^n = \sum_{n=0}^{N-1} a_n z^n \, . \, \sum_{n=0}^{N-1} b_n z^n \tag{2}$$

where a_n and b_n are the gains applied to the transducers in emission and reception, and c_n is the coarray ($Z\{c_n\}$ represents the Z-Transform of the sequence c_n). Returning to the unit circle ($|z| = 1$, $z = e^{jkdu}$) and considering equation 1 then the radiation pattern of the system in continuous wave is directly the DFT of the coarray [10].

In synthetic aperture systems, each scanned image is obtained after several firing sequences of the elements. According to this, the coarray can then be expressed as a sum of several sub-coarrays. Each of these sub-coarrays will be obtained as the convolution of two sub-apertures that represent the weights of the active elements used to emit and receive the signals each time.

Figure 1 illustrates the coarray generated by TFM method, which has been applied in ultrasound area since the late 60's and early 70's [11, 12]. As we briefly introduced in Section 1, it consists on the sequential emission with each one of the array elements in turn, and the reception in each shot with the full transducer aperture. As we can see, its coarray is fully populated what ensures a grating-lobe free radiation pattern.

The image quality achieved when TFM is employed is the highest possible, but it has, as its counterpart, the huge volume of data which is necessary to acquire. Thus, it requires more storage resources and processing capability than other techniques, which makes difficult its

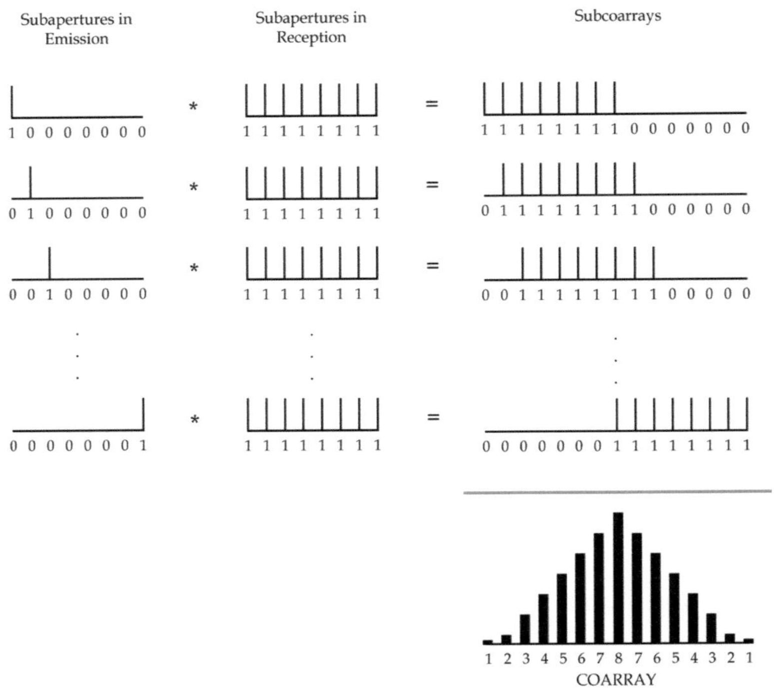

Figure 1. Firing sequences of the elements in TFM, and its corresponding generated coarray

practical implementation with todays' technology. To illustrate this, consider the following example: a 15 cm depth image, 40 MHz sampling rate, 64 channels, 1500 m/s medium velocity and 2 bytes per sample. Each firing generates approximately 1 MB of pulse-echo data, what supposes 64 MB of data to generate a single image frame when TFM is applied. For a frame rate of 20 images per second, it would be necessary to acquire and process 1.2 Gbytes of data per second.

The bandwidth of most I/O standards available today put in evidence that any of current data protocols can not deal with TFM requirements. Supposing a good efficiency and use of the resources (around 80)%, USB 2.0 port (released in April 2000) would be able to transfer less than one image per second (48 MB/s). A similar situation occurs if USB 3.0 (released in November 2008) is employed, being the maximum transmission speed up to 480 MB/s allowing to transfer around 7 images per second, even far respect to the maximum number of images which could be theoretically achieved. Finally, the most recent standard released in February 2011, known as Thunderbolt port and developed by Intel [13], combines PCI Express and DisplayPort into a new serial data interface that can be carried over longer and less costly cables. Thunderbolt has twice the transfer speed of USB 3.0 over copper wire (960 MB/s) giving us transferences of 14 images per second.

Therefore, it is clear that a reduction of data volume is desirable. In this sense, applying the coarray concept permits us to propose system designs that use less channels simultaneously working in emission and reception, but maintaining the same level of image quality. The key point for this is to use the coarray to search for solutions of minimum redundancy. This approach in conjunction with parallel computing techniques will offer an increment of acquisition velocity maintaining the highest quality and producing high frame rates with low power consumption. This topic will be the main focus of next two sections.

2.1. Minimum redundancy coarray solutions

Coarray analysis identifies which emitter-receiver combination completes each of its elements. In the TFM method seen before, we find that some of the elements are formed by a single signal (in concrete boundary elements) while the others increase progressively until reaching coarray centre with a value of N elements (Figure 1). Thus, we can consider as a minimum redundancy coarray that in which each element is composed of only one signal. Therefore, using the minimum possible number of signals the aperture's diffraction properties can be improved by manipulating the gain of the elements. With this goal in mind, it is possible to establish several strategies which maintain a balance between the number of parallel channels and the number of shots during acquisition processes.

2.1.1. 2R-SAFT acquisition strategy

2R-SAFT technique [14] has some particular advantages that make it very useful for ultrasonic imaging systems. 2R-SAFT uses only one element to transmit and two elements to receive. As it is shown in Figure 2, all elements are consecutively activated as single emitters, without the use of any beamformer in emission. At each shot, two consecutive channels are used as receivers requiring to store two signals per emission.

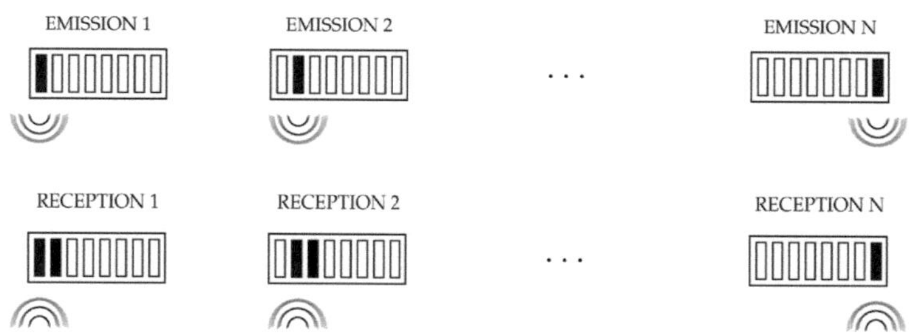

Figure 2. Firing sequences of the elements in 2R-SAFT

Thus, when the ith element is used to emit a waveform, i and $i+1$ elements are used for receiving signals. For the last element of the array, only one signal is recorded. By employing an emitter in each shot all the received signals are completely uncorrelated, containing only information of a single transmitter-receiver pair.

Figure 3 shows the coarray generated when 2R-SAFT is employed. As we can observe, the coarray is fully populated ensuring the suppression of grating lobes in the radiation pattern which produces good quality images [14, 15].

2.1.2. Accelerated-SAFT acquisition strategy

Here we present a minimum-redundancy technique we have denominated Accelerated-SAFT or, in its short form, kA-SAFT. The k subscript refers to the acceleration factor carried out during the acquisition stage which can go from 2x to Nx depending on the number of

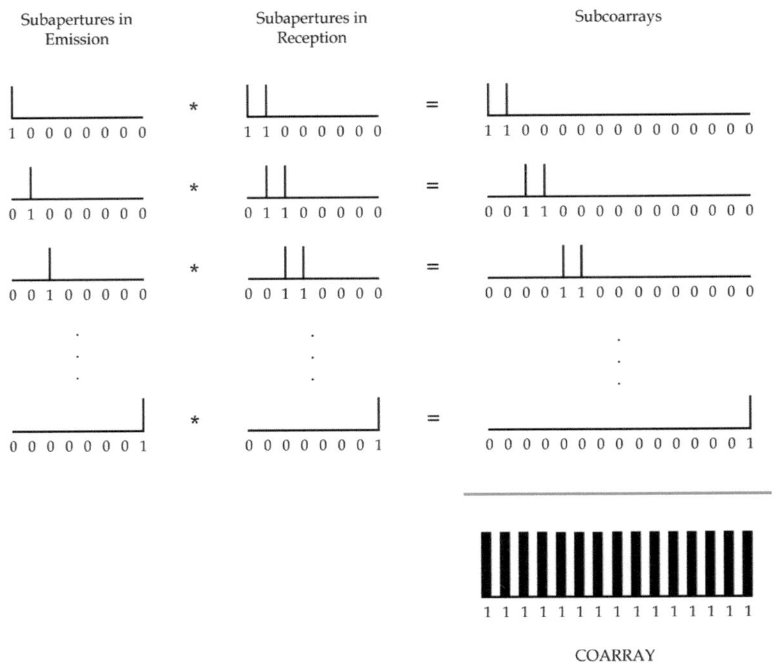

Figure 3. Coarray sequences for 2R-SAFT

channels used for the reception. This strategy increases a little bit the cost involved in the acquisition system respect to 2R-SAFT, but at the same time, reduces the number of shots by k times.

The kA-SAFT uses n_A consecutive elements to receive and a single element to emit which is centred in the active subaperture. As shown in Figure 4, the elements on emission are sequentially activated with a shift of $\frac{n_A}{2}$ elements. At each shot n_A consecutive channels are used as receivers, needing to store n_A signals per emission except for the first and the last array elements where half of the signals is acquired.

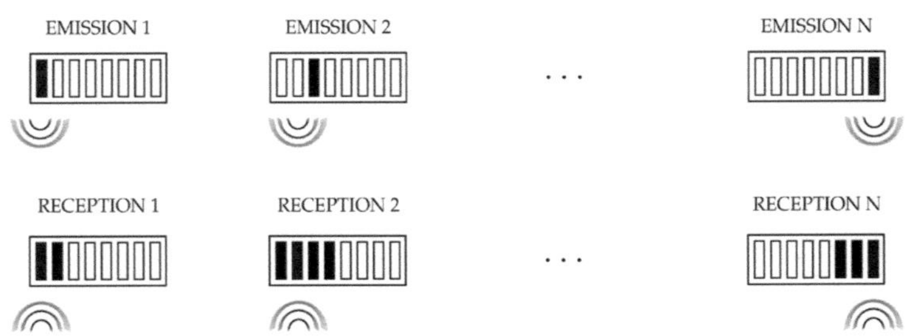

Figure 4. Firing sequences of the elements in kA-SAFT being k = 2x and $n_A = 4$

In this sense, when the ith element is used to emit the elements that are going to use as receivers are given by:

$$Elements_{rx} = \left\{ i - \frac{n_A}{2} + j \right\} \qquad 0 \leq j \leq n_A \tag{3}$$

Figure 5 shows the coarray generated when kA-SAFT is employed for the case of $n_A = 4$. As we can observe, the coarray is identical to that obtained with 2R-SAFT (Figure 3) preserving all its advantages but multiplying by 4 the frame rate in acquisition.

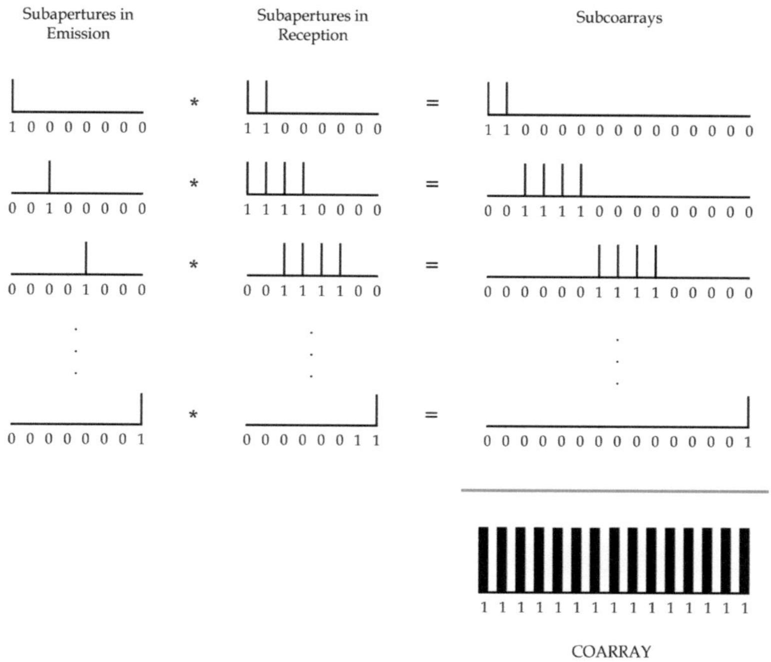

Figure 5. Coarray sequences for kA-SAFT being k = 2x and $n_A = 4$

2.1.3. Experimental results

We present some experimental results that have been done on a tissue phantom (Model 040GSE - CIRS Inc.) with 0.5dB/cm attenuation, where several cysts and wires of 0.1mm diameter are located at different depths (Figure 6). We have used a 2.6MHz phased array transducer with $N = 64$ elements, 0.28mm of pitch (Vermon Inc.) for the measurements. We will use the Total Focusing Method as a reference model to examine the cysts and wires in the tissue covering an area starting from 25mm to 80mm depth, and we will compare it to 2R-SAFT and kA-SAFT techniques. All images have been obtained by applying the DAS algorithm. TFM uses the complete set of signals $N^2 = 4096$ while 2R-SAFT and kA-SAFT images have been calculated using $2N - 1 = 127$ signals.

In Figure 7, images for all strategies are presented. It is easily observed how Figures 7(a,b,d,e,g) are very similar in terms of quality. Consequently, the strategy to be chosen relies fundamentally on the hardware requisites.

Nevertheless, at a depth greater than 60 mm none reaches the same contrast level as TFM (Figure 7(h)), highlighting the limited signal to noise ratio suffered by all minimum

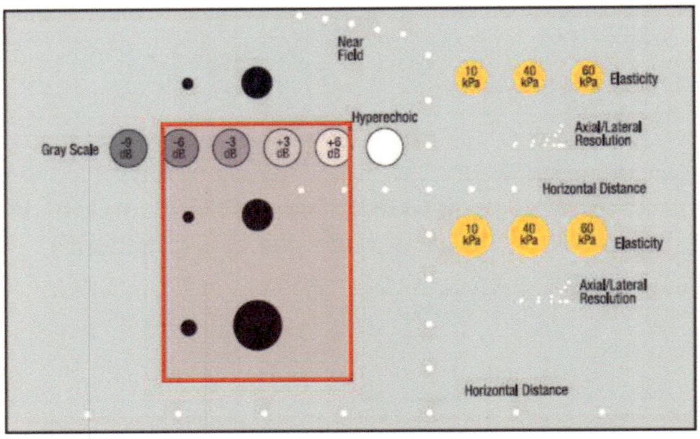

Figure 6. Region of interest analysed from tissue phantom model 040GSE by CIRS Inc.

redundancy techniques. In table 1, a comparison between the number of channels in emission and reception, number of firings, acquisition frame rates and memory buffers needed is performed for the different strategies presented. As we can see, TFM is the technique which more storage as well as more hardware channels needs. By contrast, minimum redundancy techniques requisites are more affordable and suitable for applications where size matters.

Strategy	Channels (tx,rx)	Firings	Framerate	Buffer
2R-SAFT	(1,2)	$N_{firings} = N$	$f_{frame} = \frac{f_{prf}}{N}$	$2N - 1 \times L$
2xA-SAFT ($n_A = 4$)	(1,4)	$N_{firings} = \frac{N}{2}$	$f_{frame} = 2\frac{f_{prf}}{N}$	$2N - 1 \times L$
4xA-SAFT ($n_A = 8$)	(1,8)	$N_{firings} = \frac{N}{4}$	$f_{frame} = 4\frac{f_{prf}}{N}$	
8xA-SAFT ($n_A = 16$)	(1,16)	$N_{firings} = \frac{N}{8}$	$f_{frame} = 8\frac{f_{prf}}{N}$	
16xA-SAFT ($n_A = 32$)	(1,32)	$N_{firings} = \frac{N}{16}$	$f_{frame} = 16\frac{f_{prf}}{N}$	
TFM	(1,N)	$N_{firings} = N$	$f_{frame} = \frac{f_{prf}}{N}$	$N^2 \times L$

Table 1. Comparison of the several acquisition strategies presented

2.2. Golay Codes

As we have seen, synthetic aperture images have low contrast due to the poor signal to noise ratio (SNR). Along this section, we will study how the use of pulse coding based on Golay codes [16, 17] can help to improve the dynamic range and SNR, in order to achieve an image quality comparable to that of Total Focusing Method.

2.2.1. Golay encoding for ultrasonic excitation

Golay complementary pairs have been widely used for transducer excitation because the sum of its auto-correlation function has a main peak and zero side-lobes [16]. A complementary pair is composed of two binary sequences, $A[n] = [a_0, a_1, \ldots, a_{N-1}]$ and $B[n] = [b_0, b_1, \ldots, b_{N-1}]$, of the same length N such that $a_i, b_i \in \{-1, +1\}$.

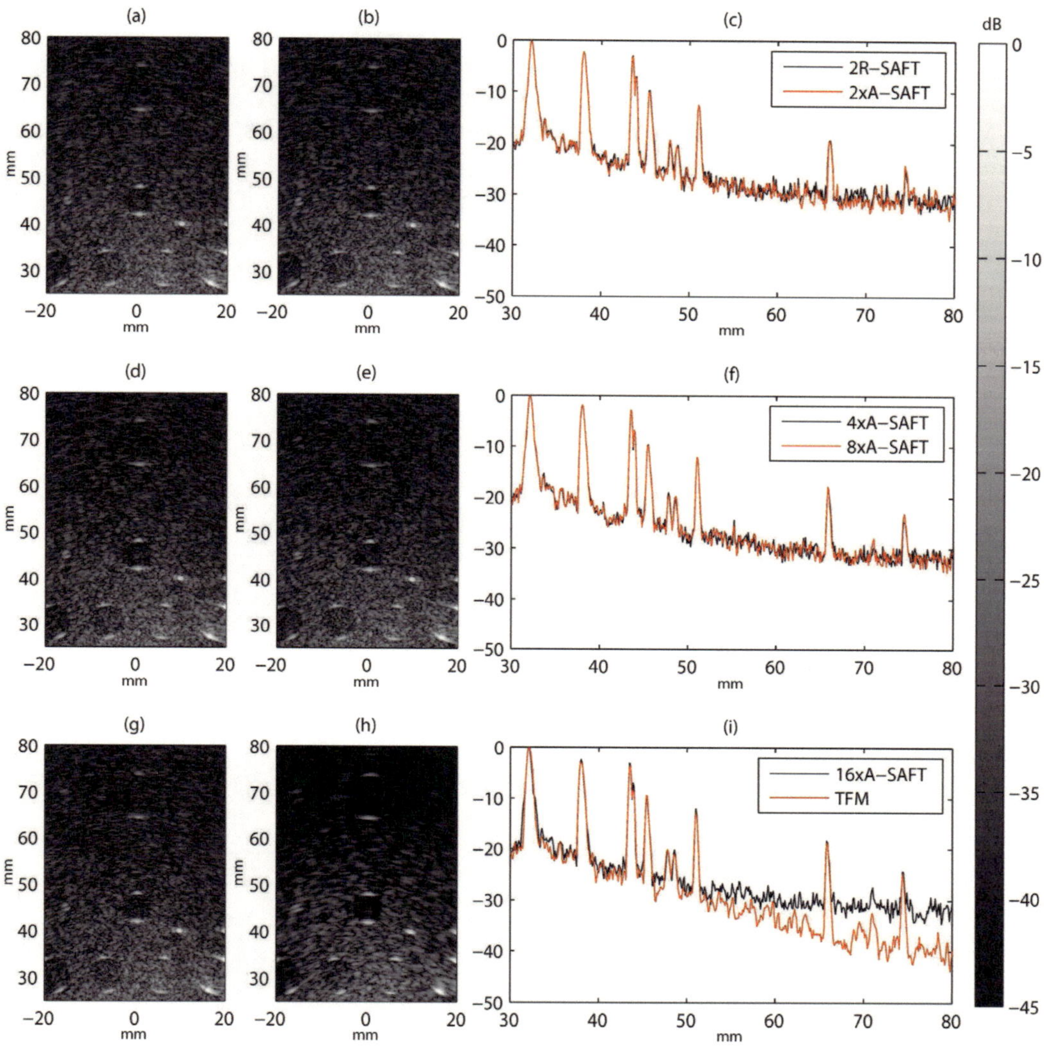

Figure 7. Experimental images from tissue phantom. (a) 2R-SAFT, (b) 2xA-SAFT, (c) Lateral profiles comparison between 2R-SAFT and 2xA-SAFT, (d) 4xA-SAFT, (e) 8xA-SAFT, (f) Lateral profiles comparison between 4xA-SAFT and 8xA-SAFT, (g) 16xA-SAFT, (h) TFM, (i) Lateral profiles comparison between 16xA-SAFT and TFM

The auto-correlation functions of $A[n]$ and $B[n]$ have side lobes with equal magnitude but opposite sign. The sum of these independent auto-correlation functions provides an ideal delta function according to:

$$C_A[n] + C_B[n] = \begin{cases} 0, n = 0 \\ 2N, \textit{otherwise} \end{cases} \tag{4}$$

where $C_A[n]$ and $C_B[n]$ are the auto-correlation functions of $A[n]$ and $B[n]$, respectively, for any integer n satisfying the equation 4. The construction of Golay code pairs is done recursively with the *"negate and concatenate"* method, a technique used by Golay [16] to create longer pairs from shorter hand-constructed given pairs. Specifically, if $A[n]$ and $B[n]$ are the N-digit binary representations of a complementary pair of codes, then a new pair of complementary codes $A'[n]$ and $B'[n]$ of length $2N$ can be formed by concatenating $B[n]$ to $A[n]$ and concatenating $\sim B[n]$ to $A[n]$ where $\sim B[n]$ is the complement of $B[n]$. Thus, $A'[n] = A[n] \mid B[n]$, and $B'[n] = A[n] \mid\sim B[n]$.

One of the major drawbacks of Golay codes is that two shots are needed for each emitting element in order to complete both A and B codes respectively. In our work, Golay codes of length equal to 8 bits have been used, being $A[8] = [+1+1+1+1+1-1-1+1]$ and $B[8] = [+1-1+1-1+1+1-1-1]$, producing a gain of 24dB according to equation 4.

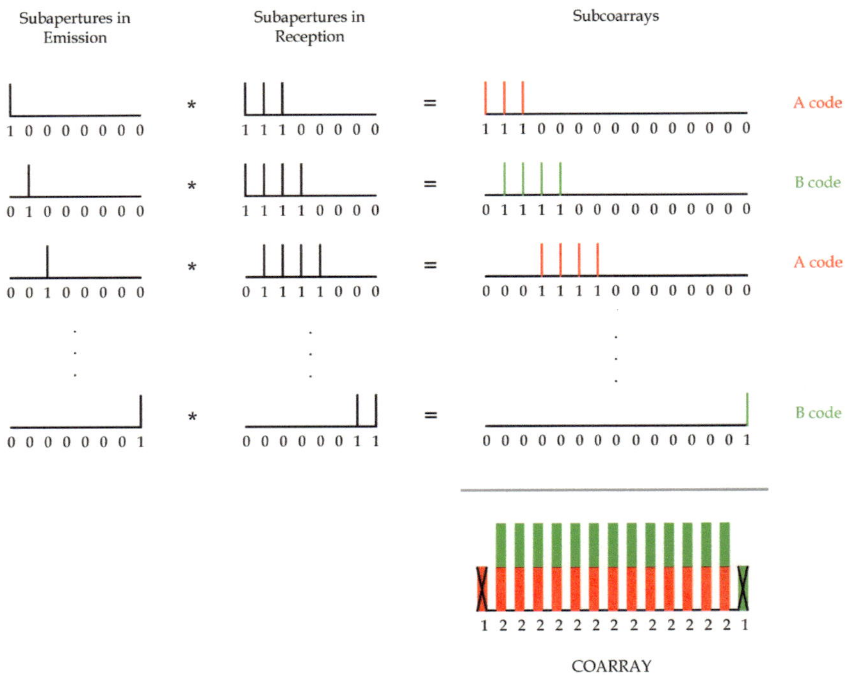

Figure 8. Golay encoding integration example

2.2.2. Coarray for Golay encoding

Golay codes, described previously, and minimum redundancy techniques can be combined. In order to illustrate how this can be done, Figure 8 shows an example using a 4R-SAFT (four receivers) [15] plus Golay codes. Here, two signals per coarray element are acquired and because Golay encoding needs to fire twice, A or B codes are alternated between shots.

This process is mathematically identical for the formerly presented strategies 2R-SAFT and kA-SAFT but with some particularities:

1. The number of channels in reception (sensors) must double the original number, in order to have two signals per coarray element for A and B codes.
2. The amount of acquired data signals also doubles the original, because of the first point.
3. The original firing rate is preserved, which means achieving identical performance at the expense of doubling the hardware involved in the reception process.

2.2.3. Experimental results

With the use of Golay codes to image the same area than in previous results, the panorama has changed. As before, TFM image has been composed from the complete set of signals $N^2 = 4096$, but now 2R-SAFT and kA-SAFT have been calculated using $4N - 2 = 254$ signals. From Figure 7 in section 2.1.3, where the corresponding images with no encoding were analysed, it can be seen how the reduction in the number of signals employed produces a loss of dynamic range respect to TFM method. Thus, with the use of Golay codes in Figure 9 we can observe how the contrast and level of detection have substantially increased. Now, both 2R-SAFT and kA-SAFT techniques distinguish the complete set of defects. Thus, in relation to TFM the number of signals is drastically reduced from N^2 to $4N - 2$, accelerating acquisition and processing velocities and the system's frame rate.

3. Ultrasonic imaging system

3.1. General system's overview

As we have said, our goal is centred in the design of ultrasonic imaging systems based on solutions which require fewer resources and storage capacity than conventional systems. Thus, in Figure 10 is schematically represented our vision of the system, which is composed by three parts:

1. **The array or probe**. It is usually composed by 64, 96, 128 or even more transducers depending on the type of application.
2. **Acquisition subsystem**. The hardware subsystem used for transducer excitation and data acquisition (represented by the box in the center). Nowadays, several electronic manufacturers have in their catalogues electronic boards and systems, which are small and can be easily used for our purposes. For example, National Instruments has 32-channel digitizer module capable of sampling on all channels at 50 MS/s with 12-bit resolution. The module is optimized for ultrasound applications [18]. Additionally, both multiplexer and bipolar programmable pulser are required. Specific architectures depending on the type of acquisition strategy will be studied in the next section.
3. **Image generation subsystem**. It is the software system which can take place in any computational device (PC, laptop, ...) shown on the right side of Figure 10. These processes include the digital signal pre-processing of the received signals and filtering; beamforming of the image, delaying and adding signals according to emission and reception lenses, post-processing the image and its representation to properly show data on the screen. To achieve these tasks, the use of GPU's great power for parallel computing will allow us to quickly and efficiently accelerate the algorithms.

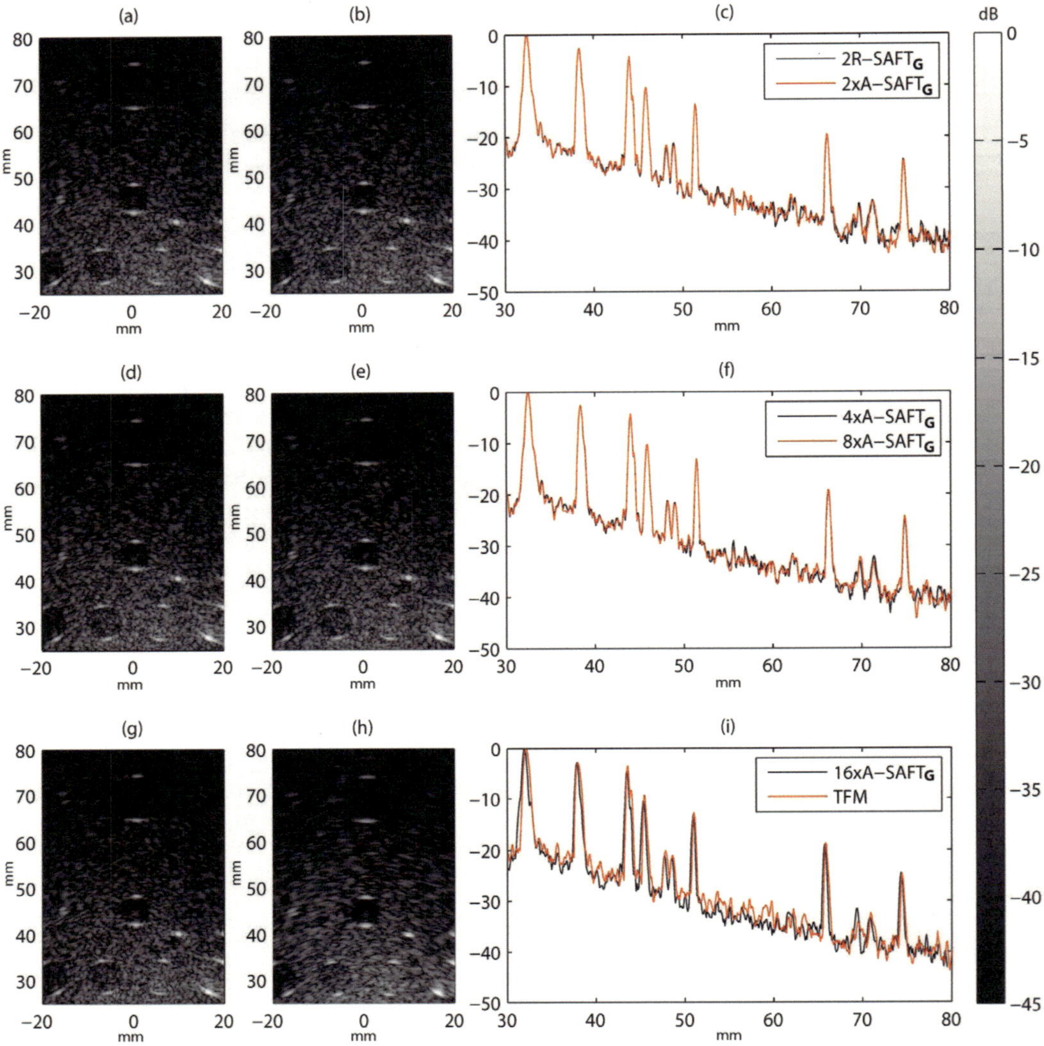

Figure 9. Experimental images from tissue phantom. (a) 2R-SAFT + Golay, (b) 2xA-SAFT + Golay , (c) Lateral profiles comparison between 2R-SAFT + Golay and 2xA-SAFT + Golay, (d) 4xA-SAFT + Golay, (e) 8xA-SAFT + Golay, (f) Lateral profiles comparison between 4xA-SAFT and 8xA-SAFT + Golay , (g) 16xA-SAFT + Golay, (h) TFM , (i) Lateral profiles comparison between 16xA-SAFT and TFM

3.2. Acquisition subsystem

In this section, two acquisition architectures are exposed. On one hand, a minimal system for 2R-SAFT strategy which allows a low-cost and small imaging system and, in the other hand, the architecture which implements 8xA-SAFT plus Golay encoding strategy and uses more hardware but yields better quality images. Which strategy to use depends on the concrete application. Any of these configurations can be carried out using boards systems available in the market.

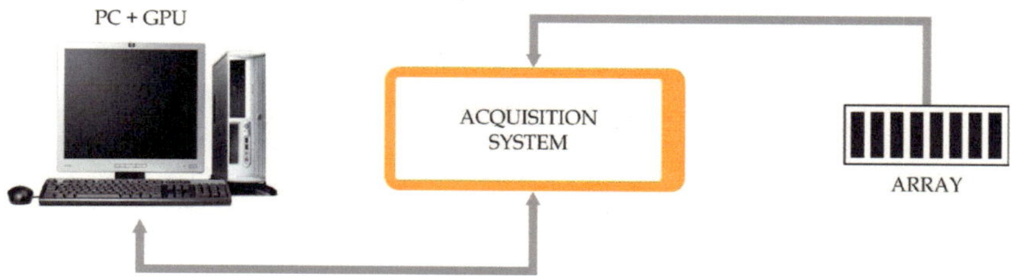

Figure 10. Hardware/Software system proposed

3.2.1. 2R-SAFT architecture

As we study in section 2.1.1, it is basically composed of one channel in emission and two channels in reception. Figure 11 shows the complete architecture for 2R-SAFT implementation. As we can see, a multiplexer is connected to the transmission channel for sequentially activate each element as an emitter, and a second multiplexer will be on charge of connecting the selected elements to both reception channels.

All the acquisition process is managed by a hardware control system which is located in a field-programmable gate array (FPGA). In addition, a local memory is also used to store every received signal. Finally, the signals are transferred to the imaging system using any communication interface (USB, Ethernet, PCI Express). In the imaging system, raw data is stored in a RAM memory of $2N-1$ signals of capacity to be used for compose and beamform the ultrasonic images using a GPU.

3.2.2. 8xA-SAFT with Golay encoding architecture

As we see in sections 2.1.2 and 2.2, and in order to combine 8xA-SAFT with Golay codes, we will double the number of channels in reception to maintain the number of original firings. Thus, in this case the system is composed of one channel in emission and 32 channels in reception as Figure 12 suggests. A multiplexer connects the transmission channel to elements for sequentially activate one of them, in steps of 8 elements, to transmit an A or B code for odd or even shots respectively. A second multiplexer will be on charge of connecting the 32 reception channels to the receiving aperture ensuring that every coded signal is stored in a local memory. Therefore, two signals per coarray element are overlapped, each one belonging to an A or B code respectively. Additionally, an offset is added to the coarray structure in order to centre its elements, and the boundary coarray elements are removed from it as we illustrated in section 2.2.2.

Now the software imaging system requires a bigger memory and an additional decoding stage, where the complete set of signals is deconvolved, generating a $2N-8$ data set. Later on, as usual, the data will be beamformed using the graphics processing unit.

3.3. Image generation subsystem: Parallel beamforming

In recent years, computing industry has been opened a way to parallel computing. Nowadays, all consumer computers ship with multi-core processors. Dual-core processors (CPUs) were introduced in personal systems at the beginning of 2006, and it is currently common to find them in laptops as well as 8 and 16-core workstation computers, which

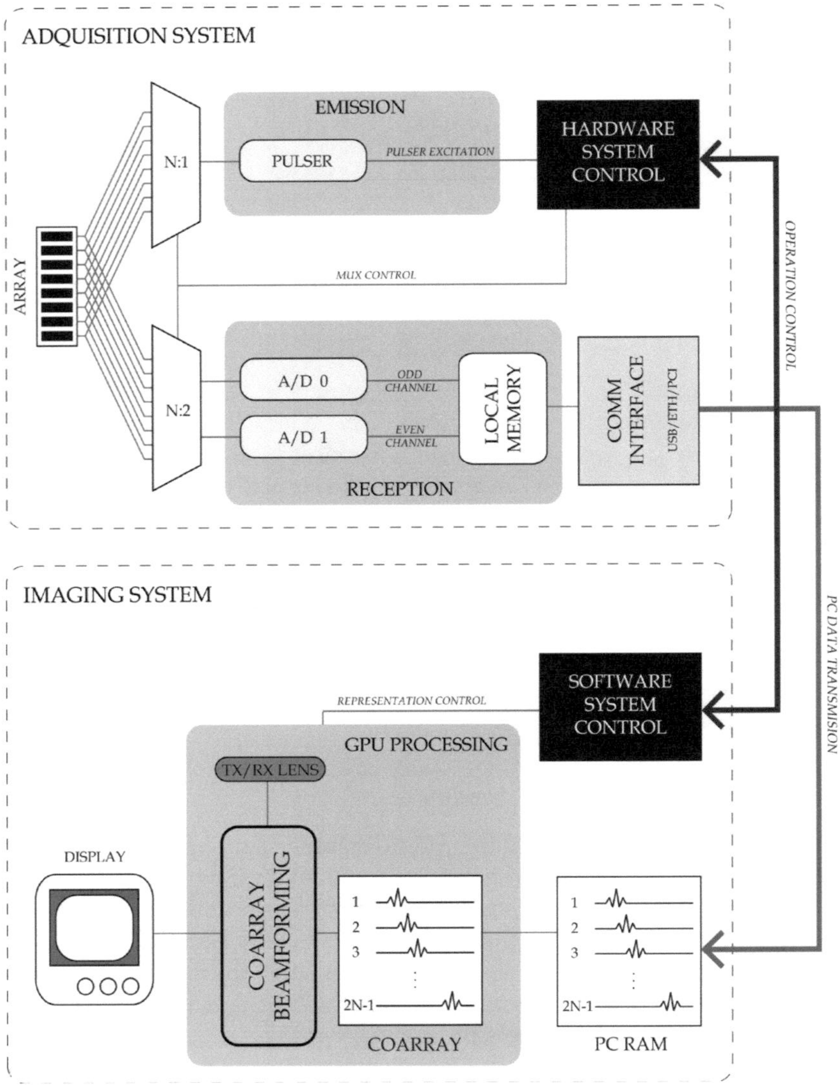

Figure 11. 2R-SAFT Minimal Architecture

means that parallel computing is not relegated to big supercomputers or mainframes computers. However, Graphics Processor Units (GPUs), as their name suggests, came about as accelerators for graphics applications, predominantly those using the OpenGL and DirectX programming interfaces. Although originally they were pure fixed-function devices, the demand for real time and 3D graphics made them evolve into increasingly flexible highly parallel, multithreaded processors with extremely high computational power and very high memory bandwidth converting them into massively parallel machines.

Unlike earlier GPU generations, where computing resources were partitioned into vertex and pixel shaders, nowadays they can be programmed directly in C using CUDA or OpenCL [19], APIs which include a unified shader pipeline, allowing each and every arithmetic logic

http://dx.doi.org/10.5772/55910

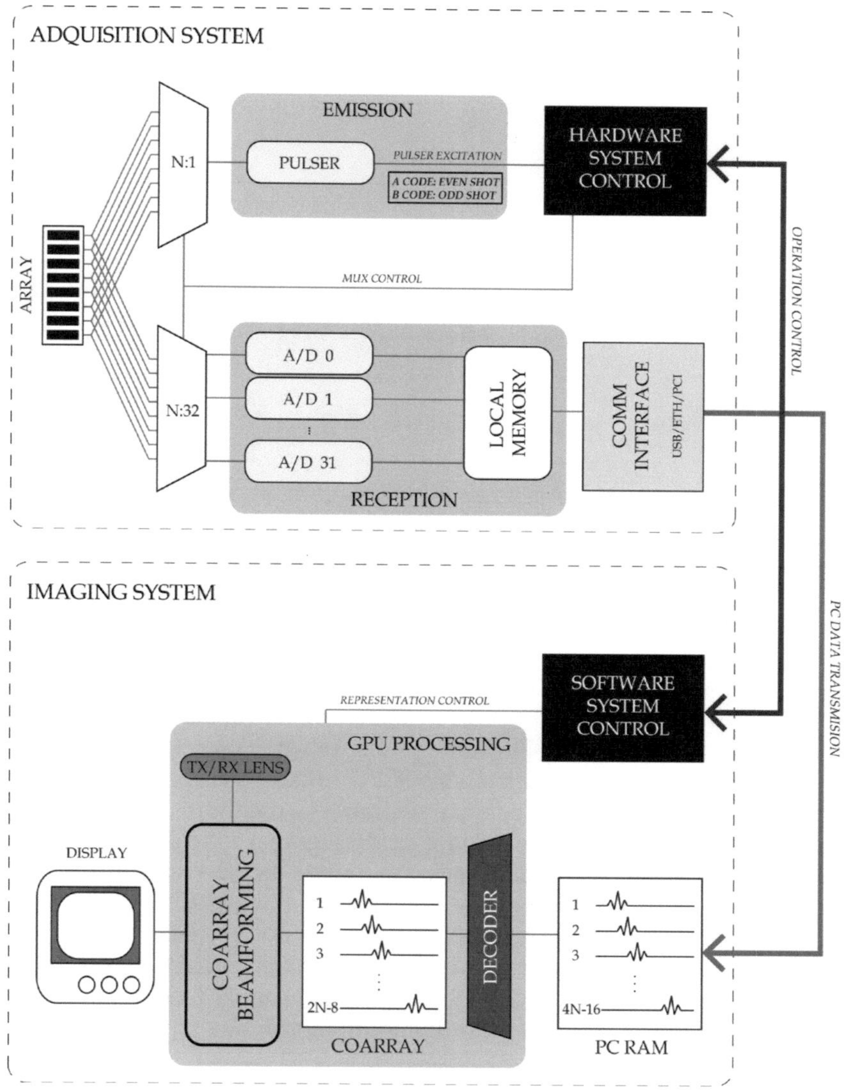

Figure 12. 8xA-SAFT Architecture with 32 channels in reception needed for Golay encoding

unit on the chip to be used by a program intending to perform general-purpose computations (GPGPU). Furthermore, the execution units on the GPU allow arbitrary read and write access to memory as well as access to a software-managed cache known as shared memory. A CUDA program consists of one or more phases that are executed on either the host (CPU) or a device such as a GPU. The phases that exhibit little or no data parallelism are implemented in CPU code. The phases that exhibit rich amount of data parallelism are implemented in the GPU code. The parallel functions (called kernels) typically generate a large number of threads to exploit data parallelism. It is worth noting that CUDA threads are of much lighter weight than the CPU threads. CUDA programmers can assume that these threads take very few cycles to generate and schedule due to efficient hardware support. This differs from

CPU threads which typically require thousands of clock cycles for their generation and their scheduling.

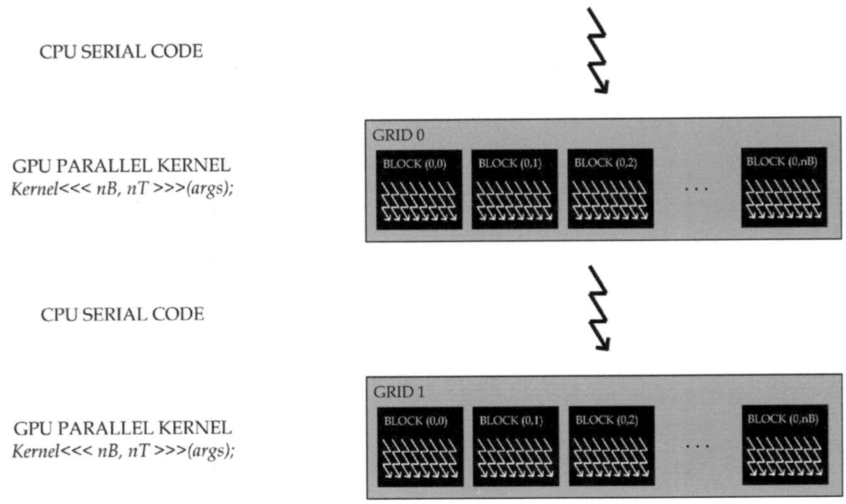

Figure 13. CUDA program execution diagram

The execution of a typical CUDA program is illustrated in Figure 13 where it is observed that the execution starts with host (CPU) execution. When a kernel function is invoked (or launched), the execution is moved to a device (GPU), where a large number of threads are generated to take advantage of huge data parallelism. All the threads generated by a kernel during an invocation are collectively called a grid. Figure 13 shows the execution of two grids of threads. A grid is a 1D, 2D or 3D structure of blocks, and a block is a 1D, 2D or 3D structure of threads. Thus, the program code is composed by classical functions, which run on CPU using only one thread of execution; and kernels, which run on GPU using multiple parallel threads. When all threads of a kernel complete their execution, the corresponding grid terminates, and the execution continues on the host until another kernel is invoked. It is not our purpose to fully cover all the aspects involved in CUDA Architecture. Thus, an extended discussion about the CUDA hardware and programming model is available in multiple sources in the literature [19–21].

Therefore, in this section we will examine different ways to implement the beamforming process on the GPU using the CUDA programming model. From the model, it is extracted that functions which are executed many times independently over different data are the ideal candidates for this kind of computing. In this sense, several algorithms have been implemented to cover the fundamental parts of a conventional Delay-and-Sum Beamformer (DAS) and they have been also evaluated for their performance. This analysis helps to give a better understanding of the GPU architecture and how to write applications for it.

Schematically, Figure 14 show the main stages of a general beamformer. As we can appreciate there are three main operations to be done: pre-processing of signals, beamforming and post-processing. In the software system we propose (Figure 10) all beamforming procedures take place in the GPU.

http://dx.doi.org/10.5772/55910

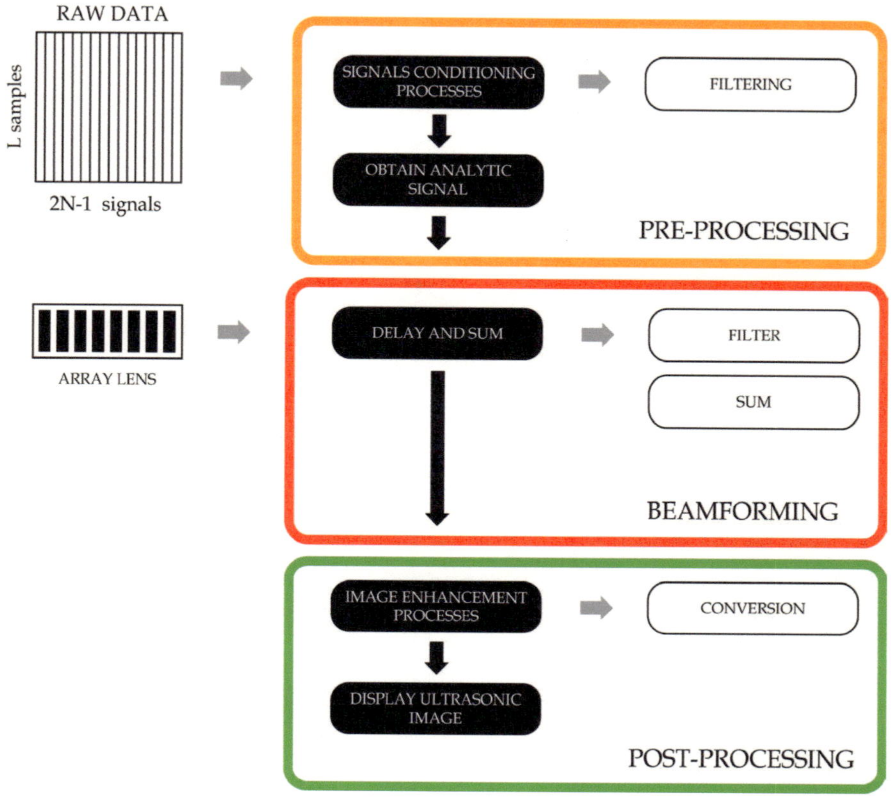

Figure 14. Schematic diagram main parts of a general SAFT beamformer

Implementing the imaging algorithm on GPU systems primarily involves the parallelization of the core algorithm into small independent threads which can be executed by the GPU in runtime. Thus, the imaging process occurs in multiple stages, which follows closely to that has been detailed in Figure 14. Thus, in order to maximize GPUs efficiency and reduce image generation time as much as possible, a specific solution for every different task have been designed. Figure 15 shows how these tasks have been parallelized on the GPU.

The first step consists on copying the complete set of acquired signals from CPU memory to GPU memory. We already know that this transaction is slow, and therefore it is recommended to copy all signals at the same time rather than doing it signal by signal.

3.4. Pre-processing

The pre-processing of the complete set of signals is a fundamental part of the image generation process. Supposing $X_{tx,rx}(t)$ the received signal from any emitter tx and receiver rx pair, a function $H(t)$ is applied to every signal as the following expression suggests:

$$Y_{tx,rx}(t) = X_{tx,rx}(t) \cdot H(t) \tag{5}$$

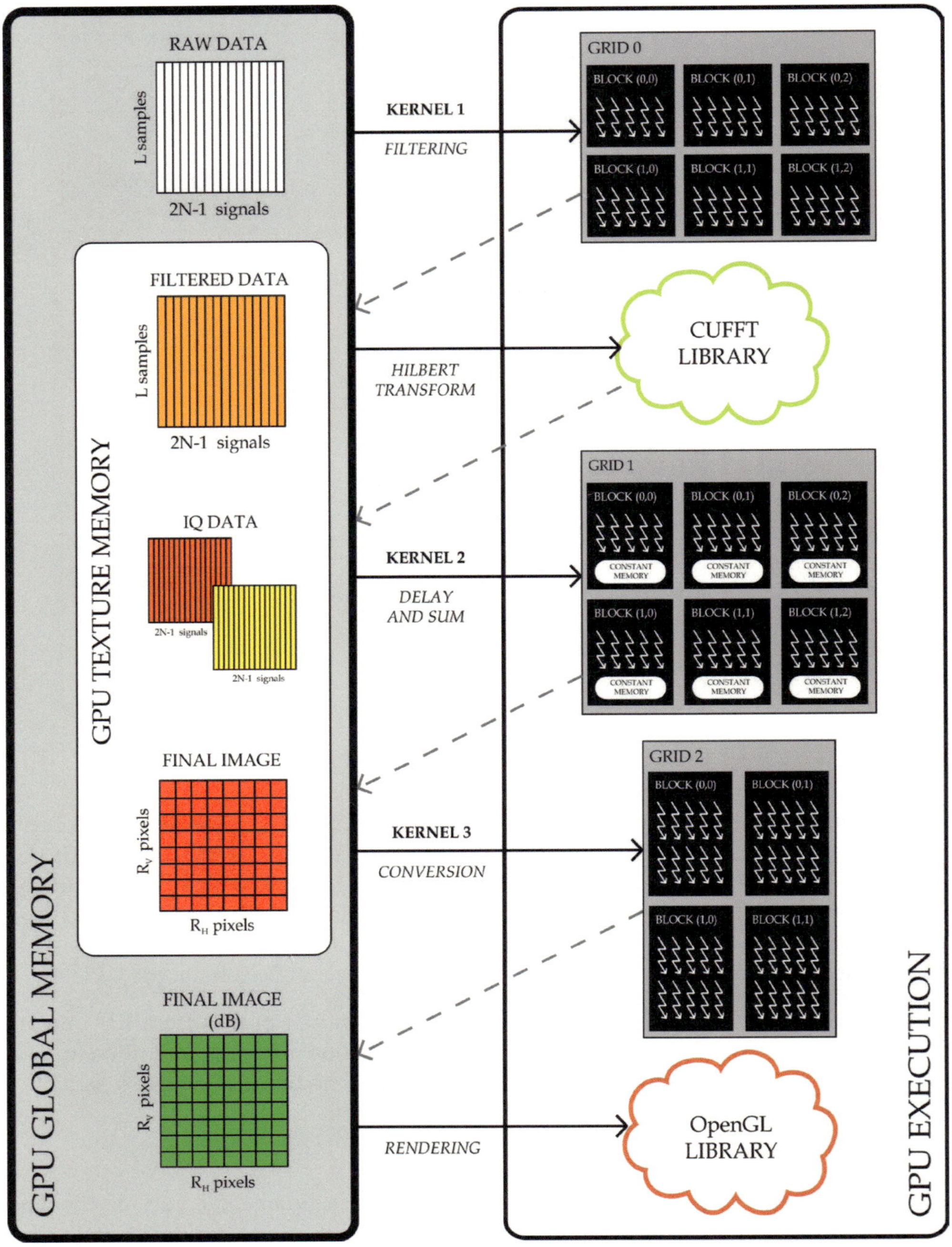

Figure 15. System beamforming loop parallelized on GPU for SAFT implementation

http://dx.doi.org/10.5772/55910

and

$$H(t) = H_F(t) \cdot H_{IQ}(t) \tag{6}$$

where $H_F(t)$ is a signal conditioning process where a filter is applied in order to remove the offset level introduced during the acquisition system and to reduce the noise.

Additionally and for convenience, the acquired signals can be decomposed into their analytic signals form [22] (in-phase I and quadrature components Q) . Thereby, the second function $H_{IQ}(t)$ is the Hilbert Transform in order to reduce errors and artefacts which appear at the envelope detection stage. Then, the signals $X_{tx,rx}(t)$ can now be expressed as:

$$X_{tx,rx}(t) = I_{tx,rx}(t) + jQ_{tx,rx}(t) = \mathbf{X}_{tx,rx}(t)e^{j\phi_{tx,rx}(t)} \tag{7}$$

where $\mathbf{X}_{tx,rx}(t)$ is the modulus and $\phi_{tx,rx}(t)$ its corresponding signal phase.

3.4.1. *Parallel implementation*

In order to carry out a parallel implementation of these operations, the proposed parallelism strategy lies in a signal-oriented parallelization. This means that a GPU computational thread will be associated to each stored signal sample. Thus, considering signals with L samples, the computational grid of the kernel will be formed as shown in Figure 15 being the number of blocks in x-dimension $BX = \lceil \frac{L}{T_{BX}} \rceil$ and the number of blocks in y-dimension $BY = 2N - 1$. As we know, the number of threads per block T_{BX} is an empirical value and the designer should evaluate what is the best according to the GPU resources. Typical values are 32, 64 or 128 threads per block, generally any power of two, and attending to our tests we have chosen 256 as the optimal value.

There is no limitation on filter length because its coefficients are stored in texture memory, which resides in the device memory and is cached in texture cache to optimize read accesses. Thus, each thread reads from memory the filter coefficients and L samples of a signal, convolving them to obtain a filtered sample.

Later on, the Hilbert Transform is applied to every filtered signal so we can obtain their analytic signals. In this case, FFT algorithms provided by CUDA (CUFFT libraries [20]) are used to compute the IFFT of the product of the corresponding signal and the Hilbert Transformer FFTs, as it is defined in [23]. With these libraries, there is no need to define a new kernel nor specify grid and block dimensions, since they are responsible for properly parallelizing and splitting the algorithm, computing the FFT of the data set directly on the GPU. In our particular case, a total of $2N - 1$ FFTs of L points are calculated in parallel. The whole resultant I/Q (in-phase/quadrature-phase) signals pairs (Figure 15) are stored in texture memory, and they are passed to the next stage via global device memory.

3.4.2. Optional stage: Decoding

When Golay encoding is used during acquisition, it is necessary to first merge and deconvolve the $4N - 16$ received signals, where 50% of signals belong to A and B codes respectively. This can be done very fast making a parallel implementation where the parallelism strategy is also signal-oriented. In this sense, the previous kernel can be modified in order to include the sum of both signals in parallel before the application of the filters coefficients to finally obtain $2N - 8$ signals.

3.5. Beamforming: Delay and Sum

All time-domain imaging algorithms are based on the principle of delay-and-sum beamforming. Typically, these algorithms emulate an acoustic lens by applying appropriate time delays to the array elements in order to focus or steer the beam as desired. SAFT beamformers focus the beam at every point in the image, giving better defect detectability as we mentioned [2, 4, 5, 7]. DAS beamforming is not difficult to implement and permits the use of arbitrary array geometries what makes suitable for a wide range of applications.

According to the Hilbert transformation of the first step, two processing streams have been created where two parallel images will be calculated following these equations:

$$A_I(x,z) = \sum_{i=1}^{N} \sum_{k=1}^{N} I_{tx_i,rx_k}(D(x,z)) \tag{8}$$

$$A_Q(x,z) = \sum_{i=1}^{N} \sum_{k=1}^{N} Q_{tx_i,rx_k}(D(x,z)) \tag{9}$$

where $A_I(x,z)$ and $A_Q(x,z)$ are the in-phase and quadrature images respectively, and $D(x,z)$ is the focussing delay for the spatial point (x_p, z_p) in the grid which is calculated as follows:

$$D(x,z) = \frac{\sqrt{(x_p - x_{tx})^2 + z_p^2} + \sqrt{(x_p - x_{rx})^2 + z_p^2}}{c} \tag{10}$$

being x_{tx} and x_{rx} the coordinates of the transducer elements tx and rx, respectively.

Henceforth, we will focus on the all the operations involved in Delay-and-Sum algorithm, studying the diverse alternatives and their parallel implementation as well as the best way of their optimization.

- **Lens calculation**. A fundamental part of beamforming is calculating the differences in wave arrival time between array elements. Therefore, each signal sample has to be properly delayed according to the distance from the spatial point to the emitter or receiver array elements. The calculation of delays is achieved using equation 10. Although in a conceptual form is a delay, what is actually done is a mapping to the memory buffer (at the sampling frequency) where the corresponding sample value of the signal is retrieved. Therefore, the number of delays to be calculated is usually large and it is given by:

$$Memory|_{lens} = R_H \times R_V \times 2N - 1 \tag{11}$$

where $R_H \times R_V$ are the dimensions of the desired ultrasonic image. Thus, the lens calculation can be afforded using two different approaches:

- *Load pre-calculated delays.* The delays are pre-calculated before beamforming and they are recovered from a look-up table inside the image generation process. The necessary memory to store all the delays is not a significant problem, but the main drawback is the requirement of high bandwidth to make the process faster as well as the fact of updating the table each time. Thereby, this would be a good solution for no in-vivo inspections, where the scenario is known and the delays are calculated only once for the complete acquisition.
- *Calculate delays on-the-fly.* The delays are dynamically calculated inside the beamforming process. This task, which can be at first computationally more expensive than the first alternative, is however not a heavy computational problem because of the great power of actual systems. In this regard, dynamic calculation of the lenses inside the threads will simplify other operations on images, such as scrolling and zooming.

Which approach to choose relies on the rest of the beamformer implementation. Thus, in order to take full advantage of the GPU it is needed to have a balance between bandwidth use and arithmetic operations. In this regard, it has been proved that it is faster to obtain the values for the lenses inside the kernels instead of having them stored in the device memory. Therefore in our proposal, it makes sense to calculate the delays on-the-fly.

- **Filtering**. In a real implementation, we sample the elements at a rate just above the Nyquist criteria. Although this preserves the frequency content of the signal, this does not give enough steering delay resolution. The solution is to perform a digital interpolation, increasing the steering-delay resolution. In this particular case, linear interpolation and polynomial interpolation can be easily implemented. The results obtained are practically identical, although the cost associated to each solution differs being the polynomial interpolation time the double of linear interpolation. For this reason, we decided to simply interpolate across two consecutive samples. The penultimate operation is the application of a window function which is multiplied with the data from each channel in order to reduce mainly the level of sidelobes.
- **Sum**. The final step in the ultrasonic generation process is to obtain the accumulated sum of all the signals samples which contribute to a given spatial point.

3.5.1. Parallel implementation

The delay-and-sum process is applied to the complex signals obtained in the previous stage. We have identified different strategies to implement the ultrasonic image generation process in a GPU depending on how the algorithm is parallelized with respect to threads and blocks and relative to the use of GPU resources.

As Figure 16 shows, the parallelization is carried out by launching a thread per image pixel. To this end, a computation grid ($GRID_1$) with $BX = \lceil \frac{R_H}{T_{BX}} \rceil$ and $BY = \lceil \frac{R_V}{T_{BY}} \rceil$ blocks of $T_{BX} \times T_{BY}$ threads is defined on the kernel, where R_H and R_V are the desired image resolution in horizontal and vertical directions, respectively. Each thread is responsible then for calculating the coordinates for the spatial point (x_p, z_p) of a specific image pixel and calculating the lens to focus at this point.

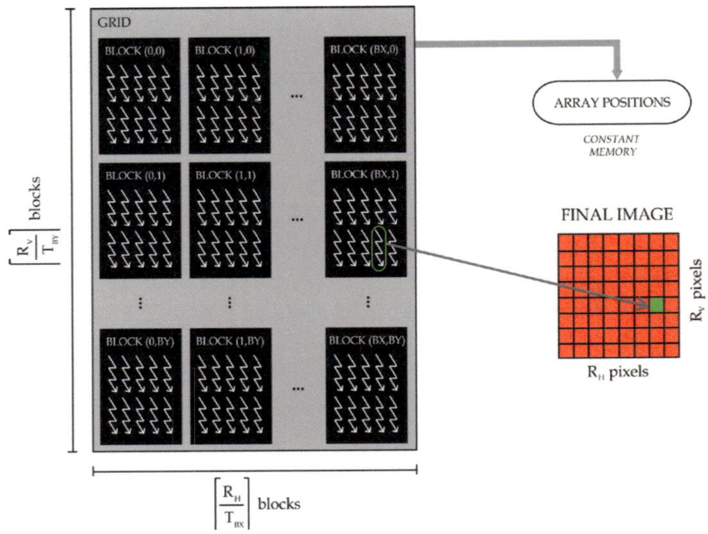

Figure 16. One thread is responsible for a image pixel

In this case, the lens is formed by the $2N-1$ times of flight of each emission-reception pair combination. Thus, in order to accelerate all these calculations, the transducer elements coordinates are stored in constant memory in each GPU multiprocessor. In addition, the computed distances from an array element to an image pixel are reused to save time avoiding duplicate calculations. The lens obtained allow us to index in the complex signals stored in texture memory, and real and imaginary parts are interpolated when needed. To this respect, lineal interpolation was implemented obtaining good performance. Then, the $2N-1$ resultant complex samples are multiplied by the corresponding apodization gains and added together. Finally, the resultant image (final image in Figure 15) is also stored in texture memory, for a quick data access to the post-processing stage.

3.6. Post-processing

The post-processing stage involves firstly calculate the envelope (in essence the modulus) of the beamformed images, according to the following expression:

$$A = \sqrt{{A_I}^2 + {A_Q}^2} \tag{12}$$

where A_I and A_Q are the *In-phase* and *Quadrature* images derived from the beamforming process. This operation prevents the appearance of diverse artefacts associated with the Hilbert Transform.

Likewise, (an optional) stage in the process is in charge of normalizing and converting the image to decibels scale. Although this is not a complex task, it cannot be carried out in the previous stage because we need to know what the maximum value for the image:

http://dx.doi.org/10.5772/55910

$$A|_{decibels} = 20\log_{10}\left(\frac{A}{max(A)}\right) \tag{13}$$

Finally, the generated ultrasonic image (Final image (dB) referenced in Figure 15) is directly displayed on the screen using the OpenGL libraries, which provide specific functionality for graphics representation.

3.6.1. Parallel implementation

The parallel implementation of the envelope calculation is carried out inside the beamforming kernel. This is because at the end of the pixel calculation, we have the final output values for both I and Q components. Thus, we avoid writing twice and we only obtain a single image. For the optional conversion to decibels scale, a new kernel (Kernel 3 in Figure 15) is defined which uses a grid with $\lceil\frac{R_H}{B_x}\rceil$ and $\lceil\frac{R_V}{B_y}\rceil$ blocks of T_{BX} threads having a thread per image pixel as before.

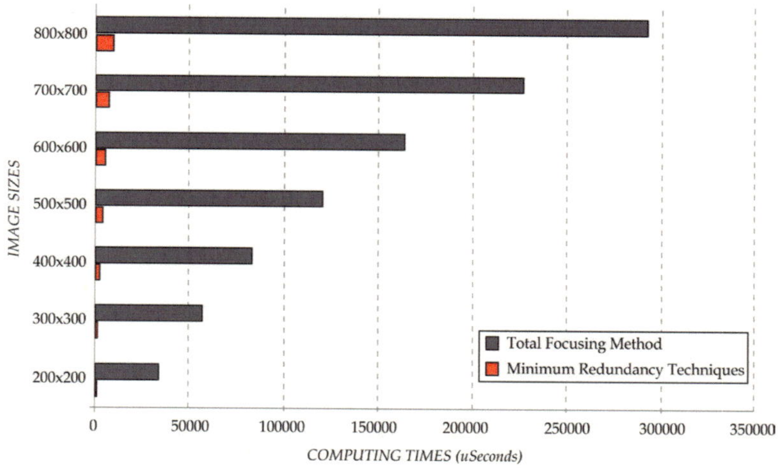

Figure 17. Computing times for TFM and MR solutions using GPU in μseconds

3.7. Performance

A NVIDIA Quadro 4000 graphics card was used to test the beamforming time achieved with the system proposed here. This card has 256 cores and 1GB global memory. It was installed in a computer with a four-core 2.66GHz Intel Q9450 processor and 4GB RAM. GPU-based implementation of the beamformer was done and tested for all acquisition strategies exposed along this chapter. In Figure 17 computing times considering image sizes starting from 200×200 to big size 800×800 for both TFM and minimum redundancy solutions are presented where it is evident than despite using the great power of GPU's the TFM solution is a very intensive procedure.

In Figure 18, the frame rate obtained for different image sizes when 2R-SAFT and kA-SAFT are employed is presented. In particular, attending to the case of an image with 500×500

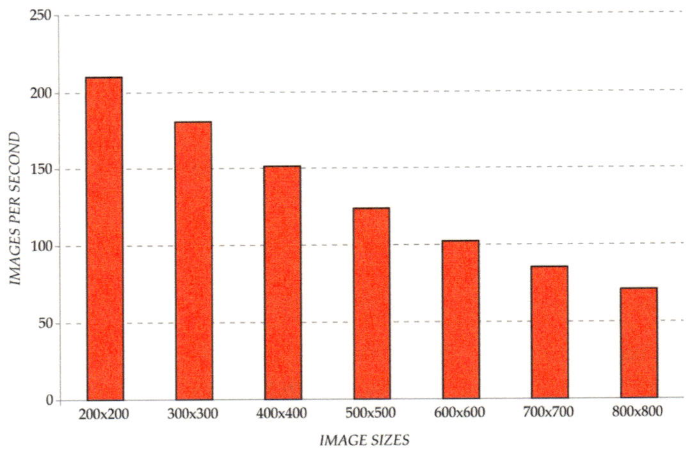

Figure 18. Images per second achieved using GPU for different image sizes for 2R-SAFT and kA-SAFT

pixels, the GPU is able to get 135 images per second, which is in nearly to the acquisition system's rate. The evidence here is that we are using a smaller dataset than that obtained with TFM method but preserving the image quality with all GPU cores completely dedicated to fast computation.

4. Conclusion and future developments

This work has presented how the use of coarray paradigm makes possible the design of ultrasonic imaging systems with reduced hardware requirements. The system is divided into two subsystems, hardware and software respectively. The first one is focused on the development of the data acquisition system, whose design is done analysing the compromise between parallel electronic resources and acquisition time. The second one exploits GPU technology to implement the beamformer via software, compensating the emission and reception distances to each image point, providing the maximum possible quality at each image pixel.

Two solutions, based on the availability of instrumentation in the market, are presented attending to this design following the minimum redundancy coarray model. In one case, it has been emphasized the miniaturization of the hardware (with only two channels in reception), and in the second case the focus has been the reduction of the acquisition time at the expense of increasing and parallelize reception channels (up to a maximum of 32). From the point of view of image quality, both beamforming techniques present similar results. Consequently it is possible to adapt the design of our system to several implementation models depending on the final application requirements.

The problems associated to the low level of the transmitted signals and the signal losses through the material have been analysed. As a solution, we have introduced pulse compression techniques in order to increase the signal to noise ratio. In addition, we have studied the implementation cost of this technique and it has been compared with the TFM technique (based on the FMA capture), verifying that the results are very similar.

Finally, we have made a detailed description of the beamforming process in GPU and it has been quantified the advantage of using the GPU as a processing tool from the image

http://dx.doi.org/10.5772/55910

frame rate point of view. So by using a simple graphics card equipped with NVIDIA CUDA technology, rates that go up to 200 images per second were obtained depending on the image size chosen. Therefore, this solution allows the development of high quality imaging systems with low requirements and excellent capabilities in a compact architecture.

Acknowledgments

This work has been supported by the Spanish Ministry of Science and Competitiveness under the project DPI2010-19376.

Author details

D. Romero-Laorden, J. Villazón-Terrazas,
O. Martínez-Graullera and A. Ibáñez

Centro de Acústica Aplicada y Evaluación No Destructiva (CSIC), Madrid, Spain

References

[1] Caroline Holmes, Bruce W. Drinkwater, and Paul D. Wilcox. Post-processing of the full matrix of ultrasonic transmit–receive array data for non-destructive evaluation. *NDT & E International*, 38(8):701–711, December 2005.

[2] Caroline Holmes, Bruce W. Drinkwater, and Paul D. Wilcox. Advanced post-processing for scanned ultrasonic arrays: application to defect detection and classification in non-destructive evaluation. *Ultrasonics*, 48(6-7):636–42, November 2008.

[3] Alan J. Hunter, Bruce W. Drinkwater, and Paul D. Wilcox. The wavenumber algorithm for full-matrix imaging using an ultrasonic array. *IEEE transactions on ultrasonics, ferroelectrics, and frequency control*, 55(11):2450–62, November 2008.

[4] Mustafa Karaman, Pai-Chi Li, and Matthew O'Donnell. Synthetic aperture imaging for small scale systems. *IEEE Transactions on Ultrasonics, Ferroelectrics and Frequency Control*, 42(3):429–442, May 1995.

[5] Jørgen Arendt Jensen, Svetoslav Ivanov Nikolov, Kim Lø kke Gammelmark, and Morten Hø gholm Pedersen. Synthetic aperture ultrasound imaging. *Ultrasonics*, 44:5–15, December 2006.

[6] Carlos J. Martín-Arguedas, O. Martínez-Graullera, G. Godoy, and L. Gómez-Ullate. Coarray synthesis based on polynomial decomposition. *IEEE transactions on image processing*, 19(4):1102–1107, 2010.

[7] Carlos J. Martín-Arguedas, D. Romero-Laorden, O. Martínez-Graullera, M. Pérez-Lopez, and L. Gómez-Ullate. An Ultrasonic Imaging System Based on a New SAFT Approach and a GPU Beamformer. *IEEE Transactions on Ultrasonics, Ferroelectrics and Frequency Control*, 59(7):1402–1412, 2012.

[8] Geoffrey R Lockwood, Pai-chi Li, Matthew O'Donnell, and F. Stuart Foster. Optimizing the Radiation Pattern of Sparse Periodic Linear Arrays. *IEEE Transactions on Ultrasonics, Ferroelectrics and Frequency Control*, 43(1):7–14, 1996.

[9] Svetoslav Ivanov Nikolov. *Synthetic aperture tissue and flow ultrasound imaging*. PhD thesis, Technical University of Denmark, 2001.

[10] Bernard D. Steinberg. *Principles of Aperture and Array System Design*. Wiley, New York, 1976.

[11] John J. Flaherty, Kenneth R. Erikson, and Van Metre Lund. Synthetic aperture ultrasonic imaging systems, Patent number 3548642, 1967.

[12] Christoph B. Burckhardt, Pierre-André Grandchamp, and Heinz Hoffman. An Experimental 2 MHz Synthetic Aperture Sonar System Intended for Medical Use. *IEEE Transactions on Sonics and Ultrasonics*, 21(1):1–6, 1974.

[13] Intel Corporation. Thunderbolt™ technology. http://www.intel.com/thunderbolt, (accessed 6 July 2012).

[14] Carlos J. Martín-Arguedas, O. Martínez-Graullera, and L. G. Reduction of grating lobes in SAFT Images. In *IEEE International Ultrasonics Symposium*, number 1, pages 721–724, Beijing, China, 2008.

[15] Carlos J. Martín-Arguedas. *Técnicas de apertura sintética para la generación de imagen ultrasónica*. PhD thesis, Universidad de Alcalá, 2010.

[16] M. Golay. Golay's complementary series. *IRE Transactions on Information Theory*, pages 273–276, 1961.

[17] Andrzej Nowicki, Igor Trots, Wojciech Secomski, and Jerzy Litniewski. Golay's codes sequences in ultrasonography. *Archives of Acoustics*, 28:313–324, 2003.

[18] National Instruments. 32-channel digitizer module for ultrasound applications. http://sine.ni.com/nips/cds/view/p/lang/en/nid/208657, (accessed 1 October 2012).

[19] Wen-Mei W. Hwu and David B. Kirk. *Programming Massively Parallel Processors : A Hands-on Approach*. Morgan Kaufmann, 2010.

[20] NVIDIA Developer Zone. Software development kit 4.2 version, https://developer.nvidia.com/cuda-education-training, (accessed 1 October 2012).

[21] Jason Sanders and Edward Kandrot. *CUDA by Example*. Addison-Wesley, 2010.

[22] A. V. Oppenheim and W. R. Schafer. *Discrete-Time Signal Processing*. Prentice-Hall, Englewoods Cliffs (NJ), 1989.

[23] S. Lawrence Marple. Computing the Discrete-Time "Analytic" Signal via FFT. *IEEE Transactions on Signal Processing*, 47(9):2600–2603, 1999.

Chapter 10

Breaking Through the Speed Barrier — Advancements in High-Speed Imaging

G. P. P. Gunarathne

Additional information is available at the end of the chapter

http://dx.doi.org/10.5772/56378

1. Introduction

1.1. Origin, expansion and applications of ultrasonic imaging

History and the discoveries of the use of ultrasound can be traced back to late 18th century, but one of the major steps toward the practical use of ultrasound may be attributed to Lewis Nixon who invented the very first sonar type listening device in 1906 as a way of detecting icebergs [1]. Rapid developments of the use of ultrasound occurred since then, particularly after world war II; initially for underwater (sonar) and industrial uses, followed by developments for medical applications [2, 3]. Today, the technology is widespread in Medicine, Non Destructive Testing (NDT) and Sonar in many specialised areas such as: industrial and medical imaging, study and classification of the properties of material and biological tissues, seismic explorations high-intensity applications etc. and the applications are growing. These rapid advances are directly related to the parallel advancements in electronics, computing, and transducer technology together with sophisticated signal processing techniques.

Irrespective of the field of applications, arguably one of the most important applications of ultrasound is "Imaging", which is the chosen subject of this chapter. However, it is important to note that imaging as applied to the three main application areas mentioned above; namely, NDT, Sonar and Medicine have fundamental similarities and also differences. For example, the speed of sound in water in the case of sonar and biological tissues are comparable (~1450m/s) but sonar is extremely long range.

In the case of NDT, the speeds of sound in industrial materials are generally very much higher, although the penetration distances are comparable to that for medical imaging. On the other hand, sonar and medical imaging primarily relies on one form of ultrasound propagation, namely, compressional waves while in solid material, there are multiple propagational modes, such as compressional, shear, surface, creep, lamb and torsional waves etc. These different modalities have widely different characteristics and they can coexist with possible mode conversions depending on the particular geometry and test scenario. In NDT, the co-existence or co-generation of this multimode propagation can be both advantages in some situations, and equally become a nuisance in other cases.

In processing and assessing an ultrasound image, one of the most striking differences between industrial NDT and medical imaging is that in the case of the latter, there is good pre-anatomical knowledge of the part of the anatomy being examined; often with the possibility of supplementary data obtained from other forms of imaging such as MRI, CT scans etc. However, for NDT inspection, the target features (shapes, sizes and orientation etc.) are almost always largely unknown, thus the interpretation is largely based on the reliability of the images being produced. This is a major challenge in industrial imaging applications. On the positive side, the targets being imaged in NDT applications e.g. a crack in a structure generally tends to appear as a good acoustic discontinuity yielding good Signal-to-noise ratio (SNR) compared to that from a tissue boundary, since the latter is dependent on small impedance contrast.

1.1.1. Dynamic range considerations

For all imaging applications, the signal dynamic range is an extremely important consideration. Usually this could be very high; far above that may be accommodated by display equipment. For medical Imaging, the dynamic range of signals could be of the order of order of 100dB covering both backscattered signals from tissues and specular reflections. (However, the range of interest is of the order of 40 to 50 dB, which is the range covered by backscattered signals). Although impedance contrast is generally high in NDT and sonar, dynamic range of signals can still be very large depending on the application, not necessarily because of high attenuation as in the case of biological tissues but because of the size of the targets such as micro-defects in NDT or beam divergence in the case of sonar. In the case of sonar, the range is extreme and the signals of interest could be of the order of several hundred millivolts to sub-micro volts. The dynamic range can be evaluated for homogeneous media, such as water, by considering signal loss between targets of same strength placed at different axial distances (R_1 & R_2) form equation 1 below, which helps formulating compensating strategies.

$$Loss(dB) = 20\log\frac{R_2}{R_1} + 2\propto(R_2 - R_1) \tag{1}$$

Where $\propto$ is the attenuation coefficient of the medium at the frequency of interest. Accommodating large dynamic range and depth gain compensation are therefore features common to all imaging systems; albeit for different reasons. Once the ranges and the loss characteristics are known, accommodation can be handled electronically, e.g. by using logarithmic compression and Time-varying-gain (TVG) functions to accommodate the signals within the much limited display dynamic range.

In order to understand the potential of imaging and areas of improvement, it is necessary to examine the fundamental characteristics of common imaging modalities, which is the subject

http://dx.doi.org/10.5772/56378

of the following section. The discussion does not include a comprehensive treatment of imaging techniques in use, but the ones that represent properties central to the understanding of primary limitations.

1.2. General principles

The simplest form of ultrasonic visualisation is what is known as the A-scan. Here an ultrasonic transducer generates a short pulse of high frequency sound which is coupled to the test medium. Echoes generated from any acoustic discontinuities within the path of the ultrasound beam are received, usually by the same transducer, and are displayed on a screen or a monitor as intensity modulated signals. The technique essentially provides (a) Target-depth information (b) An indication of the extent of the discontinuity and to a much lesser extent information on its orientation or shape. Since the time required for displaying the echoes is virtually equal to the time of flight of the acoustic pulse within the object medium, it gives the maximum temporal resolution for moving targets. However, the interpretation and information obtained from an A-scan (1- spatial dimension) or that derived from it is very limited, highly operator-dependent and therefore of limited use in diagnostic applications.

However, a collection of A-scans in a given plane in the test object could provide a two-dimensional map (or an image) of the acoustic discontinuities. This requires acquisition, storage and display of successive A-scan lines requiring digital data storage and processing. These line-serial scans may be generated in a number of ways: mechanically moving the transducer along a given direction; using an array of transducers which are switched on in succession to mimic a mechanical movement (linear or curvilinear array scanning). Images thus generated represent a two-dimensional (2-D) view of the target medium and are commonly known as B-scans.

Alternatively, the ultrasound beam may be electronically steered using a transducer array (phased array scanning) or by a mechanically rotating transducer. The 2-D images thus obtained are normally referred to as sector B-scans.

1.2.1. Real-time versus determinism

One of the confusing terminologies in imaging (or any other form of data presentation) is *"Real-time"*. The naturally implied meaning of the term real-time is: *"as it happens"*. This meaning is incompatible with laws of Physics since nothing can be observed at the same instant as something happens. So, image presentation can only approach this ideal of real-time, provided that what an observer sees in an image is close enough to what was happening to the object as a whole, both in time and spatial resemblance. Then the expression "real-time" can be considered appropriate. For example, an observer seeing a trajectory of a meteoroid views this in real-time because the velocity of light is at least 6 to7 orders of magnitude higher than the moving object. But this is not the case, for example, seeing a moving heart valve in an ultrasound image taking a few milliseconds to form just one frame. Obviously, the image is temporally and spatially distorted. Therefore a target that appears to be moving in a succession of image frames is not seen "as it happens" and therefore not true real-time. The term *"Pseudo*

Real-time" is a more meaningful definition in such cases where the image is seen to be live, while the velocity ratio (i.e. the speed of the target to that of sound) is significant, or forming an image frame takes significant time.

On the other hand, *"Determinism"* can be an important concept in defining a key aspect of image integrity. This can be a predominant requirement – for example in quantitative image analysis where accurate spatial information is important. The use of the term "determinism" in this context does not really mean "as it happens" (although the time interval between a moving target and its presentation as an image is usually small). Determinism essentially means that the spatial integrity of a moving target is persevered in the image to a high degree. In the case of ultrasound the theoretical limit of spatial determinism can only be reached if a single ultrasound pulse emitted by an imaging device produces a complete image field of the object within its time of flight. This is clearly not achievable with the existing line-serial imaging technology, but it is one of the main features of the new hybrid imaging system described later in this chapter.

1.3. State-of-the-art techniques

In late 1980's, the techniques for generating 3-D images from a collection of 2-D images have been demonstrated [4]. Producing a single frame of such an image may have taken about 20 minutes then, but with the advancement of computing power and processing techniques, live 3-D and 4-D volume imaging reaching pseudo-real time volumes of surface features have now come into existence [4, 5].

One of the fairly recent additions to B-mode imaging is the so called Zone-sonography [6]. A main feature in this system is the acquisition of data from a relatively low number of zone sectors, as opposed to line-by-line acquisition, thereby significantly improving the temporal artefacts inherent with the conventional methods. It has been claimed that in some cases, this approach could produce speed improvements of up to 10 times compared to conventional line-serial imaging systems [6], although the zones in themselves are produced using serial scanning.

In addition, in the case of medical imaging, various echo enhancement techniques such as Coded Excitation (CE) and Digitally Encoded Ultrasound (DEU) which improve sensitivity, penetration and contrast are now been widely used [7, 8]. CE is a pulse compression technique which is designed to differentiate and boost weak return signals from deep within the body. This is done by transmitting an encoded pulse sequence, isolating the coded return signal and amplifying only this signal, while regaining longitudinal resolution which is distributed within the insonifying pulse train [7]. Some systems using CE can also show blood flow together with the body tissue as a B-mode image, without the need for overlay as would be the case with Doppler imaging. Tissue Harmonic Imaging (THI) is another widely used technique which reduces haze, clutter and image artefacts. In this approach, higher harmonic components of the echoes generated by the tissues due to non-linear propagation are used instead of the fundamental [9].

http://dx.doi.org/10.5772/56378

It is also important to note that there has been renewed interest in some of the early developments that uses direct imaging technology such as ultrasonic cameras and other imaging modalities [10, 11].

2. Limitations of the conventional technology

2.1. Basic limitations

A fundamental limitation with all of the above existing technology, which arises from the need for line-serial scanning, is the loss of temporal resolution. Attempts to improve this aspect by increasing computing power alone cannot give the full-potential of real-time imaging and may only give improvements with largely diminishing returns.

The second limitation, for example when using linear-array technology, is the use of smaller effective aperture compared to the size of the total array aperture, hence affecting the lateral resolution achievable. These two limitations are analysed below in order to reveal the extent to which they affect potential performance in ultrasonic imaging. Although the discussion is based on using linear arrays for clarity, the same considerations are valid for other configurations.

Figure 1 below shows a linear array transducer coupled to a test medium. The test object is assumed to be homogeneous and have a depth (d). The array consists of (N) elements with a total aperture size (A). The elements are usually switched on as a group (as shown) rather than single elements to improve lateral resolution, since this depends on the effective aperture, as depicted in equation 3. The next group in the firing sequence advance by only one element thus keeping the line resolution equal to the spacing of the array elements.

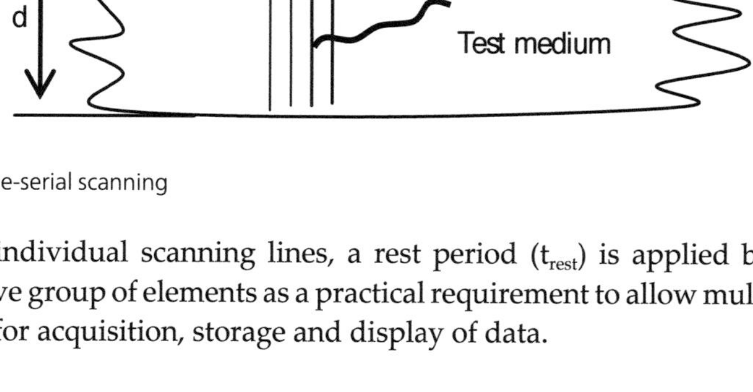

Figure 1. Line-serial scanning

Between individual scanning lines, a rest period (t_{rest}) is applied before firing the second consecutive group of elements as a practical requirement to allow multiple echoes to die down and time for acquisition, storage and display of data.

$$t_f = (N - N_G)\left[\left(\frac{2d}{c}\right) + t_{rest}\right]$$
$$\therefore \text{ Frame rate } \approx \frac{1}{t_f} \tag{2}$$

With reference to Figure 1, time (t_f) taken to produce one frame is:

where, N_G is the number of elements in the group firing at any one time and c is the speed of sound. Hence, as an example, when using an array with 150 elements, coupled to a medium in which the velocity of sound is 1.54 mm/μs, thickness 20 cm, $N_G = 50$, and neglecting t_{rest}, it can be seen that the maximum frame-rate achievable is about 75. This will be even less when t_{rest} is applied.

However, the above frame rate may sound adequate, and indeed so for many cases, but the line-serial scanning introduces a basic limitation in the case of fast moving targets such as heart valves or machinery. During the scanning time within a frame, one part of the target may have displaced significantly relative to another, causing spatial distortion, thus a frozen image of the target at any time may differ significantly from its actual position or shape. This is illustrated in Figure 2.

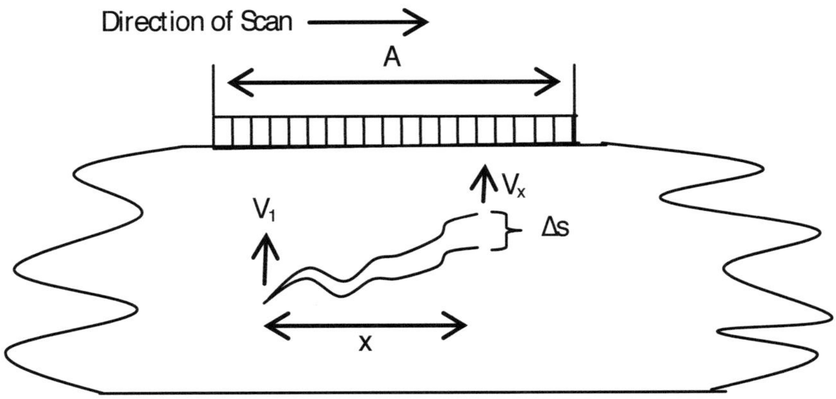

Figure 2. Formation of temporal artefacts

With reference to Figure 2, spatial distortion (Δs) could be written as:

$$\Delta s_{(x)} = \frac{x}{A} \times t_f \times v_x \tag{3}$$

where, v_X is the velocity of a point (x) on target.

The other limitation with a linear array scanner, as mentioned above, is the degradation of lateral resolution arising from the size of the aperture formed by the group of elements firing at any instant of time. The lateral resolution is limited by the beam width of the transducer or the group of elements. The diffraction limited beam width for a given transducer of aperture (D) could be expressed as:

$$\delta\theta = \frac{1.22\ \lambda}{D} \tag{4}$$

where, λ is the wavelength of sound in the medium. As can be clearly seen, for each scan line, D is determined by the number of elements within the group fired and this is clearly very much less than the total aperture size (A) of the array. Hence, the lateral resolution corresponding to that achievable with the fully available aperture is not realised.

2.2. Ideal properties of an imaging system

From the above discussion, it is clearly evident that two key properties of an ideal real-time ultrasonic imaging system is that it should be able to produce a complete image frame of the object volume from one insonifying pulse, while utilizing the full aperture available for each frame of the image. Additionally, an ideal system should produce focused images of the whole object field at the same instant of time irrespective of the distances of targets from the surface (Isochronicity) while maintaining accurate object-to-image spatial resemblance (image linearity). It is also clear that the existing technology utilising line-serial scanning cannot achieve these ideal properties and therefore alternative techniques may be needed to improve speed and high resolution capabilities beyond that feasible with conventional technology. This requires investigating non-conventional imaging modalities that can possess those capabilities, and the ways of overcoming limitations that may have precluded their use in practice. The next section presents some early developments that have some of the above key properties achieved through direct ultrasonic image reconstruction. Beyond academic interest, these techniques have not realised in large-scale use except in very specific applications due to other inherent problems.

3. Non-conventional methods

3.1. Direct ultrasonic imaging

Direct ultrasonic image visualization using alternative methods, such as ultrasonic holography, Bragg diffraction imaging etc. have been documented by many researchers in the past [12, 13, 14]. One such technique that has the above ideal properties is the Direct Ultrasonic Visualization of Defects (DUVD) system demonstrated by Hansted in the 1970's [12]. As schematically shown in Figure 3(a), this is a passive acousto-optical configuration which uses a pair of ultrasonic lenses with a common focus to form an ultrasonic image of the object field in a transparent medium from echoes received from a test object; much in the same way as an

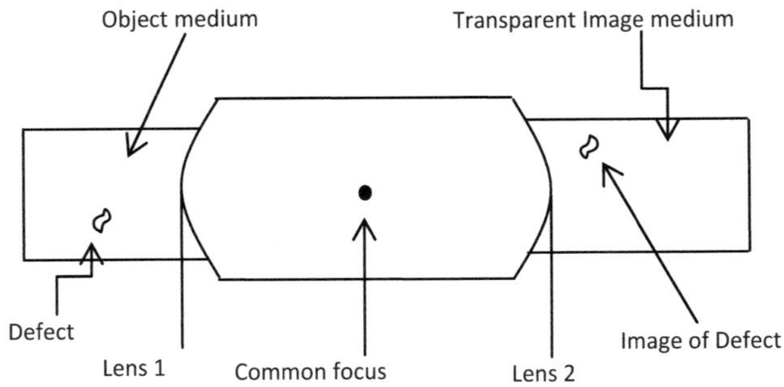

(a)

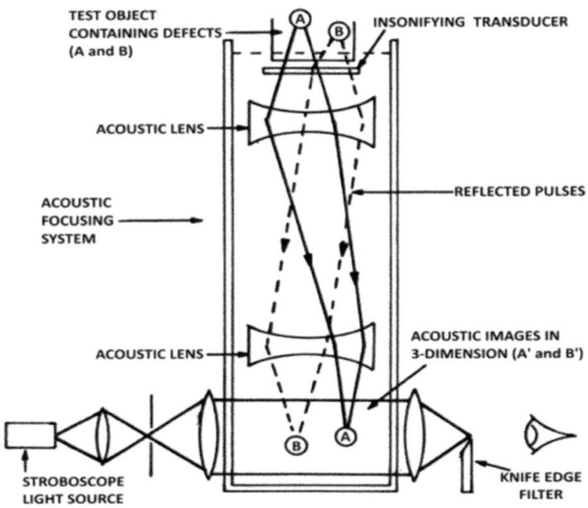

(b)

Figure 3. Direct Ultrasonic Imaging (DUVD) (a) DUVD Basic configuration; (b) A liquid coupled version of DUVD

optical lens producing an optical image. The insonifying transducer is physically bonded or intimately coupled via a liquid medium to the test object as part of Lens 1. Returned echoes are brought into focus by the acoustic lens arrangement in the image medium. The ultrasonic images thus produced is made visible by stroboscopic light which is synchronized to the transmitted insonifying ultrasound pulse, but with a fixed delay to allow the image to be formed and viewed at the point of best focus.

One of the DUVD realisations with liquid coupled lenses and a schlieren acoustooptical visualisation system developed by Hansted [12] is shown in Figure 3(b) above. It is interesting to note that the DUVD has many ideal features: It operates in Real-time; producing 3D images of the complete object field with every single insonifying pulse.

http://dx.doi.org/10.5772/56378

However, two main problems with the DUVD system shown above are: very low sensitivity and its design is such that the test objects virtually becomes part of the system; thus severely limiting flexibility as can be seen from the block diagram representation of the DUVD below (Figure 4).

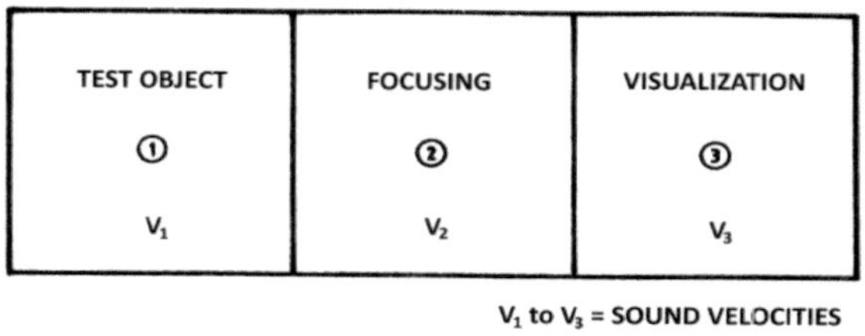

Figure 4. DUVD block schematic (Passive system). The insonifying transducer is bonded at the boundary between medium 1 & 2.

Further attempts to improve this approach have been reported by others in the late 1970's [13, 14]. But these were also passive systems and apart from theoretical interest the performance was practically inadequate.

3.2. A key development in the 1980's

3.2.1. Conceptual development

Because of the attractive features of direct ultrasonic imaging without the need for line serial scanning, a significant development was undertaken in the mid 1980's [15]. For initial feasibility studies, an active 2D version of the DUVD concept was considered. A major advancement was the introduction of amplification between a set of transmitting and receiving arrays of transducers; thereby solving the problems of low sensitivity and inflexibility inherent with the DUVD approach. This decouples the test object from the rest of the system as shown in Figure 5 below.

Since the system is now transformed from passive sonoptics to an active sampling and reconstruction technique, the design specifications were derived by detailed computer simulations and practical investigations to achieve satisfactory image quality. It should be emphasised that the requirements for image reconstruction for this system is very different to conventional imaging. It essentially involves image formation utilizing amplitude and phase of signals as represented by equation 5 and Figure 6 below.

$$P_{(x,\,y)} = \sum_{i=1}^{N} a_i \frac{exp^{-j(kr_i + \varnothing_i)}}{r_i} \tag{5}$$

where, p(x, y) represent the acoustic pressure at a point x, y in the image space as in Figure 6 below, a_i is the normalised signal amplitude, r_i is the distance to the point (x,y) from the ith element, φ_i is the relative phase of the ith element, and k is the wave number.

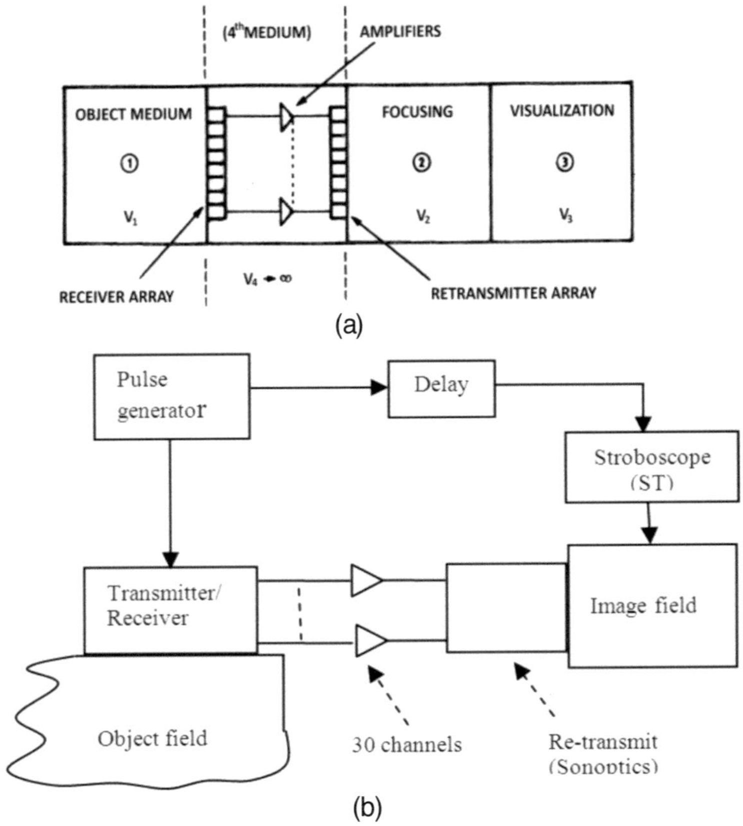

Figure 5. (a) – Active system block diagram with arrays (b) – Active system schematic block diagram

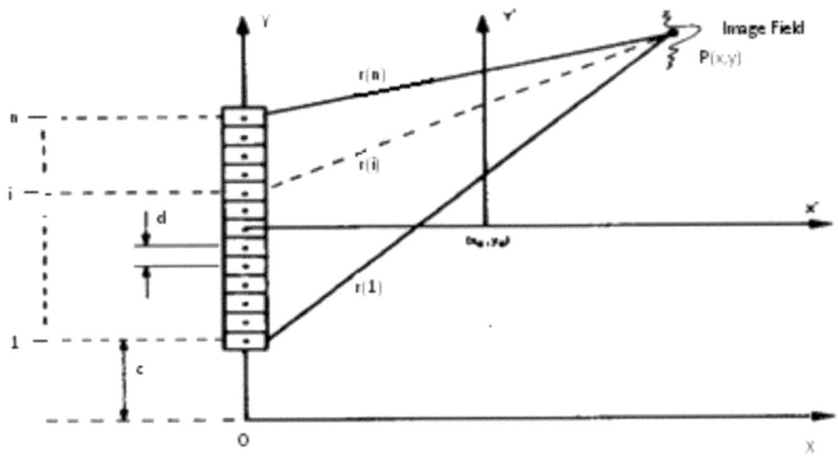

Figure 6.

Therefore in order to achieve good image quality, stringent control on the uniformity of the transducer elements in terms of their amplitudes and phase responses were essential requiring special fabrication techniques, since achieving close elemental uniformity in transducer arrays is a challenging task.

The details of the prototype design while achieving the ideal features described in section 4.1 above namely: linearity, isochronicity and maximum lateral resolution corresponding to the total acoustic aperture are presented in the Appendix.

3.2.2. *First prototype system*

For the feasibility study of the active direct imaging concept, a 2-D version of the 3-D DUVD sonoptics was chosen. However, it is important to note that as for the 3-D sonoptics, the same acoustooptical relationships could be maintained by using cylindrical lenses to give an image field similar to a B-scan. Because of the flexibility introduced by the sampling and retransmitting acoustic arrays, the operation of the lenses could be emulated by a number of different ways; e.g. by electronic focusing to represent both lenses, using solid cylindrical lenses, or by a combination of both. It should be emphasized that once the lens characteristics required are implemented, there is no further special requirement for dynamic focusing as the entire image field will be in focus at one instant of time requiring only one excitation pulse to produce the image of the whole object field.

After investigating different possibilities, the following configuration shown in Figure 7 below was used for the first prototype.

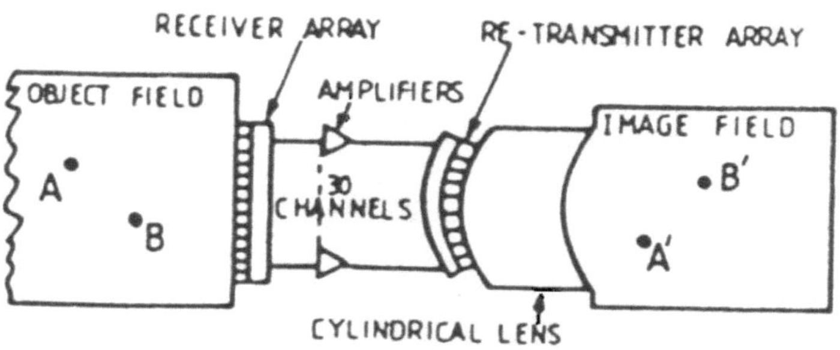

Figure 7. Active system configuration with conversion of DUVD sonoptics to maintain image linearity, Isochronicity and resolution.

Figure 8 below shows the construction of the retransmitting section of the system with retransmitting array, cylindrical lens and image medium. The design parameters were chosen to image a section of steel of depth up to 40 cm, which is well in excess of typical applications.

Figure 9 show the trolley-mounted 1st prototype system designed in accordance with the simplified block diagram shown in Figure 5. The optical assembly is equipped with an ultra-short stroboscopic light source [16] mounted on the right and a video camera for capturing

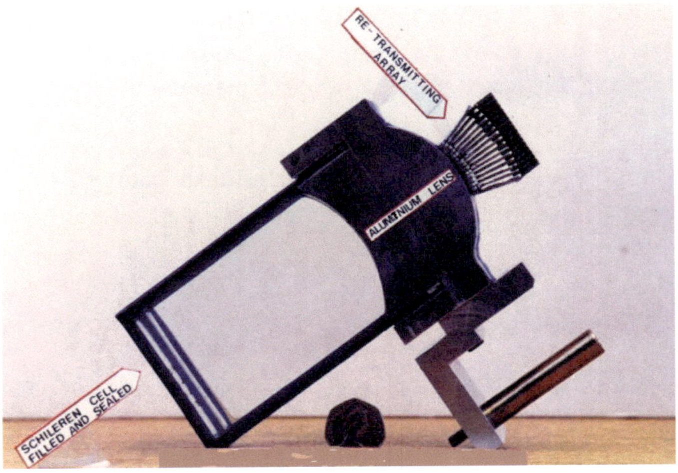

Figure 8. Sonoptical assembly including the imaging cell

images on the left along the optical axis. For experimentation, only 15 of the 30 available channels were used in this prototype.

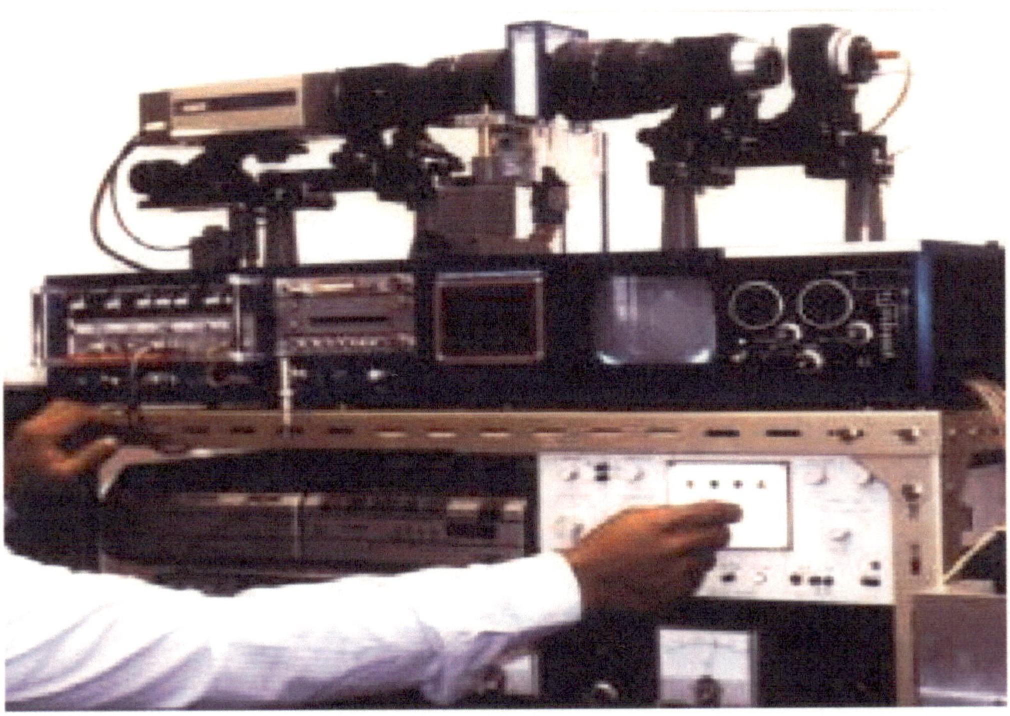

Figure 9. The active acoustooptical imaging system (1st prototype)

3.2.3. System operation

When testing, the receiving probe array is coupled to the test object medium with a liquid couplant such as oil or jelly. The test object is insonified with a short pulse of ultrasound and the delay of the stroboscopic light source is set appropriately such that the acoustic images are optically frozen in time within the optical imaging medium (schlieren cell) at the instant of best focus.

The resulting optical image of the whole object field can be seen either by naked eye or can be captured with a video camera. Since the time required to form a complete image field is now only limited by the time of flight of the acoustic signals the frame rate could reach the theoretically possible maximum limits (e.g. in excess of 1000 frames per second).

3.2.4. Results from the first prototype

Image linearity and Isochronicity

Although the system was designed with 30 channels, only 15 were used because of the difficulty of making elements of the arrays with sufficiently close characteristics as required for this imaging topology. However, as can be seen from the images, they are exceptionally of high quality in terms of image clarity and resolution. Figure 10 shows a test block with side drilled holes and the resulting image, clearly demonstrating image linearity and isochronicity as expected from the system design.

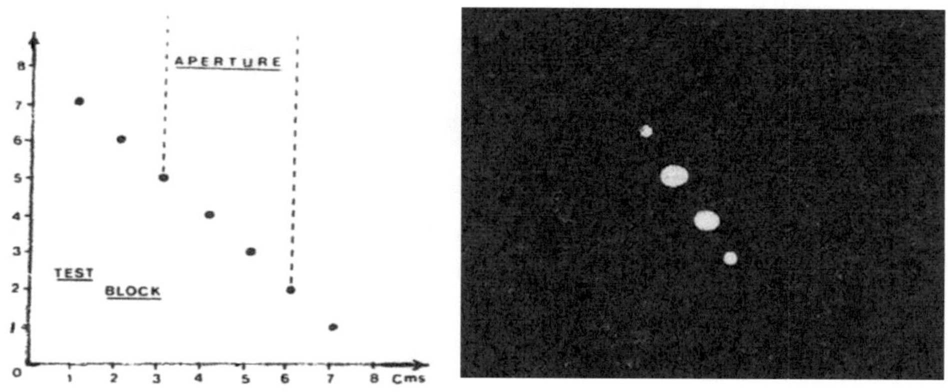

Figure 10. Images of 2mm side drilled holes.

Notice the axial magnification as depicted in equation 10 in appendix. The targets central to the array obviously have stronger return echoes, so they are somewhat saturated due to relatively low dynamic range of the channel amplifiers used. Figure 11 below show a test object, again with side drilled holes and the respective image with lateral and axial magnifications equalised. This image demonstrates exceptional image quality with object-to-image spatial relationship correctly maintained.

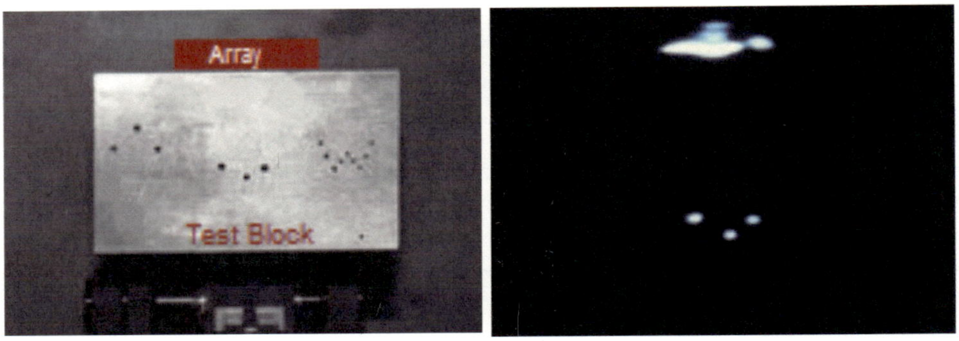

Figure 11. Imaging side-drilled holes in a test block

Figure 12 below shows an actual T-weld being tested with the prototype system and the image of a crack in the weld. This micro-crack was actually visible from the ground side surface of the test block.

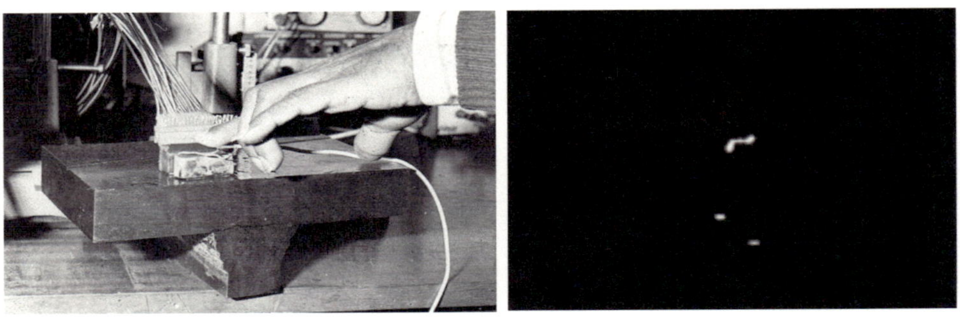

Figure 12. Image of a micro crack in a T-weld

3.2.5. Practical limitations of the first prototype

The results from the first prototype have clearly demonstrated the potential of direct ultrasonic imaging reaching performance close to theoretical limits. These include: maximum possible speed of imaging, maximum lateral resolution for the size of the arrays used, forming focused images of the whole object field covered by the transducer aperture.

However, there were still practical limitations. This system also had a small field of view approximately that covered laterally by the array aperture; in this case ~3 cm wide. This is too

http://dx.doi.org/10.5772/56378

narrow in practice since wider coverage requires moving the receiving array over the test surfaces, which are typically uneven. Since the image reconstruction is heavily dependent on the amplitude and phase information of the signals, unevenness influences the image quality to a greater extent than conventional imaging methods; although in ideal conditions, excellent results could be achieved as shown in the results section above.

4. Advancements in non-conventional methods — Development of a high-speed, computer-controlled hybrid scanner

From the performance of the acousto-optical imaging system shown in Figure 9, it was evident that to meet practical requirements and to advance the potential benefits, the following characteristics would be very desirable.

1. Ability to scan a test object for off-axis imaging, thus overcoming the limitation of small field of view.
2. Dynamic focusing along specified paths and sites to improve image quality.
3. Means of providing a degree of image enhancement.

The first property adds a much greater degree of freedom to test uneven surfaces from selected or prepared locations. The resulting images would be similar to a B-mode sector scan, but the imaging modality is such that it produces image zones for required sectors as opposed to individual line serial scanning, with just a few overlapping sectors enabling much higher frame rates to be achieved. Since there is no requirement for focusing in the image medium, as that is already taken care of by the sonoptical design, the scanning simply means that only the insonifying beam need to be steered to illuminate the object sector.

Since the image reconstruction is implemented with a sonoptical system designed with paraxial ray equations, when imaging a wide field like a sector, there is likely to be a significant degree of peripheral geometrical aberration in the image field. It should be possible to correct these dynamically, since for each image zone, implementation of an appropriately pre-calculated delay in the firing of the stroboscopic light source, channel gain/phase manipulation is possible.

Inclusion of the above properties is the basis of the development [17-19] described below. Figure 13 shows the basic block diagram of the hybrid prototype developed, incorporating scanning hardware (SCH) controlled by a microcomputer (PC). Dynamic control hardware (DCH) is intended to provide gain equalisation during off-axis imaging and time varying gain (TVG) to produce a uniform image field. Field Focus Control (FFC) ensures that the stroboscopic illumination is synchronised such that the image field is optically frozen at the instant of best focus. It is also intended to provide a degree of off-axis aberration correction with sector-dependent focusing delay control.

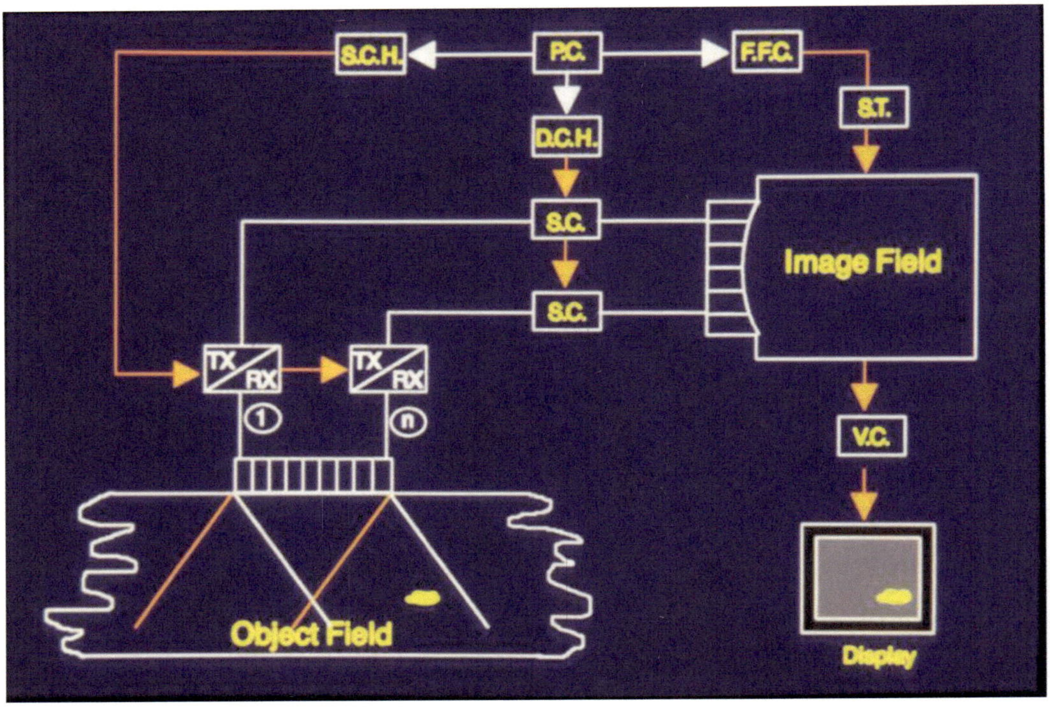

Figure 13. Basic block diagram of the hybrid scanner

4.1. Principle of operation

As mentioned previously, in contrast to conventional imaging, this system also operates on the basis of forming an ultrasonic map of the object field from received echoes inside a visible medium. Once an ultrasonic pulse illuminated the object medium, the acoustic signals intercepted by the receiving array is retransmitted into the image medium through the acoustic focusing system after conditioning and boosting signal power using signal conditioning hardware (SC). The re-transmitting section consists of an identical set of transducer array (except for the shape) to that of the receiving array, coupled to a specially designed ultrasonic focusing arrangement according to the requirements described in 8.1.1 (Appendix). Two important characteristics of this focusing lens design are that all the target echoes are brought into focus at the same instant of time irrespective of the target depth while maintaining image spatial linearity, so that a complete image frame is produced by just one insonifying pulse in real-time.

When the acoustic image field is at the time of best focus, an ultra-short stroboscopic light pulse of the order of a few nanoseconds is emitted, which produces a visible image. This can be viewed directly or captured by a video camera. Since the maximum repetition rate is now only determined by the time-of-flight of the sound pulse, the system achieves the highest speed of operation theoretically possible in ultrasonic imaging, eliminating the problem of temporal artefacts inherent with the existing systems.

Figure 14 shows a more detailed block diagram of the improved design with a possible use in testing of welds. Figure 15 shows the first prototype hybrid scanner developed.

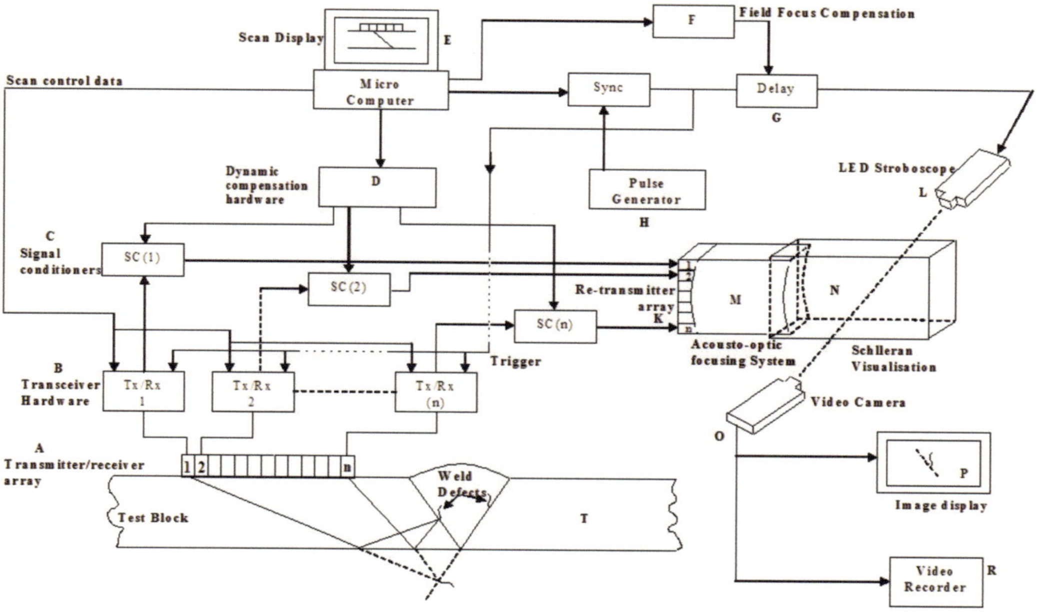

Figure 14. A hybrid imaging Topology with computer controlled scanning and acoustooptical image reconstruction (Expanded block diagram)

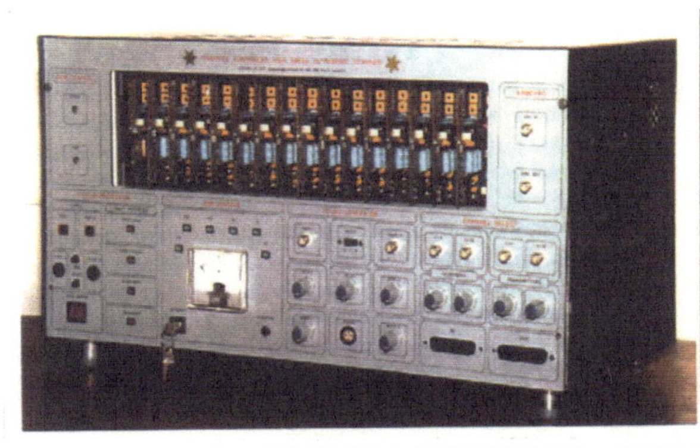

Figure 15. The first prototype of the hybrid scanner (GB2278443B)

Since the principle of acousto-optical imaging is very different to that of the conventional methods, some of the requirements of electronics and ultrasonic hardware is very different to that of the conventional systems in many ways. Since the received signals are converted back into ultrasound signals and retransmitted into an acoustic modulator to produce optical effects, the technique relies on the preservation of amplitude and phase characteristics of the signals to a high degree. Also, adequate signal power is required to produce acousto-optical modulation in the image medium to make the acoustic map of the object field visible.

For the first hybrid prototype system, the excitation pulses generated were 2MHz single sinusoidal pulses of the order of 120Vpp as shown in Figure 16 below. These pulses were shaped to obtain the near-ideal response from the transducer elements.

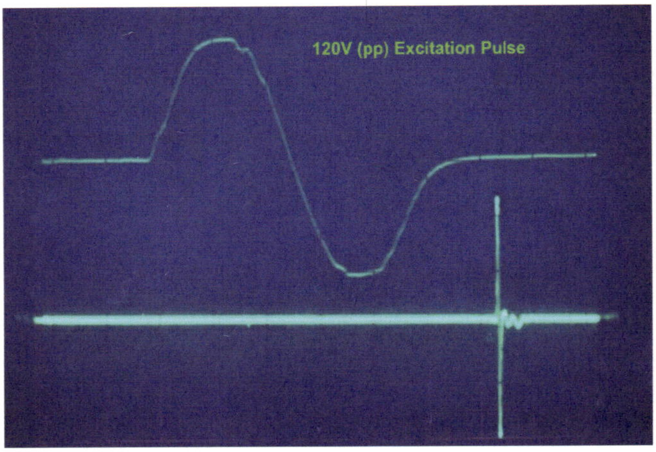

Figure 16. Single sinusoidal excitation pulse

The front-end receiving section of the hardware consists of wideband amplifiers (15 MHz) with a variable gain of up to 60dB. The output impedance is of the order of 50 Ohms with a maximum output swing capability of 120V pp. Input surge protection up to 1kV was provided with a very low recovery time to achieve minimal dead-zone. Although the above prototype scanner was equipped with 30 channels, only 8 channels were used for the feasibility study. This represented just 1.6 cm acoustic aperture. No dynamic compensation was used. However, the performance as can be seen from statically scanned images was still very good.

4.1.1. Operational modes

The system may be operated in the axial mode for very high-speed imaging or be used in the scanning mode to cover a wide field. In the coaxial mode, the system resembles in operation to that shown in Figure 10 -12, producing narrow-field linear array B-mode images covered by the aperture of the array. In the scanning mode the system is under the control of the computer and can be used to produce wide-field, high resolution B-mode sector scan images, or be programmed to scan along any specific areas of the target. In order to achieve field uniformity for off-axis imaging, scan-angle derived field-focus compensation (FFC) and dynamic compensation (DCH) may be applied. In the scanning mode, wideband insonifying pulses are beamed to target areas by phased array beam steering. However, when receiving the echoes from the targets, there is no requirement for beam forming at all, as the system essentially behaving as an active, acousto-optical imaging device operating in real time. Therefore, even in the scanning mode, this allows very high temporal resolution to be achieved since one beam produces a complete image field or image zone. Furthermore, the whole of the effective aperture is utilized for each image frame and therefore diffraction-limited lateral resolution approaches the theoretical maximum.

If the scanning angles are small, the system could produce images without the need for any compensation. This is the simplest mode of scanning operation. For larger beam angles in the scanning mode, compensation to account for the reduction in sensitivity and field uniformity may be applied by the control of insonifying energy, receiver gain and scan derived electronic phase delays, which is an area for further development.

4.2. Results from the 1st hybrid scanner prototype

As mentioned above, although the prototype was equipped with 30 channels, the number of channels used for the feasibility study was just 8 with an effective aperture of only 1.6 cm (as marked on the receiving array in Figure 17a). This was because of a problem of some of the channels breaking into oscillations due to excessive capacitive feedback at the time of experiments. Nonetheless, it can be seen from Figure 17 that the images produced are still very good for the aperture used.

As mentioned above, in the coaxial mode, the system resembles in operation to that shown in Figure 10 to 12. The speed of imaging is very high, e.g. in a test block of steel 40 cm deep, a complete image is formed within 0.15ms and the frame rate can be as high as 1kHz or more. Estimation of resolution capabilities previously obtained using the coaxial system of Figure 9 showed that the images can be produced to within one wavelength resolution in the axial direction and about 1.5 wavelengths laterally at about 60mm below the surface of the test block; thus approaching theoretical limits.

In order to test the operation in the scanning mode; a test block with side drilled holes covering a wide sector was prepared as shown in Figure 17(a). Figure 17 (b), (c) & (d) shows the images when the insonifying beam was steered statically (i.e. in manually selected angles) to image the 3 holes in the left, two in the centre and the two on the right-hand side of the test block.

Dynamic scanning was also verified. However, since the scan sector required for the above test object was very large (~120^0) peripheral geometrical aberration was significant. When statically scanned, aberration can be controlled for each angle manually by selecting stroboscopic firing delays to achieve best focus. For smaller sectors (e.g. < 60^0) aberration was not a significant factor.

Although the prototype system was designed for NDT applications, attempts to image biological moving tissues, such as heart valves, revealed excellent temporal resolution as expected. However, since the transducer arrays used did not have the required element spacing characteristics and matching properties, and the sonoptics of the prototype was designed for industrial material, the prototype could not obviously produce true B-mode images for biological tissues although the potential for advancement in this area was clearly evident.

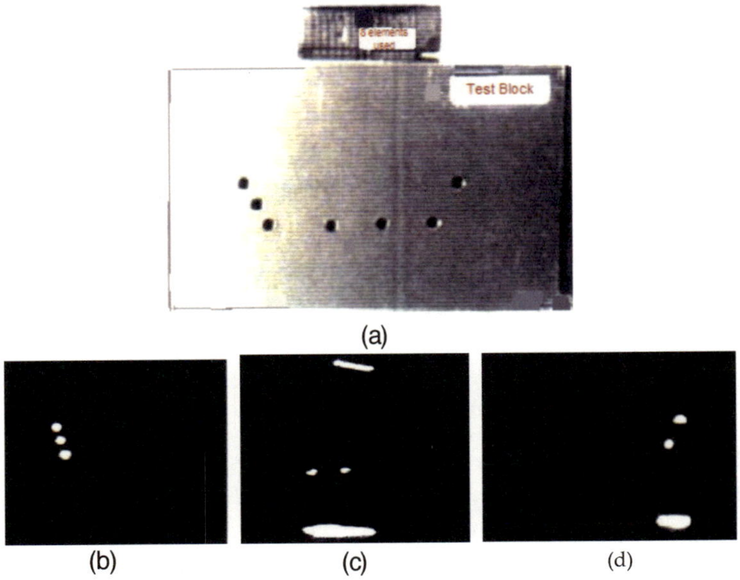

Figure 17. a) - Test Block. Statically scanned images of the test block

5. Discussion — Breaking through the speed barrier

In contrast to conventional line-serial computer based image reconstruction as used in existing systems, it has been demonstrated that the acousto-optical hybrid scanner has the potential to provide a number of important properties. These are:

- Ultimate speed of imaging as the image reconstruction is done using acousto-optical means thus *"Breaking through the speed barrier"* of the conventional line-serial imaging technology.
- In axial imaging mode, a complete image frame can be produced using a single ultrasonic pulse within its time of flight thus allowing ultimate imaging speed thus eliminating temporal artefacts when rapidly moving targets were imaged.
- In sector scanning mode image zones for each scan angle is produced allowing much higher frame-rates to be achieved, since very few scan angles are required as opposed to line serial scanning in conventional technology.
- A focused image of the whole object field is produced at the same instant of time without the need of any dynamic focusing as in the conventional technology.
- High lateral resolution, close to theoretical limits is achieved as the whole transducer aperture is used for each image frame.

As evident from the images, the signal-to-noise ratio (SNR) of the above prototype is very high. One of the reasons for this arises from the fact that true signals are coherent and the noise signals are not. Since the image reconstruction is based on amplitude and phase of signals, this

http://dx.doi.org/10.5772/56378

allows true signals from targets to be coherently re-constructed in the image medium while the noise and out of phase signals are being largely rejected as evident from Figure 18 below. However, just like all ultrasound equipment multiple reflections between closely spaced targets could still cause artefacts. Therefore, inclusion of selective insonification of the object medium as in item No. 2 above should enable the system to achieve even higher SNR while suppressing artefacts when imaging near-field targets.

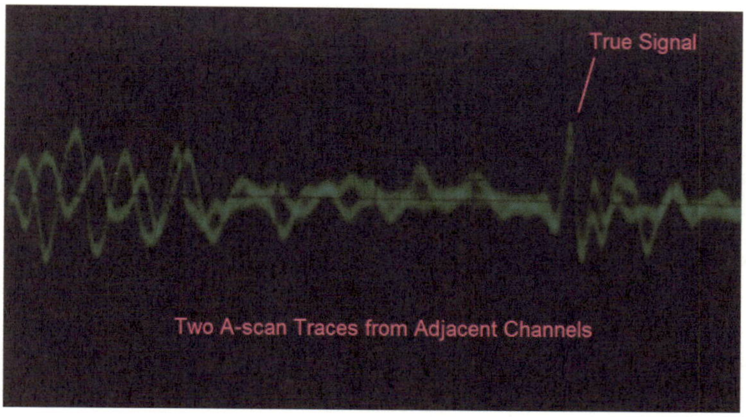

Figure 18. Noise suppression

Another important factor as mentioned in section 2 for any imaging technique is the dynamic range. In this respect, one of the typical bottlenecks is the limited dynamic range of display equipment. The present development can provide a greater display dynamic range when images are viewed with the naked eye as the acousto-optical modulator can provide a higher display dynamic range than images captured by a camera and presented on a typical conventional VDU.

6. Conclusions

Conventional ultrasonic imaging systems have inherent limitations such as low speed leading to temporal artefacts and in some cases limited lateral resolution; these being the result of line-serial scanning, lengthy processing and other limitations arising from the particular techniques used. The extent to which the above deficiencies affect performance has been analytically investigated.

In this respect, it has been shown that an alternative hybrid approach to imaging using acousto-optical image reconstruction could give clear advantages; reaching theoretical limits of performance in speed and resolution unachievable with the existing methods. This is mainly due to the combination of electronic and sonoptical image reconstruction, avoiding line-serial scanning and lengthy processing required by the conventional systems. The hybrid system reaches almost ultimate speed and resolution in the coaxial imaging mode. In the B-scan mode, it produces sector images formed by overlapping zones, but each zone requiring only one pulse to produce a complete zone image, thus gaining by far the highest speed of sector scanning compared to conventional methods.

Furthermore, the clarity and contrast of the images are high as the stroboscopic image mapping results in gating out many artefacts, problems due to reverberations and noise, to a high degree. Since the image reconstruction, by design, is based on coherent summation of signals in amplitude and phase corresponding to true targets satisfying the sonoptical focusing requirements, random noise gets suppressed without the need for further processing.

6.1. Future work

The typical results shown with the hybrid imaging system is applicable at present only to structural NDT for which it was designed. In order to produce true B-mode images for medical applications requires further work on the design of transducers and the sonoptical geometry to satisfy the conditions necessary for body tissue imaging, while accommodating the required dynamic range. In particular, it should be noted that the technique of image reconstruction is based on amplitude and phase integrity of signals; thus the inter-element uniformity of transducer elements and channels are crucial. In the case of medical imaging, the transducer element spacing is much smaller compared to NDT applications for any given frequency. For the above NDT system, the arrays were constructed using ordinary PZT transducer material. This is unlikely to be satisfactory in the case of medical transducers utilizing the above imaging techniques, since the requirements of transducer specifications are different and much tighter compared to conventional imaging to achieve good performance. Hence, transducers with piezo-composites or PVDF material may have to be developed for this application. Although the present system is designed to produce imaging in 2-D, extension of this technology to 3-D imaging in real-time is a distinct possibility which needs to be explored. This work and the development of dynamic compensation hardware will be taken forward in the next phase of development.

Appendix

Prototype design considerations

Since the active imaging system depicted in Figure 5 in section 4 above is required to produce a direct acoustic image which is made visible by synchronised stroboscopic light (Schlieren or other acoustooptical modulation technique), the design parameters for NDT applications were determined both by theoretical simulations and experimentation. For the construction of the transducer arrays, bearing in mind the tight requirements for elemental uniformity, number of parameters for a selected centre frequency of 2 MHz were determined which included [15]:

- Estimation of number of channels (30 for the initial design)
- Transducer element spacing (2 mm for the initial design)

http://dx.doi.org/10.5772/56378

- Element width-to-gap ratio
- Physical size, shape and transducer material

The primary aim was to obtain an idea of the sharpness of the images and the extent of artefacts that may be formed in a given image space. Since the transducer backings were conductive, maintaining a low level of electrical cross-coupling was required for the size of the backing thus the element gap spacing was kept around 0.3mm. For visualisation of the acoustic image formed in the modulating medium, the requirements for channel characteristics were then determined. These included practical determinations of number of parameters including:

- Typical and worst case input signal levels
- Output signal power required from each channel
- Phase linearity and bandwidth considerations
- Signal dynamic range
- Input and output impedances
- Element damping characteristics

Acoustooptical design considerations

As mentioned in section 4 above, as opposed to conventional image reconstruction, the passive DUVD system had some ideal properties for ultrasonic imaging namely, image linearity and isochronicity. Maintaining the same properties in the active system was therefore important. The requirement for image linearity as determined by Hansted [12] for the DUVD is given below.

Maintaining image linearity

Figure 19 shows the two-lens system of the DUVD.

Using paraxial ray analysis, it can be shown that in order to maintain image linearity throughout the image field, the only requirement is to make the focal point of the two acoustic lenses coincident. This however changes the lateral magnification as given in equation 10, but since this is a constant it does not affect linearity or image quality and can be easily compensated if necessary.

Maintaining isochronicity

As stated in section 4 above, iscochronicity means that when the test object is insonified with a short acoustic pulse, all the echoes from the different targets, irrespective of their special distribution within the object field, arrive simultaneously at their respective image points thus giving the system its ability to display the whole image at once.

The above capability is in stark contrast to the need for line serial scanning in conventional imaging, giving the system its speed - the highest theoretically possible speed of imaging as it

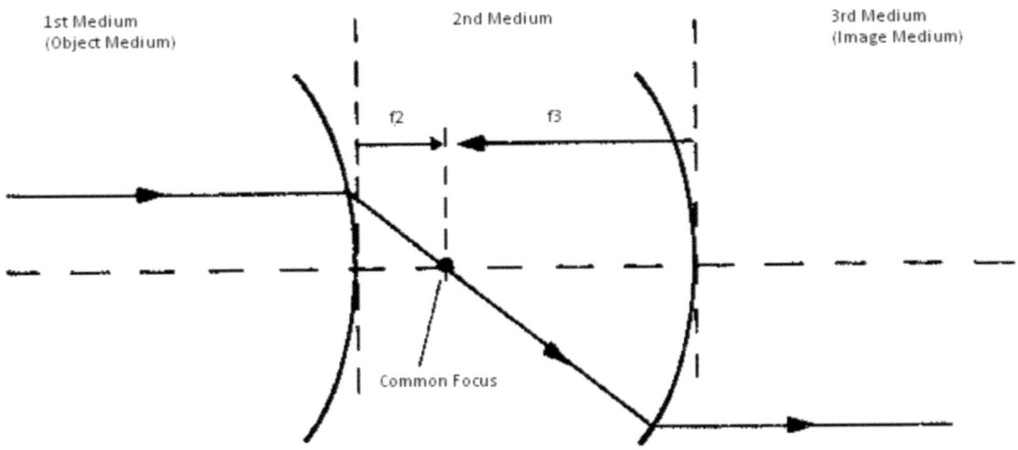

Figure 19. Maintaining image linearity

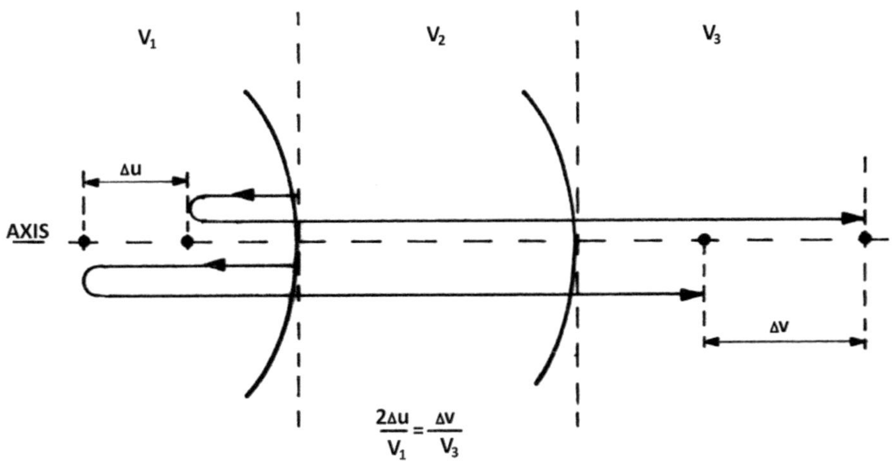

Figure 20. Requirements for maintaining Isochronicity

produces images with a single pulse practically within the time of flight of the pulse echoes in the object and image media. The conditions required for iscochronicity as determined by Hansted for his DUVD system with reference to Figure 20 is given below.

It can be clearly seen that the necessary and sufficient condition for the images of two objects in the object medium with velocity v_1 to be brought to focus at the same instant of time in the image medium with velocity v_2 could be given as:

$$\frac{2\Delta u}{V_1} = \frac{\Delta v}{V_3} \tag{6}$$

where, Δu is the axial separation of the objects in the object medium and Δv is the axial separation of the respective image points in the image medium. In terms of respective focal lengths in object and image media (f_1& f_4) the condition depicted in equation (6) is achieved for this lens combination with a common focus in the medium v_2 when f_1 & f_4 are related such that:

$$\frac{f_1}{f_4} = \frac{1}{\sqrt{2}} \tag{7}$$

Using paraxial ray analysis, it can also be shown that when satisfying the above necessary conditions, the maximum object distance (U_{max}) and maximum image distance (v_{max}) can be written as:

$$U_{\max} = \left(\frac{f_1 f_2}{f_3} \right) + f_1 \tag{8}$$

$$v_{\max} = \left(\frac{f_3 f_4}{f_2} \right) + f_4 \tag{9}$$

where, f_1 & f_2 are the focal lengths of the first lens defined by medium velocities v_1 v_2, and f_3 & f_4 are that determined by the 2nd acoustic lens.

Thus the necessary and sufficient conditions for linearity and Isochronicity for the acoustic imaging system are:

- The internal focal points must be coincident
- The external focal lengths must be related in accordance with that given in equation (7)

Using paraxial ray analysis taking also into account the conditions necessary for Isochronicity, it can be shown that there is however lateral image magnification (as mentioned above) such that:

$$M_A = \sqrt{2} M_L \tag{10}$$

Where, M_A and M_L are axial and lateral magnifications respectively. This does not affect image linearity and can be compensated if necessary.

Acknowledgements

Author wishes to express his sincere thanks to the School of Engineering of the Robert Gordon University, UK where much of the developmental work was carried out and to Mr Andrew Fairhead, ultrasound engineer of the Aberdeen Royal Infirmary, NHS Grampian, for his valuable comments and advice regarding medical imaging systems.

Author details

G. P. P. Gunarathne

School of Engineering, Robert Gordon University, Aberdeen, UK

References

[1] http://inventors.about.com/od/sstartinventions/a/sonar_history.htm (Accessed 24th February 2013).

[2] http://www.ob-ultrasound.net/history1.html (Accessed 24th February 2013).

[3] http://www.ndt-ed.org/EducationResources/CommunityCollege/Ultrasonics/Introduction/history.htm (Accessed 1st Jan 2013).

[4] Three-dimensional imaging system: Olaf von Ramm and Stephen Smith, Duke University, USA, United States Patent – 4694434 http://www.freepatentsonline.com/4694434.html (Accessed 1st Jan 2013).

[5] Portable PC-based Ultrasound scanners, Imaging Tools, Telemed http://www.hospitalmanagement.net/contractors/imaging/telemed/ visited 1st Jan 2013.

[6] Zone Sonography, Zonare Medical systems, http://cdn.zonare.com/0d87056c5a4bae2587f9710a5d669d33.pdf (Accessed 24th February 2013).

[7] Coded Excitation: GE Healthcare, http://www.gehealthcare.com/usen/ultrasound/education/products/techcodex.html (Accessed 1st Jan 2013)

[8] Digitally Encoded Ultrasound: GE Healthcare, http://www.gehealthcare.com/usen/ultrasound/education/products/techedu.html (Accessed 1st Jan 2013)

[9] Research Corporation Technologies, *"Tissue Harmonic Imaging"*: http://rctech.com/resources/downloads/THI_Overview_9-06.pdf visited 1st Jan 2013.

[10] Ultrasound C-can camera: Acoustocam, http://www.reinforcedplastics.com/view/1180/ultrasound-camera-makes-internal-composite-damage-easy-to-find/ (Visited 2nd Jan. 2013).

[11] G.P.P. Gunarathne, "Ultrasonics Imaging, Invited Presentation at the World Congress of Engineering 2007, London, UK, July 2007.

[12] P.D. Hanstead: *"Three Dimentional Imaging of Ultrasound – Direct Ultrasonic Visualisation of Defects"*, Nature 239, 1972, pp 273-274.

[13] A.J. Hayman: *"Schlieren Visualisation of Ultrasonic Images"*, PhD Thesis, City University, London, 1977.

[14] Y. Bar-Cohen, B. Ben-Joseph and E. Harnick: *"Compact Sensitive Instrument for Direct Visualisation of Defects"*, Rev. Sci. Instruments, Vol.49, 1978, pp 1709–1911.

[15] G.P.P. Gunarathne and J Szilard:*"A Real-time High Frame Rate Ultrasonic Imaging System"*, IEEE Ultrasonics Symposium, San Francisco, USA, Conference Proceedings, 1985, pp 98-203.

[16] G.P.P. Gunarathne and J Szilard: *"A New stroboscope for Schileren and Photoelastic Visualisation of Ultrasound"*, Ultrasonics, July 1983, pp 188-190.

[17] G.P.P. Gunarathne: *"A new real-time Ultrasonic Imaging System"* IEE International Conference on Acoustic Sensing and Imaging, Conference Publication No. 369, pp93 – 98, March 1993.

[18] G.P.P. Gunarathne: "A Real-time, Hybrid Ultrasonic Display/Imaging System for Medical and Industrial Applications", United Kingdom Patent: GB2278443B, July1997.

[19] G.P.P. Gunarathne: "Real-time Ultrasonic Imaging and Advancements in Non- conventional Methods" ^{2}MTC 2008 – IEEE International Instrumentation and Measurement Technology Conference, Victoria, Vancouver Island, Canada, May 12–15, 2008.